THE COMPLETE
CRYSTAL
SOURCEBOOK

A practical guide to crystal properties & healing techniques

GENERAL EDITOR: RACHEL NEWCOMBE

HarperCollins_Publishers_
1 London Bridge Street
London SE1 9GF
www.harpercollins.co.uk

HarperCollins_Publishers_
Macken House, 39/40 Mayor Street Upper,
Dublin 1 D01 C9W8, Ireland

1 3 5 7 9 10 8 6 4 2

Published by HarperCollins_Publishers_ in 2021

Copyright © HarperCollins_Publishers_ 2021

General Editor: Rachel Newcombe
Authors: Rachel Newcombe and Claudia Martin
Cover and interior designer: Peter Clayman
Picture researcher: Claudia Martin and Peter Clayman
Proofreader: Carron Brown
Indexer: Ben Murphy

A catalogue record for this book is available from the British Library

ISBN: 978-0-00-847959-6

Printed and bound in India

Note from the Publisher
Any information given in this book is not intended to be taken as a
replacement for medical advice. Any person with a condition requiring
medical attention should consult a qualified practitioner or therapist.

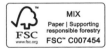

This book is produced from independently certified FSC™ paper
to ensure responsible forest management.

For more information visit: www.harpercollins.co.uk/green

THE COMPLETE
CRYSTAL
SOURCEBOOK

A practical guide to crystal properties & healing techniques

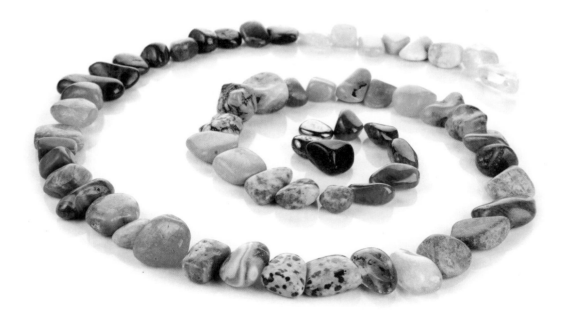

Thorsons

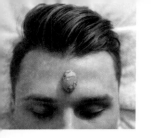

CONTENTS

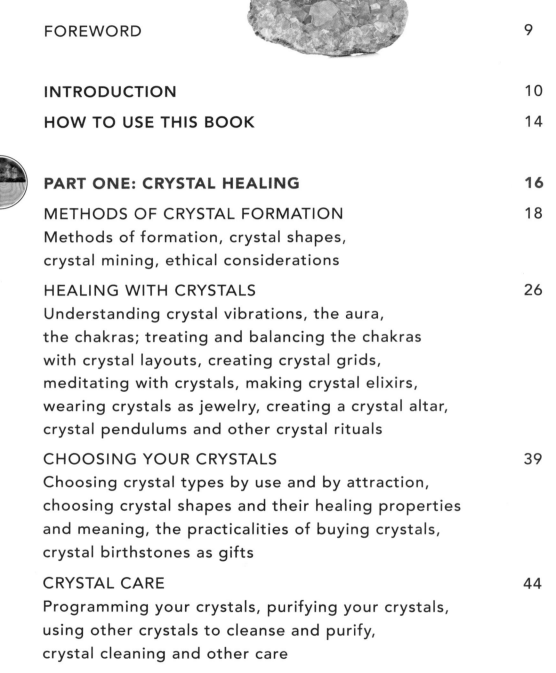

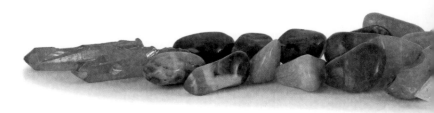

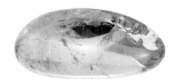

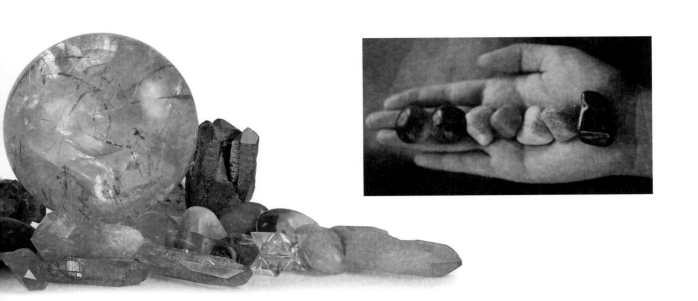

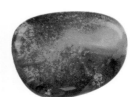

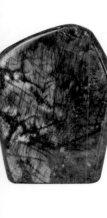

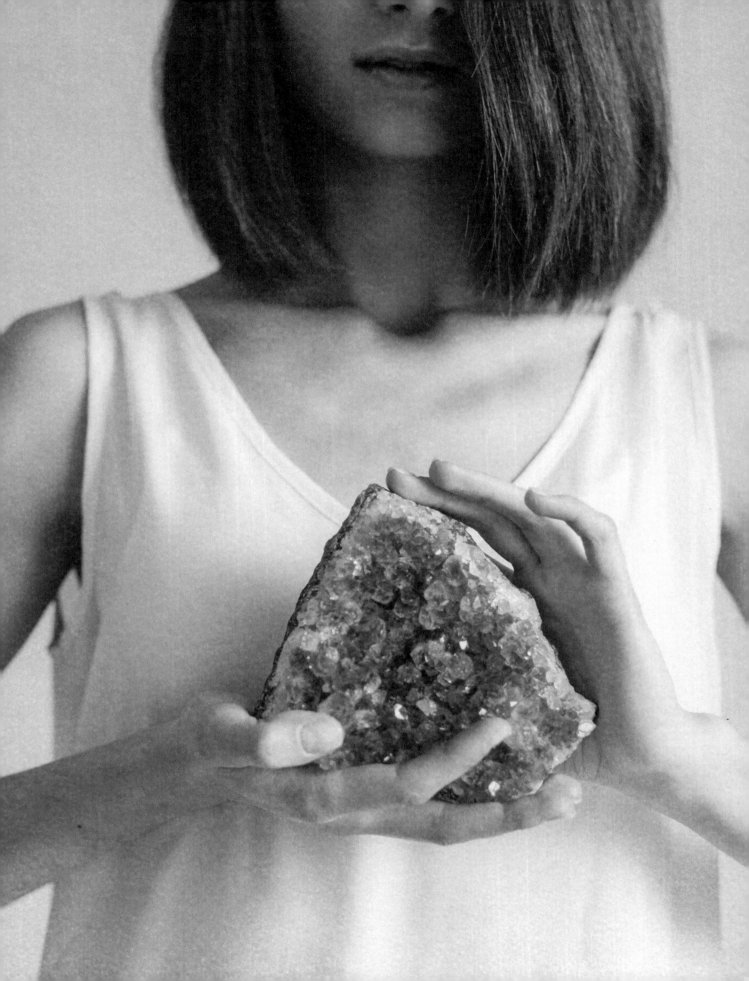

FOREWORD

Welcome to the world of crystals!

The Complete Crystal Sourcebook is designed to be a practical guide to crystal properties and healing techniques and is full of ideas on how and why you should utilize the power of crystals.

From understanding crystal vibrations and discovering different crystal shapes, wearing, programming, and purifying your crystals, to discovering how they could positively influence your health and well-being, there's a huge amount of crystal knowledge to explore within the pages of this book.

We strongly believe that crystal healing should never be regarded as an alternative to conventional medicine. Instead, it should be viewed as a holistic technique that can be used alongside it. Crystals work in a different way to modern medicine, focusing more on energy and vibrations, and can provide help, comfort, and support in other ways.

There's a lot you can achieve by using crystals in your daily life and well-being habits, and they could prove beneficial as extra support for certain health conditions and ailments. Do keep in mind that crystals should never be used as the first port of call for major illness, health problems, emergencies, or new symptoms for existing conditions—always see a medical professional first—and that some crystals can be toxic, so precautions should be considered and these crystals need to be used with care.

If you're in any doubt about how best to work with crystals, seek out the help and advice of a trained crystal therapist.

We hope you enjoy your crystal journey! Have fun exploring the beautiful rainbow of crystals, experimenting with using them, and, most of all, discovering if they could benefit your life.

INTRODUCTION

Crystals form in the earth over hundreds and thousands of years and are prized for their beauty, unique qualities, and healing powers. They have been used for centuries in various cultures and traditions, for both decorative and healing purposes. For example, the ancient Egyptians used crystals such as lapis lazuli and turquoise in jewelry and were buried with quartz crystals to promote safe travel to the afterlife, the Romans wore protective amulets made out of crystals, and there's even a mention in the Bible of the High Priest of the Israelites wearing a breastplate studded with crystals.

The ancient Greeks rubbed crushed hematite crystals onto the bodies of soldiers before they went into battle to help protect them, the ancient Egyptians used crystals for healing, and in India the Vedas Hinduism scriptures include details of the healing properties of crystals as part of Ayurvedic medicine.

As you can see, the idea of harnessing the power of crystals isn't new. Even today, crystals are used in numerous ways that you may be unaware of. In modern technology and medicine, for example, crystals are used for their piezoelectric properties—or the ability to produce electricity and light via compression. Quartz crystals can be found in electronic products, such as watches, radios, computer chips, and sonar devices, and they're used in ultrasound machines in hospitals.

In terms of health, crystals offer a holistic way of adding an extra dimension to your healing. Used alongside conventional medicine, crystals can work on the chakras and aura, helping the mind and spirit and providing an uplifting way of rebalancing your well-being.

Sunlight, moonlight, and still or running water are the best ways to purify and charge your crystals to rejuvenate their energy.

Once you have selected the right crystal for you, it is essential to cleanse, purify, and program your stone so that it is in prime condition.

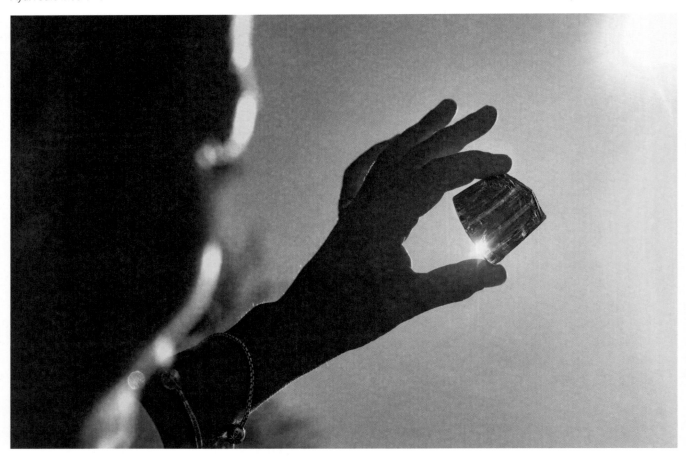

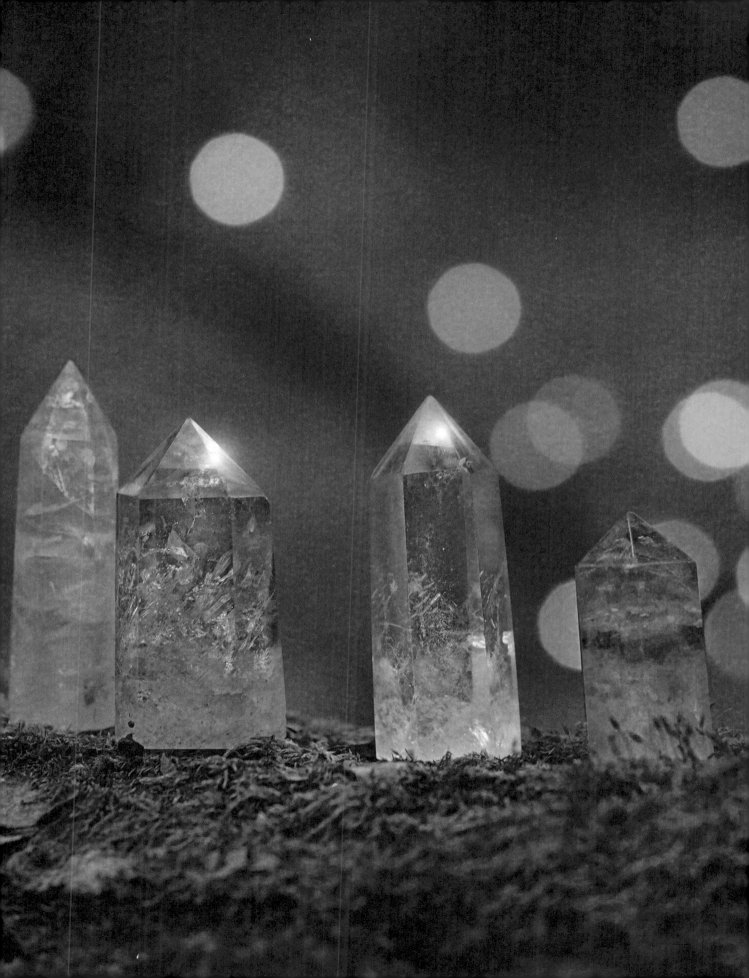

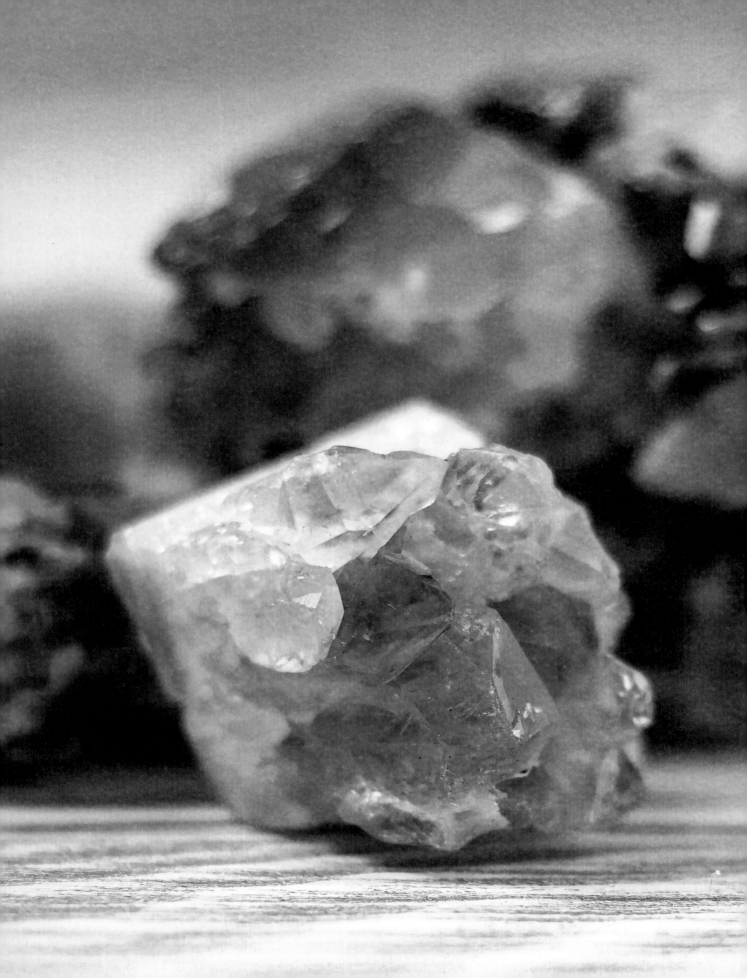

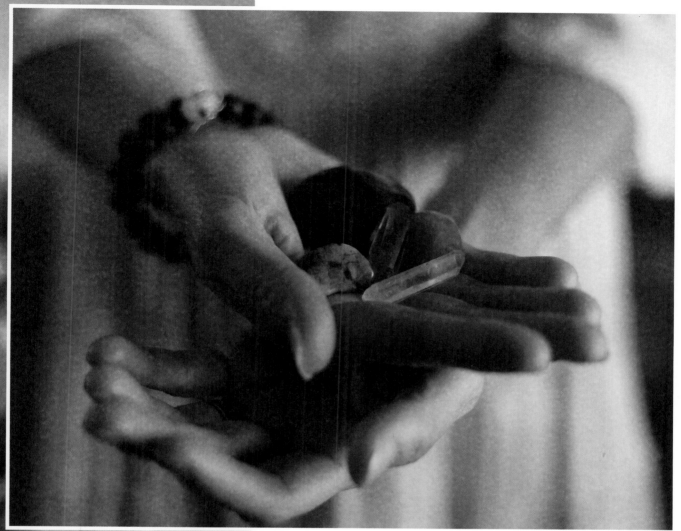

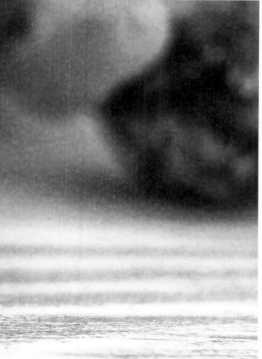

The color can significantly impact a crystal's healing properties. Green crystals encourage love and nurturing, resonating with the heart chakra. Purple crystals resonate with the crown chakra, linked to intuition and spirituality.

Spend time choosing the crystals that "speak" to you and your current circumstances. This is likely to change over time, but you may find some crystals remain core for you.

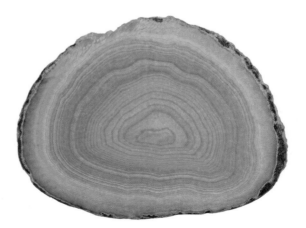

Agate can come in a range of colors but tends to show vivid color variations and is often polished to a high shine. Agate heightens concentration and memory.

HOW TO USE THIS BOOK

This is designed to be your essential sourcebook on crystals and how to use them holistically. If you're looking to heal your mind and spirit, rebalance your chakras, or cleanse your aura, this is your go-to source. The book contains a wealth of information about every aspect of crystals and can be read from cover to cover or dipped into when you need guidance and inspiration.

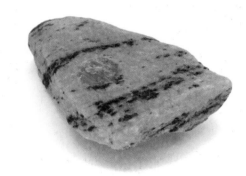

PART ONE: CRYSTAL HEALING

—

Part one offers an introduction to the art and nature of crystal healing. You'll discover the basics of crystal formation, how to understand crystals and care for them, and learn how you can use them for healing purposes. It covers techniques such as using pendulums, rebalancing your chakras, and creating a sacred crystal altar.

Introduction to elements of crystal healing, including when each treatment is best used

The properties and most effective uses of each crystal by color and shape

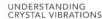

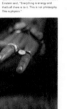

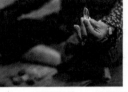

UNDERSTANDING CRYSTAL VIBRATIONS

PROGRAMMING YOUR CRYSTALS

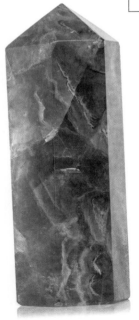

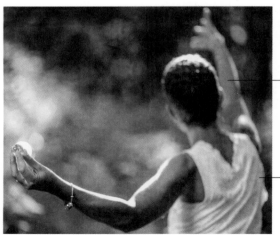

Methods for cleansing, purif and programming your cryst

Information on individual crystal's properties, crystal grids, and body layouts

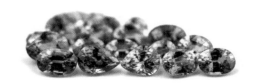

PART TWO: CRYSTAL DIRECTORY

Part two offers an extensive directory of over 200 crystals, including some that are likely to be familiar to you and some lesser-known varieties. The directory is arranged into color groups and you'll discover a range of different types of crystals in a rainbow of shades. There's information on aspects such as their appearance, formation, attributes, healing potential, and how you should care for them, as every crystal has its own unique qualities.

The crystal color is described by healing properties and broken down into individual crystal's descriptions

Clear descriptions of each crystal's appearance, rarity level, formation, attributes, healing action, effective combinations, and care is given

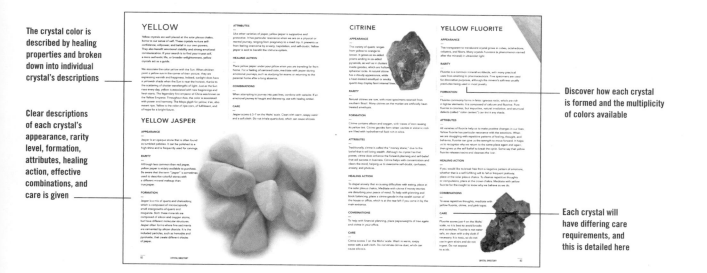

Discover how each crystal is formed and the multiplicity of colors available

Each crystal will have differing care requirements, and this is detailed here

PART THREE: CRYSTAL REMEDIES

Part three covers crystal remedies and ideas for how crystal healing can be used alongside conventional medicine and other treatments. It's split into sections covering related topics, such as the brain and nerves, bones and muscles, digestive system, and positivity. You'll discover which crystals could be beneficial for each ailment, crystals you could use in grids and layouts, plus additional therapies that you could use to improve your health and well-being.

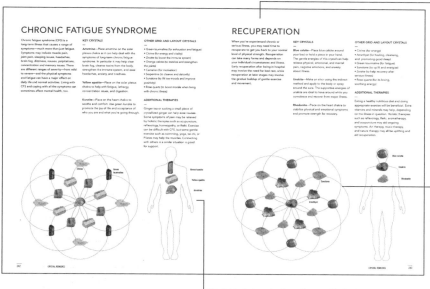

The Crystal Remedies section is clearly broken down into an index of ailments and their corresponding treatments

Crystal grids show the best placement of specific crystals on a grid for ultimate focus and specific intention. Find crystal grid templates to work with in part four

Crystal body layouts show where on the body a specific crystal should be placed for best results

PART FOUR: REFERENCE

Finally, if you're keen to explore crystal healing further, part four contains some useful resources, blank crystal grid templates to use, and further reading to follow up with. Plus, there's a useful glossary of key terminology.

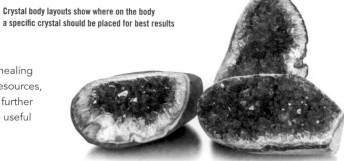

CRYSTAL HEALING

PART ONE

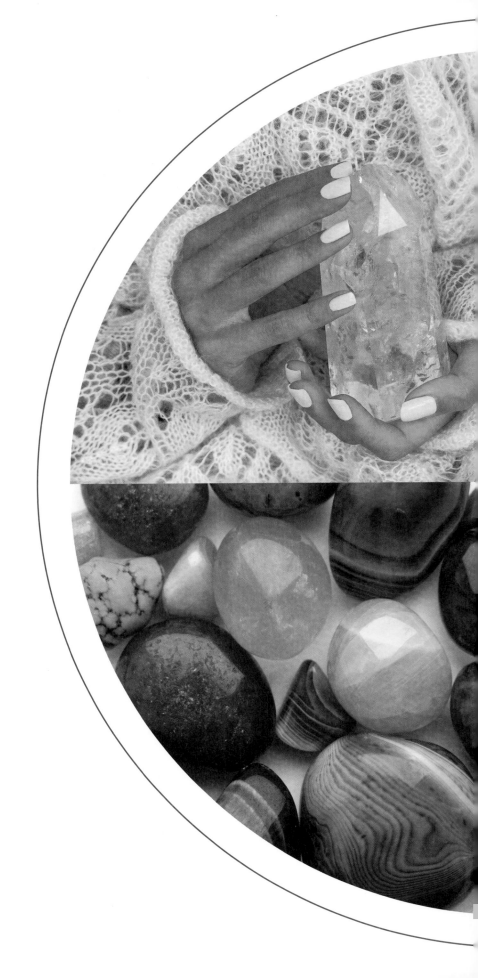

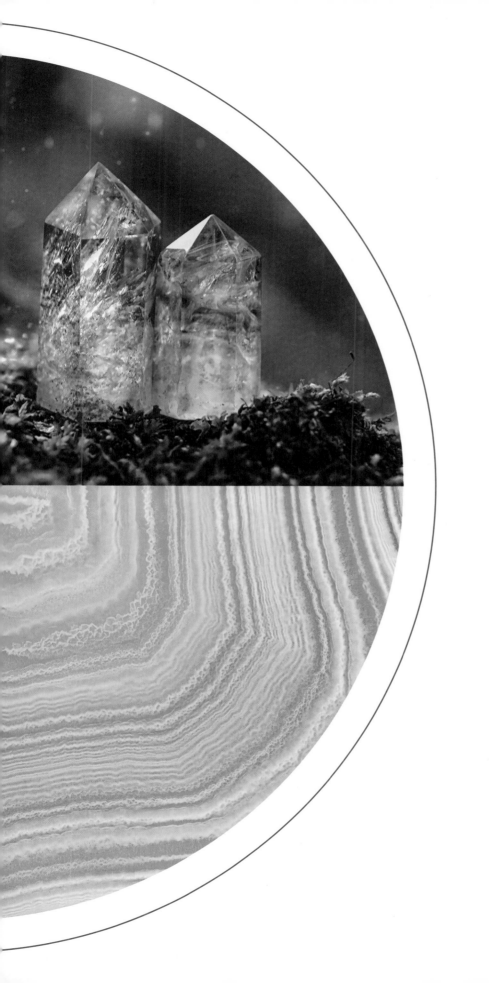

METHODS
OF FORMATION

Crystals are formed deep in the surface of the Earth, over hundreds, thousands, and millions of years. Crystals are essentially made of molecules and atoms and they're formed in several different ways.

Some crystals are formed when liquids, such as lava or magma, cool and harden, others form when water evaporates and comes into contact with other elements or are built up in layers over time. Factors such as temperature, pressure, and the location within the depths of the Earth can all affect how crystals form.

Amethyst, for example, is formed when a concentrated solution of silicon dioxide, containing traces of iron, becomes trapped inside a lava bubble. When the water evaporates, the silicon merges with oxygen to form a crystal—it's the traces of iron that give it its distinctive purple color.

Diamonds are formed from carbon atoms and are the hardest gemstone known on Earth, while emeralds are formed from the mineral beryl and get their color from elements such as chromium and vanadium. Crystals such as tourmaline are formed due to gas penetrating rock.

The ingredients of crystals are complex and vary considerably, which helps produce the wide array of different shapes, colors, and sizes of crystals. Even some crystals from the same family, such as sapphire or jasper, can have different colors or patterns, depending on the unique way in which they were formed and the interactions between different chemicals in the earth.

Crystals are formed deep inside the surface of the earth through pressure, temperature changes, and the elements.

Crystals vary in hardness, too, which is why the Mohs' scale of mineral hardness was formed to rate crystals depending on how hard they are in comparison to others. All crystals have a special inner crystal structure, which is formed by the atoms and molecules. It's this unique crystalline structure that can absorb, focus, and emit energy.

CRYSTAL STRUCTURE FORMATION
—

Crystals are built by nature into geometric forms. The atoms are cleverly arranged into repeating structural patterns, also known as crystal systems or lattices, that are all geometric at heart.

At their core, all crystals are made up from seven different forms:

• Triangles
• Squares
• Rectangles
• Hexagons
• Rhomboids
• Parallelograms
• Trapeziums

These different forms combine to create different three-dimensional shapes:

• Triangles form trigonal shapes
• Squares form cubic crystals
• Hexagons form hexagonal crystals
• Rectangles form tetragonal crystals
• Rhomboids form orthorhombic crystals
• Parallelograms join to form monoclinic crystals
• Trapeziums join to form triclinic crystals

These unique three-dimensional crystal lattices aren't visible to the human eye, but they do become apparent if you examine a crystal under a microscope.

Even though crystals from the same family, such as amethyst, may look different on the outside and be a different shape or color to other pieces, when viewed under a microscope their inner lattice structures are the same.

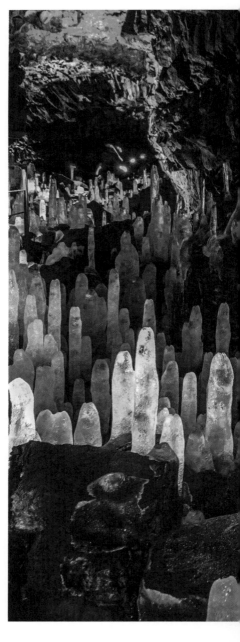

This is one of the key ways in which crystals from the same family can be identified, especially when there are color variations.

Understanding the structure of crystal formations has also helped scientists identify new crystals that are discovered. Amazingly, new crystals are still being found—and it's likely that not all of the Earth's hidden treasures have yet been revealed! For example, in 2020, a new crystal named kernowite was identified from a rock mined in Cornwall, UK. The green crystals were originally thought to have been a type of liroconite until the actual composition of the stone was studied in detail.

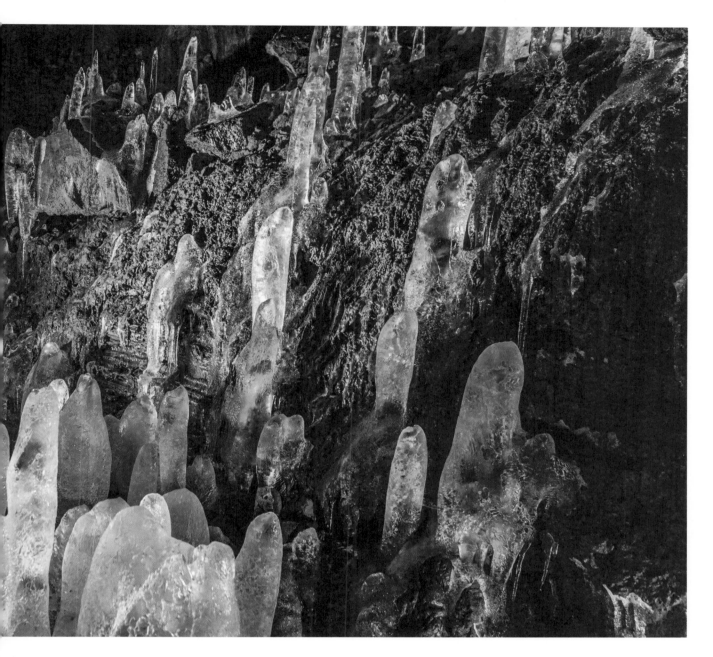

CRYSTAL SHAPES

Crystals come in a wide variety of different shapes, some of which are natural and reflect how they were discovered and brought out of the earth, while other shapes are artificial and carved.

When you're working with crystals, the shape is an important factor, as certain facets and shapes can have particular benefits and be used to direct or draw away energy.

SINGLE POINT

A single point is a crystal that has one end that's pointed, defined, and faceted. The other end will tend to be rougher, asymmetric, and undefined, or carved with a flat base. Crystals such as clear or smoky quartz can often be found as single points.

Crystal points can be natural or carved into shape and are often used in healing for directing energy. When they're pointed inward toward the body, they can direct energy toward the body. When they're pointed outward away from the body, they draw unwanted or negative energy away from the body.

These incredible crystals have formed inside the Raufarholshellir lava tunnels in Iceland.

DOUBLE TERMINATION

A double termination is a crystal with two clearly defined points, one at each end. Double-terminated crystals can be natural, or they can be carved and created.

Having points at both ends means that double-terminated crystals can be used for balancing work, both directing and drawing away energy.

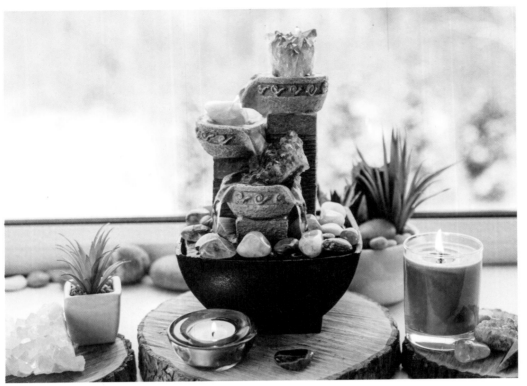

FREEFORM
Freeform crystals are pieces that don't fall into any of the other shape categories. They can be naturally freeform in shape or cut in this way. Many freeform crystals are stunning shapes in their own right, highlighting the beauty and uniqueness of natural gemstones. Freeform crystals can be used for healing purposes, or simply enjoyed for their beauty.

A crystal altar can be created as a sacred space to display your favorite crystals, healing tools, or other items of meaning. What you choose to include and how you choose to set it up is entirely up to personal preference.

CLUSTER
As the name suggests, a cluster is a group of crystal points embedded together. The crystals can be large or small, or a mix of shapes and sizes. Clusters can look very attractive and are often used as decorative accessories, but they serve a useful purpose for cleansing a room, too.

SQUARE
Square crystals can be naturally formed or created. Pyrite and fluorite are two of the crystals most often found in a natural square or cubic shape. Square-shaped crystals are beneficial for grounding purposes.

GENERATOR
A generator crystal has six equal-faceted sides and a distinct sharp point. They can be large or small, rounded or thin, and can be naturally discovered or specifically cut to produce this shape. Generators can be used to recharge other crystals and amplify their energy, as well as used for healing purposes. It's also possible to find a cluster generator, with lots of large, long, defined points.

TUMBLED
Tumbled crystals are pieces of rough gemstone that are tumbled in a special machine to make them smooth and polished. They tend to be smaller in size and are very tactile. Tumbled crystals can be good to use when creating grid layouts, plus their smaller size makes them ideal for carrying with you. As a bonus, tumbled crystals are often a more affordable option and a good way to get started on your crystal journey.

PALM STONES
Palm stones are a created crystal shape. They tend to be oval or round, are normally polished and smooth, and are designed to be the right size and shape to fit comfortably in the palm of your hand. Palm stones are perfect to hold when you need extra emotional support, or to use when you are meditating.

This rhodochrosite is an example of a companion crystal.

GEODE
A geode is a hollow, spherical rock that looks inconspicuous from the outside, yet when cracked open it reveals a cavity packed with crystals. Every geode is unique, with its own array of different-sized crystals inside, and they can be spectacular pieces to have on display. A geode can be placed in a room to help the flow of energy.

SEER STONE
A seer stone is a crystal that's been naturally tumbled by water, for example, as a result of being in a river. They tend to have a smooth, frosted surface on the outside (rather than being polished and shiny, like machine-tumbled crystals). A window on the crystal is revealed by cutting across the top of it. Traditionally, seer stones are used for scrying—gazing into the crystal for meditation or to gain insight and revelations.

COMPANION
A companion crystal is so-called when two crystals have grown and melded together. One crystal may be inside the other, or a smaller crystal may be growing from a larger companion.

Varieties of quartz, including rose quartz, can often display the phantom shape.

PHANTOM

A phantom crystal is a gemstone that appears to have the ghostlike structure of another crystal inside it. Sometimes it's even possible to have multiple phantoms inside larger crystals. A phantom is created when a crystal forms on top of an existing crystal. Varieties of quartz, such as clear, smoky, or rose quartz, as well as calcite, fluorite, and tourmaline, are most likely to develop the phantom shape.

PYRAMID

Pyramid crystals have four sides meeting in an upward point and a base. They can be naturally found in this shape or cut to become a pyramid with a squared-off base. Pyramids are a symbol of ancient and sacred geometry, and in crystal form they can focus and amplify energy.

This lapis lazuli is a stunning example of a cut pyramid shape.

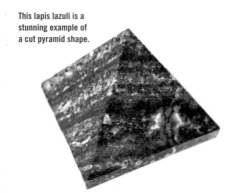

WAND

Wand-shaped crystals are long, rounded crystals with points—they can be both single or double terminated. Although it's possible to find some natural wand-shaped crystals, most are carved, polished, and shaped into a pristine-looking wand. Wand crystals are traditionally used as healing tools and,

Wands can be used to transmit energy through their points.

according to legends, are said to have been used in Atlantis. When working with crystals, wands can be used to transmit energy through their focused points. A variety of different crystals are available in a wand shape, including fluorite, rose quartz, and selenite.

SPHERE

Spheres or balls are carved crystals that are formed into smooth, round, and polished spheres. Clear quartz is traditionally associated with crystal balls, but many different types of crystals can be carved into spheres of all sizes.

EGG

Egg-shaped crystals are gemstones that have been carved into an egg shape. They're often popular with gemstone collectors as the smooth and tactile shape of an egg shows off the patterns and designs of different gemstones very well.

HEART

Heart-shaped crystals are carved gemstones and can be large or small in size. When polished, crystal hearts have a smooth, shiny surface and are ideal to hold in your hand when meditating, or to be given as a gift to a loved one. Rough, natural, unpolished crystal clusters can also be effectively carved into heart shapes, with stunning results.

This transparent amethyst palm stone is designed to fit comfortably in the palm of the hand for meditation and emotional support.

CROSS

Crystals can naturally form into a cross shape, where one crystal has formed at right angles to another. But crystals can also be carved and polished into cross shapes, which may be comforting to hold when meditating.

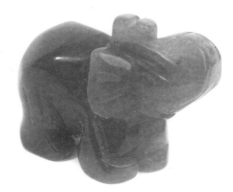

This jade elephant is an example of a carved shape that is used as a connection to the angelic realm, or simply for display.

ANGELS AND ANIMALS

Other popular carved shapes for crystals include angels and an array of animals. Angels can be used to bring a sense of connection to the angelic realm. Animal crystals make cute decorative ornaments, but they can also serve as a good introduction to different gemstones.

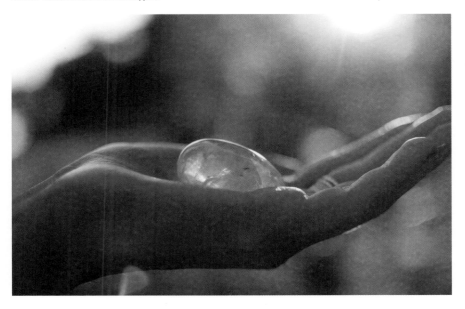

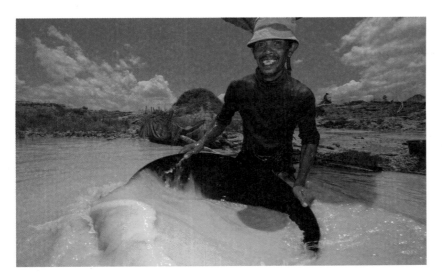

This diamond miner in Indonesia shakes his mining tray at a traditional diamond mine in South Borneo.

CRYSTAL MINING

In order to be able to buy crystals, they first need to be found and mined. There are various different methods of crystal mining used across the world, with the techniques used dependent in part on the type of crystal being sought and the area in question. Sometimes machinery is used, but in poorer areas, crystals may largely be mined using tools and hardworking individuals.

UNDERGROUND MINING—TUNNELLING
This involves making a tunnel from the surface down to where the crystals are located. This is a popular method when seams of gemstones are spotted, often near the surface, which provide a trail to gemstone sources. When the tunnel has been created, the crystals are either mined by hand using tools such as a pickax to cut through the stone, or, in bigger mines, by a blasting technique.

UNDERGROUND MINING—CHAMBERING
Another approach to underground mining is chambering. This involves creating a vertical shaft down into the rock, then driving tunnels into the shaft at various different points and levels. The crystals are then mined, usually via a blasting technique, and taken up to the surface using the shaft.

Amber catchers working in the Baltic Sea.

OPEN-PIT CAST MINING
Open-pit or open-cast mining doesn't tend to be used for the majority of crystals. However, it is a technique used to mine for diamonds, as well as precious metals such as silver and gold. It's an approach that's favored when the gemstones aren't too far under the surface of the ground.

PANNING AND RIVER DIGGING
The idea of crystal mining tends to automatically conjure up an image of miners digging underground, but many types of crystals can also be found lodged in the beds of lakes and rivers. For example, crystals such as opal, garnet, jasper, amethyst, topaz, and even ruby have all been found in certain rivers and lakes across the world.

Panning, also sometimes called wet digging, is a traditional technique that involves collecting crystals while painstakingly washing stones, rocks, and dirt from a riverbed. It can be associated with panning for gold, but in rivers rich with gemstones, it's possible to find a wide variety of crystals using this technique. Panning pans tend to be circular in shape, with a flat base and sloping sides. The pan is filled with gravel, stones, and rocks from a river bed and then it's immersed in the water. A shaking method is used to disperse lumps of clay and allow miners to pick out large stones or rocks. The idea is that heavy pieces will eventually fall to the bottom of the pan, while lightweight gravel or other material will be washed off the surface. Where rivers have run dry and are likely to contain crystals, miners dig in the dry riverbed to find them.

SEA MINING
Some crystals can be found on the bed of the ocean, so a sea mining technique is used. Amber, for example, can be found in the Baltic Sea (it's also mined from underground in other areas). Sea miners use nets to fish out the amber from the sea.

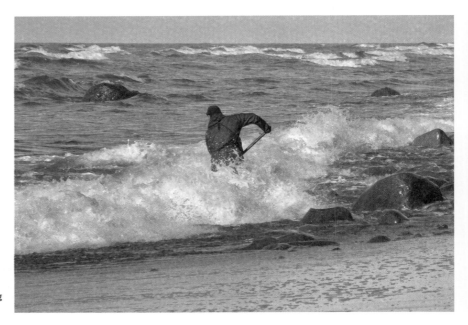

ETHICAL CONSIDERATIONS

When it comes to the business side of mining and selling crystals, sadly not all mines around the world operate ethically. There are issues regarding how the crystals are mined, whether they are regulated or not, and how workers are treated. In a world where ethical issues are increasingly high on the agenda, it's good to factor in ethical crystal concerns when you're buying and working with crystals.

MINING PRACTICES
In the case of diamonds, an international certification scheme exists to ensure that standards are met in the mining process, giving consumers knowledge when they buy. As yet, there's sadly nothing similar for crystal mining, but there perhaps should be.

Mining practices across the world differ on a huge scale and it's often very hard to know exactly how the crystals you're buying were obtained. For example, were they mined by a reputable company, was consideration given to the environmental impact that the mining could have on the land, and were workers' rights adhered to?

Some countries do have regulations in place, such as the Fair Labor Standards Act (FLSA) in the US, so you can be assured that if you buy gemstones sourced in the US, the miners of them should have been treated well.

CRYSTAL MINERS
Some of the countries that are rich in crystals are relatively poor, so they don't have the ability to mine with machinery, maintain good work conditions, or pay appropriate wages.

For example, in countries such as Madagascar, where the earth is abundant with crystals such as tourmaline, citrine, labradorite, carnelian, rose quartz, and amethyst, the majority of mining is done by hand, rather than by machine. There are some reputable mines, but others are less so, and as a result many of the workers are paid minimal fees for backbreaking work and long hours. Plus, there are often whole families involved in crystal collection, including children.

ASK BEFORE YOU BUY
If you're concerned about where your crystals come from and whether they were ethically mined, look for companies that specify details about where the crystals they sell are obtained from.

A reputable seller who cares about ethics will do their best to source their products with care. They'll build relationships with their suppliers, and maybe even individual mines, and be happy to share their knowledge with their customers.

Some sellers will give details about the country and area from which the crystal originated, while others will give specific details about exactly which mine it was from. The more details available for you to peruse when purchasing, the better choice you're able to make about whether the crystals you're buying are ethically sourced.

You can ask for details at crystal shops in person, or online. If you're not keen on buying crystals online (many people like to hold them first) and don't have a shop near you, look out for gemstone fairs and events, where you can meet numerous sellers and select the ones that have the best ethical practices.

DIY CRYSTAL HUNTING
Another way to be sure of where your crystals have come from is to hunt for them yourself!

This doesn't mean randomly digging for crystals wherever you are, but rather going to a specialist mine where you can pay to hunt for crystals. There are various mines offering this service in the US and it can be a fascinating insight into the process involved, as well as highly rewarding when you find your own crystals.

ALWAYS BE AWARE OF CRYSTALS THAT ARE CHEAP—THEY MAY BE CHEAP FOR A REASON AND COME FROM NON-ETHICAL SOURCES.

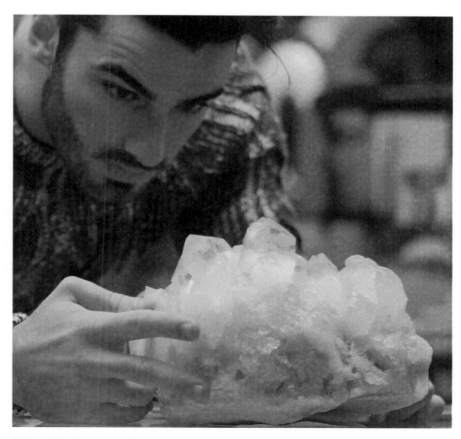

Closely consider the source and ethical implications of your crystals before purchase.

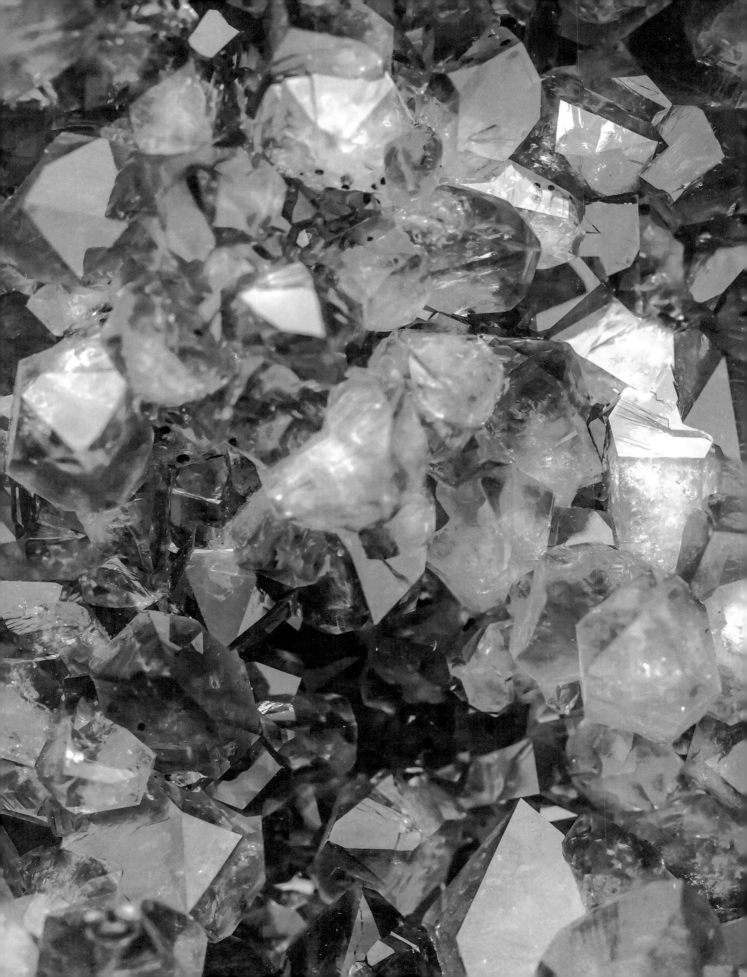

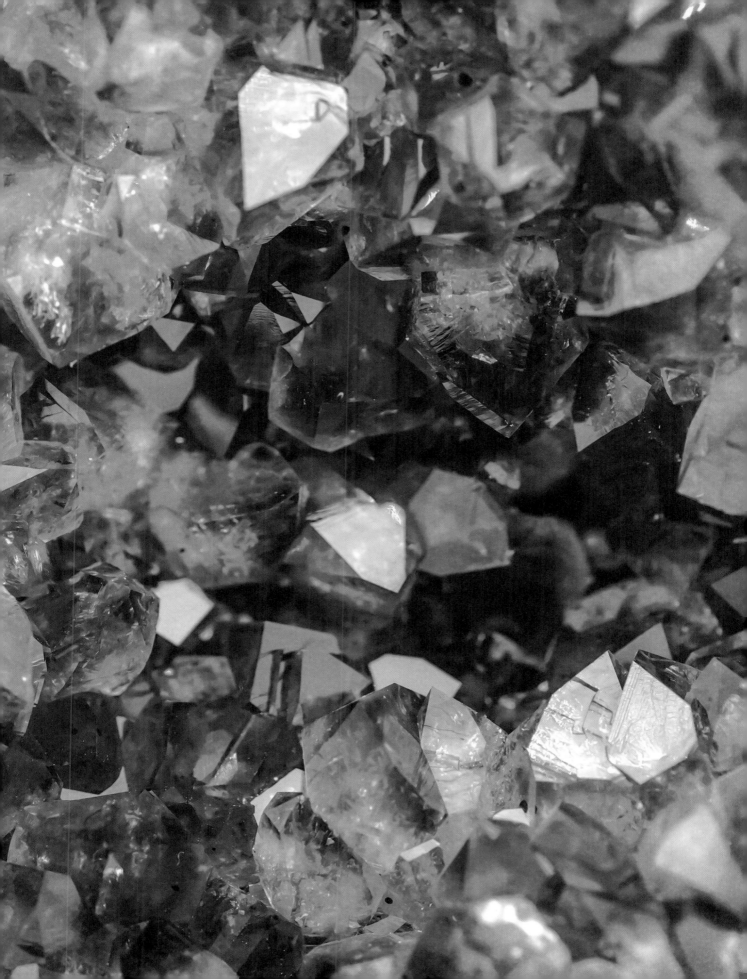

UNDERSTANDING CRYSTAL VIBRATIONS

Crystals are special. They're not just beautiful rocks and gems that are lovely to look at, they have hidden qualities, too. All crystals have a unique energy or vibration and can absorb, focus, store, transmit, and transmute electromagnetic energy.

Crystals are formed from an organized structure of repeated geometric molecular patterns, and it's this structure that gives them a strong vibration.

It's not just crystals that have a vibrational frequency – humans do, too. But while the vibration of crystals remains strong, constant, and powerful, due to their unique structure, our vibrations can go up and down and be influenced by a range of factors.

For example, your mood and how you feel can be affected on a daily basis by other people, by social media and what's in the news, by your past memories, daily experiences, and a host of other factors.

That's one reason why crystals can be so beneficial to use, as the vibration of crystals never ebbs, but always flows. Of course, this vibration can be dulled by dust, dirt, overuse, and negativity, but cleansing and purifying crystals can bring them back to their full potential.

The healing energy of crystals can be a powerful resource during meditation and mindfulness practice.

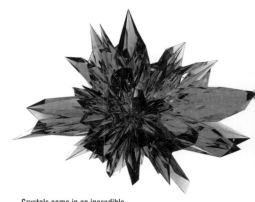

Crystals come in an incredible array of shapes and colors.

Each crystal has a different type of vibration or frequency. Their energies depend on factors such as the type and color of the crystal, and the size of the piece.

It can be hard to get your head around the idea of vibrational frequencies. But as Albert Einstein said, "Everything is energy and that's all there is to it. This is not philosophy. This is physics."

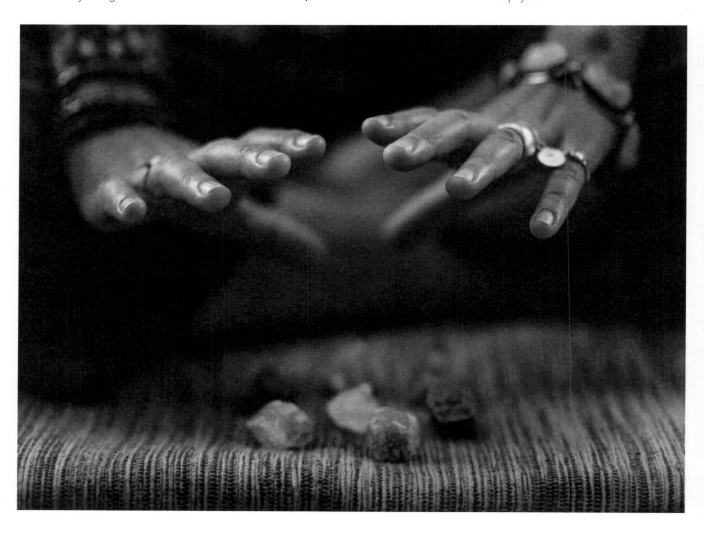

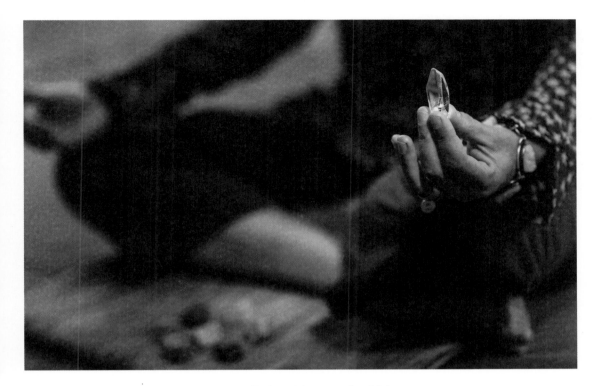

HOW TO BECOME ATTUNED TO CRYSTAL VIBRATIONS

—

The best way to become attuned to crystal vibrations is to get to know each crystal you own and to use each one. Take time to hold your crystals, cleanse and purify them, and set positive intentions for how you'd like to use them.

Meditating with crystals, or practicing mindfulness techniques, can help you become attuned to their subtle vibrations. Hold your crystals regularly and get to know the look and feel of them. Make a note of how different crystals make you feel.

Try carrying small crystals in your pocket or purse, so they're near you throughout the day. Wear jewelry made of crystals, such as necklaces, bracelets, or earrings. Having the crystals close to your body can help connect you to their subtle energy. Wearing earrings, for example, can help link the crystals to the chakras around your head, whereas wearing crystal necklaces can stimulate the throat chakra.

Enjoy having your favorite crystals on display in your home or on your desk at work, so that you can get to know their vibrations better.

Wand crystals focus energy through their points. Here, this quartz wand is being used for meditative practice.

The more you use and touch crystals, the more you have them in your home and see them in your surroundings on a daily basis, the more you'll become attuned to their unique vibrations.

SELECTING CRYSTALS

—

When selecting crystals, learn to trust your intuition and go with the crystal that feels right at that particular time. Sometimes you'll just know and instinctively pick the right crystal for your needs. On other occasions it might be that you like the way a certain crystal feels in your hand, or the way it shines in the light.

If you feel drawn to aparticular crystal, but you are unsure why, it's likely that the crystal has properties that are in tune with your body's needs.

Crystal use can be seamlessly woven into our everyday lives.

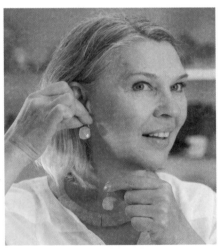

Trust your intuition when selecting crystals for wear or use.

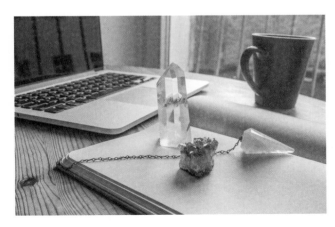

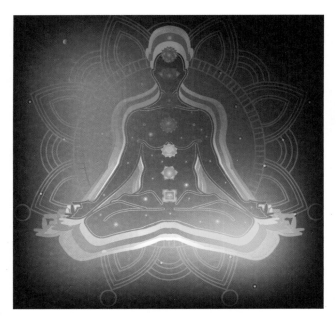

A spiritual energy known as the aura is believed to surround all living things and can be displayed in a range of colors.

THE AURA

The aura is the spiritual energy field that surrounds all living things, including human beings, animals, and plants. In most cases the aura is largely unseen, but some people are attuned to be able to see auras. When viewed, the aura is seen in the form of colors, which are believed to provide insight into your emotional, mental, and spiritual health and well-being.

While you might not be lucky enough to see an aura, most people can feel them. For example, you may well notice that some people give off a very warm, affectionate, or friendly vibe, while others are more prickly, down, or negative. That unspoken vibe that you feel is you picking up on their aura.

Your aura is formed of seven auric layers, sometimes known as auric planes. The layers are arranged inside each other, a bit like a set of Russian dolls or layers of an onion. Each layer is connected to a different aspect of your health and well-being, and the farther the auric layer is from your physical body, the higher it vibrates.

The number of layers is significant, as there are also seven main chakras or energy fields around the body and they work hand in hand with the aura. Like the chakras, each auric layer is associated with a particular role and a color.

CLEANSING YOUR AURA
—

The colors of your aura can change over time and be affected by factors such as your health, feelings, and energy. When your aura is dampened down by negative thoughts, feelings, or experiences, the colors fade and dark patches appear.

In the same way that you care for and look after your physical body, you can cleanse your aura. This helps to wash away negative energy, making your aura shine and become more vibrant again.

You can cleanse your aura in various ways, including:

• Using meditation and visualization techniques.
• Through the use of positive affirmations.
• By using crystals to help rebalance your aura layers and chakras.

A specialist aura reading or aura photograph can reveal the true state of your aura and if any particular colors stand out in your spiritual energy field.

THE SEVEN AURIC LAYERS
—

Each of the main seven auric layers around the body is associated with a particular role and color.

1. THE PHYSICAL OR ETHERIC LAYER
The physical or etheric layer is located closest to the body, approximately 0.5–2 inches (1–5 cm) away from the skin. The layer connects with the root chakra as well as the organs, glands, and meridians of the body. It is linked to the health of the physical body.
Color: Red

2. THE EMOTIONAL LAYER
The emotional layer is located 2–4 inches (5–10 cm) away from the body and is connected to the sacral chakra. It is linked to emotions, feelings, and experiences.
Color: Orange

3. THE MENTAL LAYER
The mental layer is located 4–8 inches (10–20 cm) away from your body and is connected to the solar plexus chakra. This auric layer is linked to thoughts, ideas, and beliefs.
Color: Yellow

4. THE ASTRAL LAYER
The astral layer is located 8–12 inches (20–30 cm) away from the body and connects to the heart chakra. It is linked to love, balance, and well-being. The astral layer is the first of the auric layers that is focused on more spiritual aspects.
Color: Green

5. THE ETHERIC TEMPLATE LAYER
The etheric template layer is located 1–2 feet (30–60 cm) away from the body. It acts like a copy of your physical body on the spiritual plane. It connects with the throat chakra and is linked to communication.
Color: Blue

6. THE CELESTIAL OR CAUSAL LAYER
The celestial or causal layer is 2–3 feet (60–90 cm) away from the body and is linked with the subconscious mind and the third eye chakra.
Color: Indigo or violet

7. THE SPIRITUAL OR KETHERIC TEMPLATE LAYER
The spiritual or ketheric template layer is located 3–5 feet (90 cm–1.5 m) away from the body and is linked to the crown chakra. It protects all the other layers and vibrates at the highest frequency.
Color: Bright white

THE
CHAKRAS

You are probably familiar with the seven chakras (from the Pali for "wheel" or "circle") of ancient Hindu texts. In crystal healing, we work with these focal points, as well as five additional points. Each chakra is linked with a particular color of crystal or stone.

TUNING INTO CHAKRAS
—

The chakras are the links between your aura, or energy field, and your physical body. They are part of your subtle body, which is composed of mind, intelligence, and ego. The subtle body controls the physical body. The chakras are connected to each other by energy channels known as Nadi, through which the energies of the physical body and subtle body flow. Through day-to-day living, or emotional or psychic attack, the chakras can become disturbed, blocked, or stuck open, leading to physical illness, psychosomatic conditions, and spiritual upset. By restoring the chakras to equilibrium, we can work toward peace of mind and body.

Each chakra links both to a specific body part and to an area of spiritual, mental, and emotional life. A simple overview of the chakras and their functioning is to say that the chakras below the waist relate to the physical body and our ability to function practically in the world. The upper torso chakras relate to our emotional functioning, which can also create psychosomatic conditions. The head chakras correspond to our mental and intuitive faculties.

The crown and higher chakras relate to our spiritual selves.

Chakra stones or crystals can be used during stone therapy massage.

IDENTIFYING PROBLEMS
IN THE CHAKRAS
—

Chakras can become disturbed or imbalanced, leading to specific areas of physical disease or emotional, mental, or spiritual dysfunction. In addition, a chakra can become stuck open, or "blown," leaving the body and spirit undefended. The opposite condition can also occur: a chakra can become stuck in the closed position, leading to physical damage or negative emotional states. In all cases, the positioning of the correctly colored crystal over the chakra can result in a rebalanced energy flow.

ADDITIONAL THERAPIES
—

In addition to any medications prescribed by their specialist, sufferers may benefit from talking therapies, meditation, yoga, and good nutrition to ensure that any deficiencies (such as vitamin B in alcoholics) are addressed.

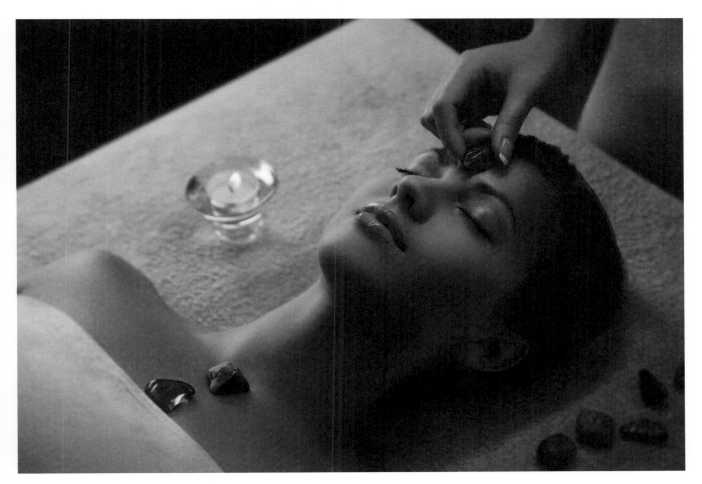

TREATING AND BALANCING THE CHAKRAS WITH CRYSTAL LAYOUTS

You can use crystal layouts to effectively treat and rebalance your chakras. One of the benefits of crystal layouts, especially if you're new to working with crystals and subtle energy healing, is that they work on all the chakras at once. The chakras are interdependent, so if one chakra is out of balance, it can affect all of the others, too.

Working with crystal layouts is a good approach for beginners, as it can help you get to know your crystals and also how the chakras feel. In time, you'll feel more confident to focus on individual chakras and will instinctively know when one needs more attention than another.

A crystal layout is, as the name suggests, simply a way of laying out your crystals. In this case, crystals that correspond with each of the chakras are placed on or around your body.

BASIC CHAKRA BODY LAYOUT
—

For this chakra body layout you'll need to lie down. So, first find a quiet and comfortable place on the floor or on a bed and lie flat on your back. If it's chilly, get a blanket to keep you warm and turn off your cell phone so you're not disturbed. You'll get the best out of this exercise if you have time to yourself to focus on it. If you're not comfortable with complete silence, find some calming music to have on in the background. Set the scene by dimming the lights and having essential oils or scented candles burning in the background.

There's no set time limit for how long you should do your crystal layout—anything from 5 to 20 minutes is sufficient. But the longer you practice, the more you're likely to feel the benefits. As a beginner, it's helpful to note down how it makes you feel and whether there are any particular areas of your body that feel different afterward. It will help you get to know how you respond to certain crystals.

For this chakra body layout, lay in a quiet, comfortable place on your back to begin.

CHAKRA CRYSTAL LAYOUT
—

You'll need to choose seven crystals that represent the colors of each of the chakras. If you don't have many crystals, use what you have available. However, a good starting point for a chakra crystal layout includes crystals such as:

Root chakra—smoky quartz, red jasper, black tourmaline, bloodstone.

Sacral chakra—carnelian, orange calcite.

Solar plexus chakra—citrine, yellow calcite, yellow jasper.

Heart chakra—rose quartz, green aventurine.

Throat chakra—blue lace agate, angelite, lapis lazuli, turquoise.

Third eye chakra—amethyst, sodalite, iolite.

Solar plexus chakra—clear quartz, moonstone, selenite.

Once you have chosen your seven crystals, lay them out on and around your body as follows:

Root chakra—place the crystal on the floor or bed, between your legs.

Sacral chakra—place the crystal between your hip bones.

Solar plexus chakra—place the crystal between your lower ribs and belly button.

Heart chakra—place the crystal in the middle of your chest, level with your heart.

Throat chakra—place the crystal on your throat.

Third eye chakra—place the crystal in the middle of your forehead, between your eyebrows.

Crown chakra—place the crystal on the floor or pillow, by the top of your head.

If you're worried about the crystals falling off, you may wish to use surgical tape to gently stick the crystal in place while you're performing the layout.

When all of the crystals are in place, close your eyes, relax, breathe deeply, and allow the crystals to do their work. You might find it beneficial to say an affirmation out loud or in your head to confirm to the crystals that you're open to healing. For example, you could say, "I am open to the healing power of these crystals," or, "I thank these crystals for rebalancing my chakras."

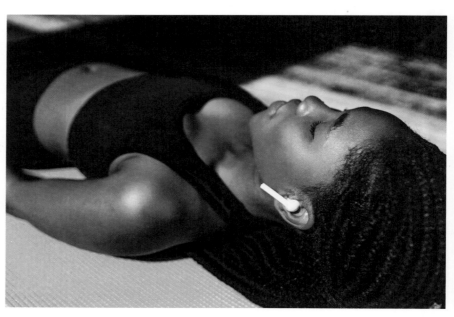

CREATING CRYSTAL GRIDS

Crystal grids are a special technique you can use to amplify the power of crystals. A grid is an arrangement of crystals in a geometric pattern that is designed with a particular purpose or intention in mind. When a selection of crystals is brought together and used in a grid, the individual energetic properties of the crystals are magnified, producing a more powerful effect. Their energies work together in harmony and they produce more energy than they would if used individually.

Crystal grids are traditionally based on sacred geometry patterns of geometry, but you can use any geometric pattern you have an affinity with. Grids vary in size and complexity, from large multilayered grids to small and simple shapes, with each grid pattern carrying different energies. Crystal grid templates can be found in Part 4, from page 290.

Some simple grids to start with include:

• A circle, with one focus crystal in the center and other crystals placed around the outside of a circle shape. A circle grid represents unity, wholeness, and protection.
• A square, with one crystal in the center and four more positioned in each corner of the square shape. A square grid can be beneficial for helping set and maintain boundaries.
• A triangle, with one crystal in the center and three more on the points of the triangle. A triangle grid shape helps represent structure and order.
• A spiral-shaped grid, with crystals located all along the spiral. The spiral shape represents reaching out, expanding, and growing.
• A five-stone cross grid, with one crystal positioned in the center, and the other four around it, positioned in the north, south, east, and west points. A cross grid shape can be used to enhance physical and spiritual connections.

The key to a successful grid is to choose the appropriate grid layout, a clear purpose, and the right crystals to achieve this.

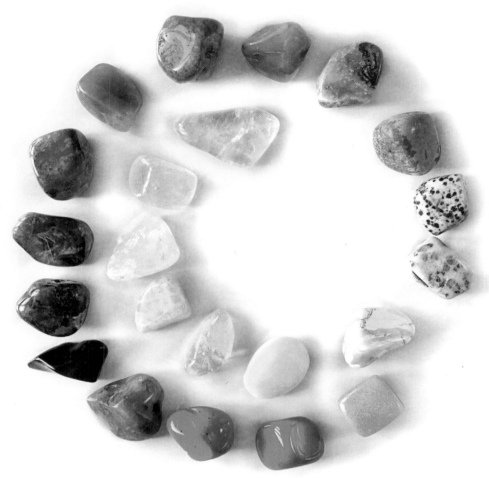

HOW TO SET UP AND ACTIVATE YOUR CRYSTAL GRID
—

To set up your crystal grid, follow these steps:

• Set your intention for the grid. For example, do you want to focus on creating energy, building emotional strength, developing self-acceptance, or improving communication?
• Choose appropriate crystals, using the guides in Part 2 and Part 3 to help your selection. Select a focus stone that is appropriate for the outcome you're seeking, plus some active or anchor crystals for the key points on the grid. Additional stones can be added as amplifiers between the main crystals.
• Choose a grid layout and decide where you're going to position your grid. Ideally, it needs to be located where it won't be disturbed (take into consideration inquisitive pets or children) but is easily accessible for you. You may find it useful to lay the crystals out on a tray or board that can be placed on a shelf.

Some people find it useful to have a full set of chakra healing stones in a variety of colors.

• Cleanse and purify your crystals using a method of your choice (see page 48).
• Start by placing your focus crystal in the center of your grid, then add the active stones in their positions. Finally, add any amplifiers between them.

If you've set a clear intention and aim for your grid, it should start to function as soon as it is laid out. But you can make it more powerful by adding an additional step and activating all the crystals.

Use a clear quartz crystal wand and place it above the central focus stone. Move the wand clockwise in a small circle over the central stone, while stating your intention for the grid. Repeat the action on all of the active crystals, going back to the focus stone after you do each active crystal. As you get to grips with crystal energy, you may be able to feel subtle energy changes as you move over each stone.

MEDITATING WITH CRYSTALS

Meditating with crystals is an ideal way to get to know your crystals and learn to attune to their energy.

Meditation is the practice of sitting quietly and stilling the mind. Small crystals can be held in your hand while you meditate, while larger crystals can be placed in front of you to look at and meditate on.

Meditation is accessible for anyone—you don't need any specialist training to do it (although you can learn it via classes if you wish). You just need to find some time to yourself where you can sit quietly, breathe deeply, and be calm. Think about whether you could make meditation part of your regular self-care routine, as regular practice can be beneficial.

GETTING STARTED
—

Before you meditate, cleanse and purify the crystal you're going to use (see page 48). Set the mood by turning off your cell phone so you're not disturbed, then find somewhere warm and comfortable to sit. If you sit on a chair, have your back straight and feet flat on the floor.

Start by closing your eyes and taking a few deep breaths, then breathe slowly for 2–3 minutes. Hold your crystal in your hands and state your intention to connect with it.

As you hold your crystal, let your body and mind attune to the subtle vibrations of the crystal. Use the time to soak up the crystal energies. You might feel sensations in your hands, see colors in your mind, hear sounds, or receive messages.

Sit holding the crystal for as long as you feel comfortable, then thank it for connecting to you. When you finish, jot down a note of how you felt.

It can take time and practice to learn to quieten and still your mind, and it's not a skill that comes naturally to everyone, so be patient. Remember, though, there's no right or wrong way to meditate.

CRYSTALS TO MEDITATE WITH
—

Any type of crystal can be used to meditate with, especially when you're getting to know a new stone. However, there are some crystals that are naturally regarded as being ideal meditation companions.

Amethyst is a good crystal for meditation if you're seeking to boost your intuition or to promote inner peace.

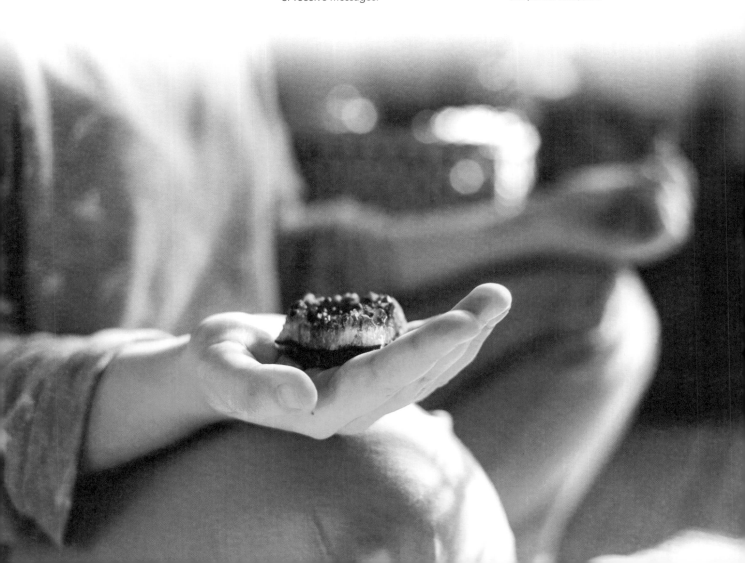

MAKING CRYSTAL ELIXIRS

Clear quartz—associated with the crown chakra, clear quartz is a good balancing crystal to use for meditation and is ideal for beginners. Quartz can help you maintain balance, raise your vibrations, and open up to energies.

Selenite—like clear quartz, selenite is also associated with the crown chakra. This calming and cleansing crystal can help to clear your mind and improve your clarity. Try starting the day with a selenite crystal meditation.

Rose quartz—this pink stone is associated with the heart chakra and has properties of love, compassion, and forgiveness. It can help promote feelings of peace and love as you meditate.

Amethyst—an amethyst crystal is associated with the third eye chakra and is a good crystal to meditate with if you're seeking to boost your intuition. The calming and healing properties can promote inner peace and reduce stress. Try ending the day with an amethyst meditation.

Smoky quartz—associated with the root chakra, smoky quartz is a good choice to use if you want to feel more balanced. If you're stressed, this crystal can help promote feelings of grounding, plus it can dispel negative energy.

MINDFULNESS WITH CRYSTALS
—

If you find meditation tricky, try mindfulness instead.

Rather than trying to clear and empty your mind of thoughts (which often causes more thoughts to appear!), hold a crystal and focus on the stone. Explore the size and shape of it, look at its structure, angles, and facets, learn how it feels in your hand, and see how the light shines through it. Practicing mindfulness is a great way to get to know your crystals better.

Experienced crystal healers and therapists may sometimes make crystal elixirs, which can be applied externally to the skin or, in some cases, consumed.

Crystal elixirs are made in two main ways: indirectly and directly. The indirect method, which is the safest and recommended way to try, involves filling a large glass bowl with water (ideally pure spring water), then placing a smaller glass bowl containing the crystals into the larger bowl.

Once the crystal bowl is inside the water bowl, it should be left for a few hours. The idea is that the water will become infused with the healing vibrations of the crystals. If you wish, you can cover the bowl with plastic wrap or a glass lid and place it outside in the moonlight or sunlight.

When the crystals have finished infusing, you can decant the water into a bottle to use for healing purposes. A dropper glass bottle made from colored glass is useful, or you could fill a spray bottle.

HOW TO USE CRYSTAL ELIXIRS
—

Indirectly made crystal elixirs are best used freshly made. You can use your homemade crystal elixirs in number of ways:

• By putting a few drops (4–6 drops) of the water under your tongue every few hours.
• By directly dabbing a few drops of the water onto your skin. (Note: if you have sensitive skin, do a small patch test first.)
• By spraying the water around you, to clear and clean your aura or to banish unwanted negative energies from a room.
• By adding the crystal elixir to a bath.

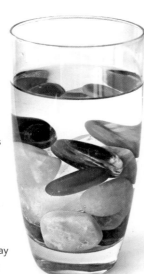

Crystal elixirs are made by infusing water with your chosen crystals and can be used in a number of ways.

If you visit a professional crystal healer, they may prescribe a crystal elixir that will last for a longer period of use. This is because the elixir will be preserved in alcohol, such as brandy or vodka.

CRYSTAL ELIXIRS—DIRECT METHOD SAFETY WARNING
—

The direct method of making a crystal elixir involves immersing crystals into water directly.

As tempting as it may be to try this approach, it's very important not to attempt making direct method crystal elixirs without having been properly and professionally trained in crystal healing. This is especially so in the case of crystal elixirs that are consumed, as well as those that are applied directly onto your skin.

Not all crystals are capable or safe to be made into elixirs. For example, some crystals don't react well when they come into contact with water. More importantly, some crystals—such as dragon's blood, which contains lead, and malachite, which has traces of copper—contain toxic elements. The toxicity can be transferred into the water and could be highly dangerous and poisonous if consumed.

SPECIAL CRYSTAL WATER BOTTLES
—

Look out for specially designed crystal water bottles, which can provide a great alternative to the indirect method.

These bottles are usually made of plastic or glass and look very much like a normal water bottle. However, they are designed with a special inner compartment where small crystals can be placed. The main bottle is then filled with water and it can be drunk from safely, as there is no direct contact between the crystals and the water. Most bottles are sold complete with the right-sized crystals to place in the compartment, such as quartz, rose quartz, and citrine.

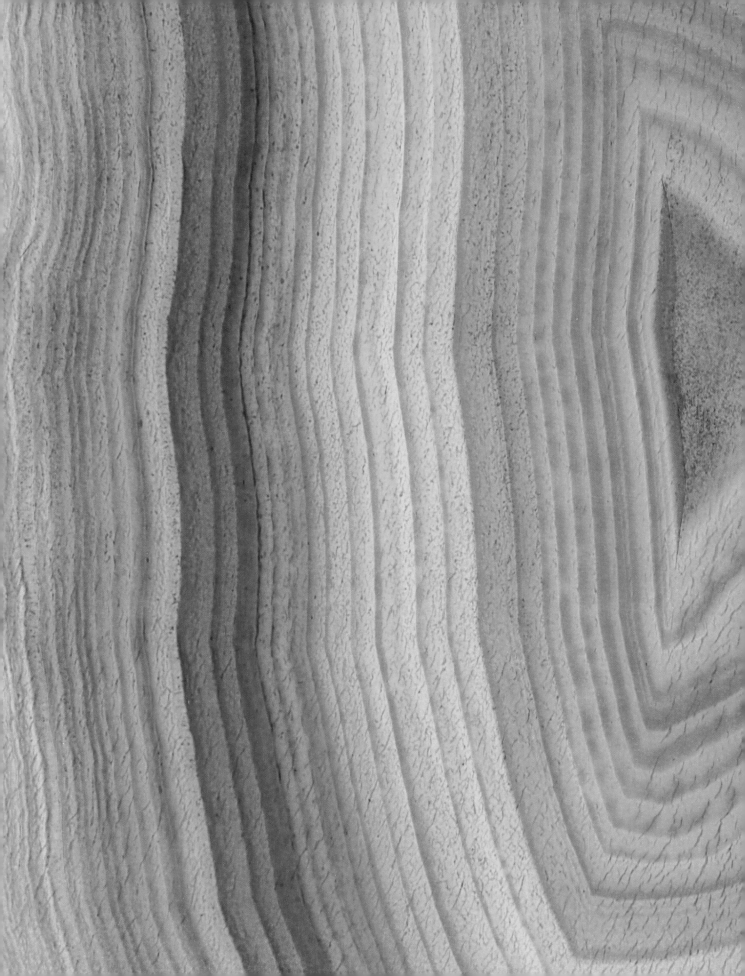

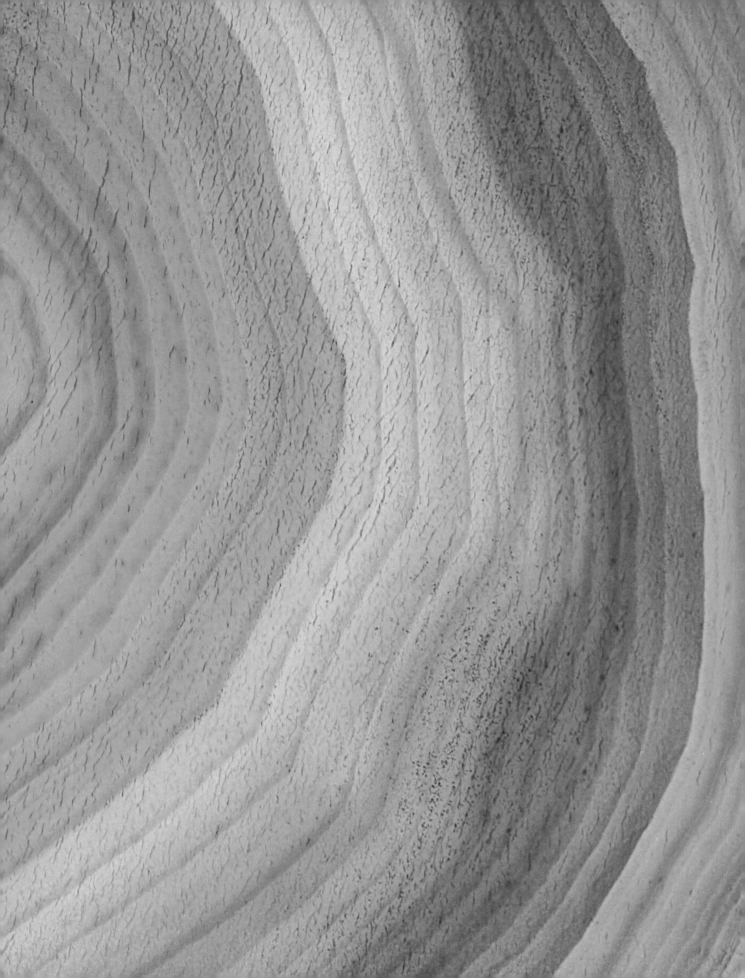

WEARING CRYSTALS AS JEWELRY

One of the many benefits of crystals is that they make perfect jewelry. People have been wearing jewelry made from crystals for centuries, including precious and semiprecious gems, and it never goes out of fashion.

Crystal jewelry doesn't just look good—wearing crystals is an ideal way to keep them close to you and to draw on their healing benefits. Crystals can help balance and stimulate the chakras and your aura while you wear them.

HOW TO CHOOSE CRYSTAL JEWELRY
—
Crystal jewelry comes in a wide variety of designs and styles, from simple crystal points to wear on a chain, to elaborately designed and set faceted-cut gems. Beyond your own personal choice, the style of the jewelry isn't important, and neither is the size of the crystals. In terms of their healing potential, small crystals can be just as powerful as larger ones.

There are several methods you can use to choose crystal jewelry:

• **By color**—choose jewelry with the crystals in your favorite color, or a color that most complements your clothing.

• **By type of crystal**—choose your jewelry by the type of crystals it contains. Perhaps it's one that you love, or one that you know has qualities you desire.
• **By intuition**—use your intuition and choose crystal jewelry based on what you feel most drawn to. The chances are it could be a crystal that has properties that could be beneficial for you, even though you're consciously unaware of it. When it comes to crystals, there's a lot to be said for gut instinct!
• **By birthstone**—each month of the year has a birthstone linked to it, so many people enjoy wearing crystal jewelry made from their particular birthstone.

If you have no major crystal preference, try a multicolored chakra ring or bracelet, as this could be beneficial for generally rebalancing the energy centers throughout your body. Plus, a piece of jewelry with all the colors of the rainbow can look bright, colorful, and raise your spirits.

TYPES OF CRYSTAL JEWELRY
—
A range of different types of crystal jewelry is available, or if you're creative, you could have a go at making your own. When you're choosing or making jewelry, it's worth thinking about the placement of the crystals and how they could affect you. For example:

Necklaces—if you'd like a crystal to work on your throat chakra, a short choker-style necklace may be appropriate, whereas if you're keen to work on your heart chakra, a longer necklace may be a better option.

Earrings—carefully chosen crystal earrings can help stimulate your third eye chakra, especially those with a purple stone, such as amethyst.

Tiaras and headbands—wearing a tiara or headband with crystals on can be beneficial to your crown chakra.

Belts—a decorative belt with crystals on can be close to the root or sacral chakras.

Rings and bracelets may not be located directly next to chakras, but they can be just as beneficial for your overall well-being.

WEARING YOUR CRYSTAL JEWELRY
—
Once you've chosen your jewelry, wear it often. Having the crystals directly next to your skin will help attune the crystal to you, raising your vibrations and improving the energy in your body.

If you're wearing crystal jewelry regularly, it's a good idea to take time to cleanse and purify the crystals when you can. They can pick up negative energies, collect dust and dirt, plus residues of perfume or hair products can get on them. By purifying your crystals, you'll refresh their exterior look and color, plus give them a new burst of positive energy.

If you're wearing crystals to serve a particular aim or purpose, you could also program the crystals to boost their potential.

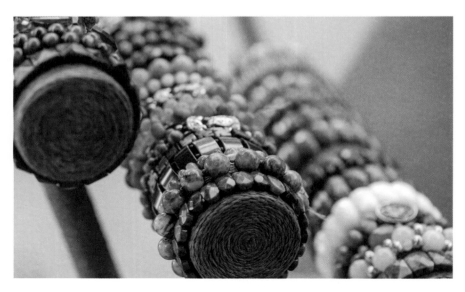

Wearing crystals as jewelry is a great way to keep crystals and their healing energy close to you.

CREATING A CRYSTAL ALTAR

A crystal altar is a sacred space where you can display your favorite crystals, healing tools, and other items that have special meaning for you. It is the ideal place to put the crystals that you're currently working with, or have set intentions for, and to sit near when you're meditating or practicing mindfulness.

Altars have featured for centuries in religious, spiritual, and cultural belief systems, but today they're a sacred space used for much more. You might like to think of your altar as reminiscent of a 3D vision board—a display that will inspire, uplift, and motivate you when you look at and interact with it.

There's no right or wrong way to create a crystal altar. First, simply find a free space to use, such as windowsill, shelf, mantlepiece, empty fireplace, or tabletop. Ideally, it should be a location where it won't be disturbed and you can leave it permanently set up. Clean and clear the space, so it's clutter- and dust-free.

Next, choose the crystals you'd like to display on your altar and cleanse and program them. It could be the crystals you're currently working with, your favorite gems, or larger display pieces, such as chunks of amethyst, rose quartz, or agate geodes.

Also, think about other items you'd like to include, such as shells, flowers, pine cones, acorns, pebbles, driftwood, favorite quotes, photos, or pieces of artwork that you find inspirational. Take time to place your chosen crystals and items on your altar until you're happy with how they look.

Once your crystal altar is created, enjoy it! Sit by it, light some candles, meditate, connect with the crystals, and soak in the energies. It's your special place.

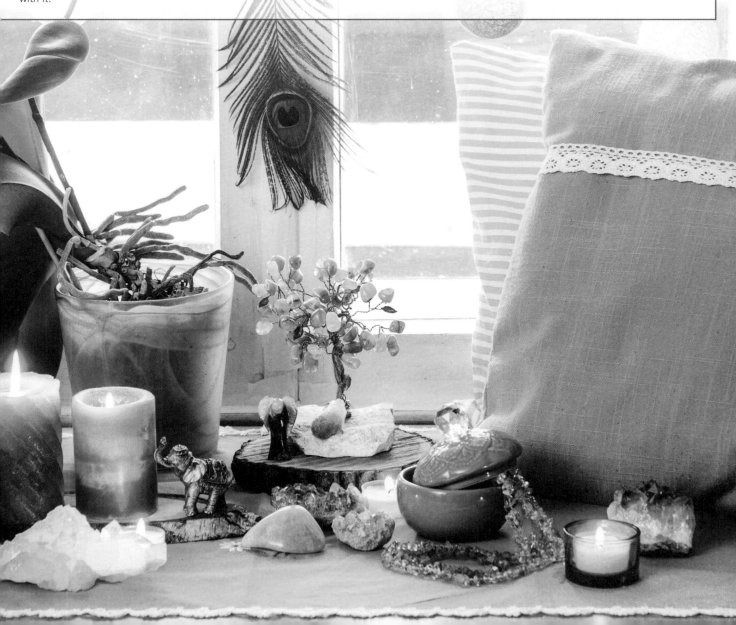

CRYSTAL PENDULUMS AND OTHER CRYSTAL RITUALS

A pendulum is a divination and dowsing tool that consists of a symmetrical, weighted object hung from a cord—specially cut crystals can be used for this purpose.

Using a pendulum enables you to tap into your intuition and higher guidance and get answers to simple yes or no questions, such as which crystals to use in grids or layouts, how long to leave them in place, or what chakras need rebalancing. The idea is that the crystal pendulum acts as a receiver and transmitter of information and moves in response to your questions. It's often described as being like bringing together the rational and intuitive sides of you—or the left and right brain—so that you can make well-rounded decisions.

Pendulums can help you access higher guidance and intuition. Cleanse, purify, and charge your pendulum with your energy prior to use.

CLEANSING AND PROGRAMMING YOUR PENDULUM
—

Any crystal can be used as a pendulum, but a good starting point is clear quartz. First, you'll need to cleanse and purify your crystal, then charge it with your own energy. To do this, simply hold the crystal in your hands, sit quietly, and state your intention to charge the crystal with your energy. If you like, say a prayer or ask spirit guides or guardian angels for their support and guidance. A short meditation while holding the pendulum can also help attune you to its energy.

The pendulum works by moving in certain directions—small circles or side to side. In order to understand and use your pendulum effectively, you'll need to ascertain which movement represents a yes answer and which a no. Hold your pendulum cord between your thumb and forefinger, with any excess cord wrapped lightly around your index finger. Still the pendulum by running your hand down the length of the cord, bringing it to rest with the tip of the crystal in the upturned palm of your hand.

HOW TO USE YOUR PENDULUM
—

Start by asking a simple question with an easy yes or no answer. For example, "Is my name X?" Relax and watch the pendulum move. Be patient—the first time you do this, you might need to repeat this step several times before you're sure of the response. You may find your pendulum moves in clockwise circles for yes and back and forth for no, but everyone is different and the way it moves may be unique to you.

If at any time the pendulum moves in an indistinct way, then it might be a signal of a "maybe" answer. Try again with a more specific question and see if you can achieve a definite response.

Once you've ascertained how the pendulum moves in response to yes or no, try it again with another question. Be sincere about what you ask and treat your pendulum with respect.

CRYSTAL RITUALS
—

Many crystal aficionados have crystal rituals they use to enhance various areas of their life. Rituals needn't be complex—just spending a few minutes a day to stop, connect, and set intentions can be beneficial.

Here are some examples of popular crystal rituals:

Sleep ritual—hold a celestite crystal before you go to bed to clear your mind, prepare your body for sleep, and enhance a calm state.

Home-protection ritual—black tourmaline has energetic shielding properties. Place a piece of tourmaline inside your front door, or outside in a sheltered porch, and imagine it forming a protective shield around your house.

Stress-release ritual—hold blue lace agate stones in each hand and state the intention that it will release stress and fill your body with calming vibes.

Manifestation ritual—hold a piece of citrine and set it with the intention to promote manifestation of prosperity into your life. Also try putting small citrine tumbled stones in your wallet to promote wealth.

CHOOSING CRYSTAL TYPES BY USE

Each crystal has its own unique qualities, so one of the easiest ways of choosing which crystals to work with is by their individual use and purpose.

Crystals, of course, don't come with an instruction leaflet detailing their uses—but help is at hand! In Part 2 of this book, you'll find a comprehensive directory of over 200 crystals, arranged by colors, with accompanying text to explain how each one can be beneficial to you. If you have a particular ailment for which you'd like additional support, turn to Part 3, which covers a wide range of conditions that may benefit from the use of crystals, to heal the mind and realign the chakras.

Like other areas of health and healing, there's not a "one-size-fits-all" solution to finding the right crystal for you. There can be multiple factors causing your symptoms, some of which you may be unaware of, and different crystals help in different ways.

For example, if you are experiencing a headache caused by sinusitis after a bad cold or due to poor posture, blue aventurine placed at the site of the pain might help. However, if your headache is due to a hangover, you'd be better off using turquoise. If eyestrain from computer use has triggered your headache, emerald might help, and if stress is the underlying cause, charoite might be more beneficial.

It can be a case of trial and error, testing out which crystal could be more beneficial in each situation. Some crystals work in conjunction with others, while others work more effectively on their own.

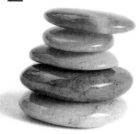

Some crystals work well in combination; others are best used in isolation.

As you get to know crystals better, you'll gradually gain an understanding of the different types and their uses and become more confident at finding the perfect stone for every purpose.

CHOOSING CRYSTAL TYPES BY ATTRACTION

Another element to choosing crystals is simply by attraction. Maybe there's a crystal that you're itching to use, one that you love the color of, one that has an amazing shape, or a stone that feels lovely to hold in your hand? Be open to trusting the stones that you feel most attracted to and use them when it feels right to do so.

Working with crystals involves tuning in to subtle energies, and there are often cases where you feel attracted to certain stones and feel compelled to choose them, even if you're not sure why. Sometimes the reasons will become apparent quickly, while on other occasions it might take a little time for the stone to reveal to you why it was so important.

Get to know your crystals by handling them often. Hold them in your hands while meditating or pick one crystal a day to hold or have in your pocket. The more you get used to them, the better able you will be to detect and feel their energies, and you'll start to notice those subtle shifts and changes in attraction as one stone becomes more relevant to what's going on in your life.

Trusting your intuition and learning to be guided by higher energies isn't a skill that necessarily comes naturally to everyone. If you're normally fueled by the need to know logically why something is right, it can be hard to trust the unknown. But it's definitely worth persevering with and, in time, you'll hopefully find yourself being attracted naturally to the crystals that are right for the occasion.

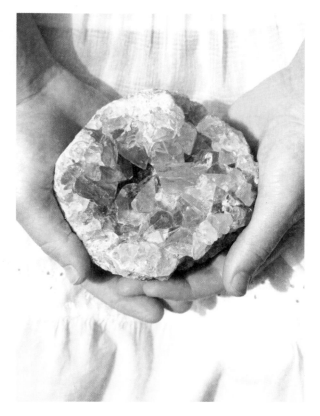

Trust yourself to choose the right crystals for you. That intuition could be due to the crystal's energy, shape, color, or something subtle that only becomes apparent with use.

CHOOSING CRYSTAL SHAPES AND THEIR HEALING PROPERTIES

The shape of the crystals plays a part in your choice, too. Crystals come in a variety of different shapes—some natural and some deliberately carved—and both types can have distinct purposes that are appropriate when working with crystals. When you combine the unique properties of individual types of crystals with the symbolic meaning of their shape, it can produce powerful results.

Here's a guide to some of the shapes you may find useful when working with crystals, and also the purposes they serve.

ANGELS
—

Choose crystals carved in the shape of angels when working on connecting to higher realms and protection. Angel-shaped crystals are available in a range of sizes, from mini to large. Small and mini carved angels are ideal to use in grids.

ANIMAL SHAPES
—

Choose crystals carved in the shape of animals to help boost a connection to your pet or a spirit animal.

BALLS OR SPHERES
—

Crystals carved into smooth finished balls or spheres represent a sense of wholeness or completion. Small balls can be used as part of grid layouts—just make sure they don't roll off!

CUBES
—

Choose a cube-shaped crystal when you're working on maintaining stability and grounding. Crystals such as black tourmaline, hematite, and black spinel are good options.

DOUBLE-ENDED POINTS
—

Choose double-ended or double-terminated crystals—those with faceted points at both ends—to both attract and emit energy.

EGGS
—

Egg-shaped crystals can symbolize creation and birth, but they are also relevant to any circumstances involving new beginnings.

HEARTS
—

Choose a carved heart-shaped crystal when you're working on boosting feelings of love. Pale pink rose quartz, which is a stone associated with love and emotions, is particularly good for working with the heart chakra.

MERKABA
—

Merkaba-shaped crystals (carved into a three-dimensional star tetrahedron) are good for spirituality work, for raising vibrations, and connecting to higher realms.

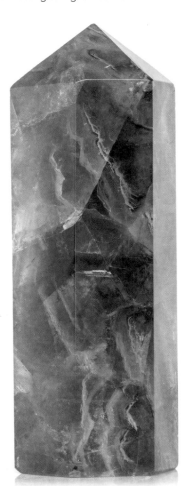

OBELISK
—

Like carved merkaba crystals, obelisk-shaped pieces are a good choice for spiritual work. They can act as a connection between the physical and spiritual realms, sending energy and vibrations heavenward.

PYRAMID
—

Choose pyramid-shaped crystals if you're looking to focus and amplify energy. As an ancient symbol, pyramids are great for creating and amplifying energy fields.

SINGLE-POINT
—

Choose single-point crystals that have a carved or faceted point at one end to enable you to direct and focus energy. When the point is directed toward you or an area of your body that you're working on, energy will be drawn toward you. When the point of the crystal is facing away from you, energy will be drawn away from you.

TUMBLESTONES
—

Tumbled gemstones are so versatile. They are comfortable and convenient for placing on or around the body, with their small size meaning that they're not too heavy. They're great for using with grids and tend to be an affordable starter option if you don't have many crystals yet. Plus, you can easily pop a tumblestone or two in your purse or pocket, so that you can carry them with you and have their energy near you.

WANDS
—

Like single points, crystals carved into wand shapes can be used to direct and transmit energy to a specific point.

LEFT: This green fluorite wand can direct healing energy to a specific area.

RIGHT: Whether through daily or occasional use, crystals are embedded with their own individual energy. A variety of crystal shapes, colors, and types can allow for a greater range of healing properties, like a well-stocked crystal apothecary.

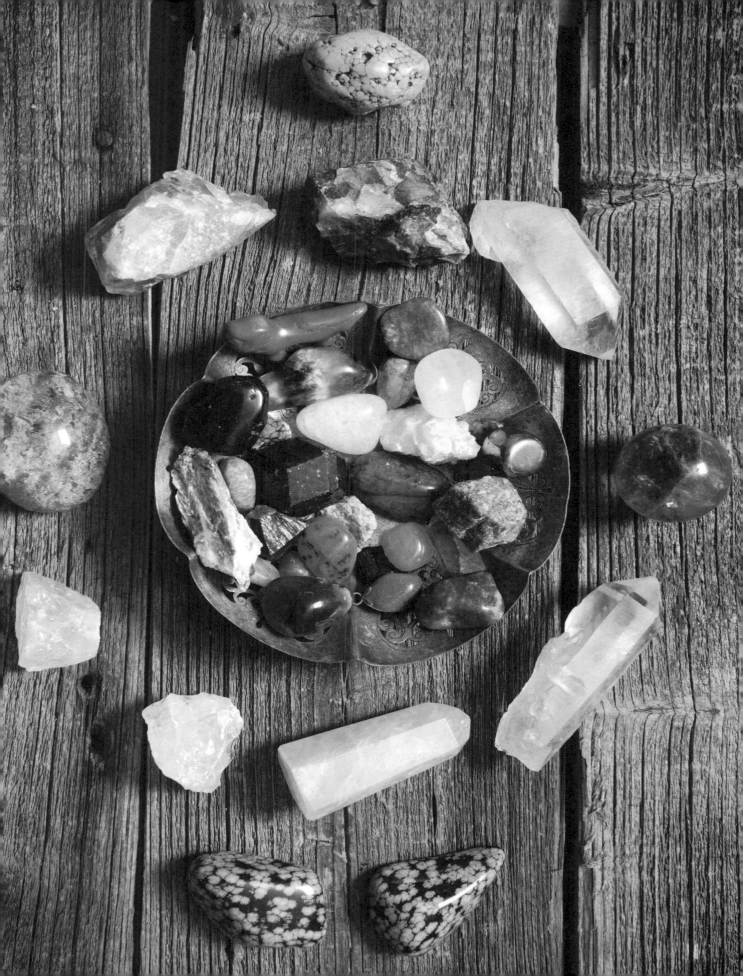

THE PRACTICALITIES
OF BUYING CRYSTALS

When it comes to buying crystals, ideally the best method is to choose them in person. This enables you to look at the array of crystals available, get hands on, to touch and feel the crystals, sense their energies, and use your intuition to decide which crystals are calling at you to buy them.

Look for specialist crystal shops, or one-off fairs or events near you, and go along to buy your crystals. It might help to equip yourself with a shopping list of crystals you're interested in, as this can enable you to target your buying and prevent you getting carried with spending!

If you can't find any specialist crystal shops in your area, the next best option is to buy online or by mail order. There are a variety of specialist websites selling online and you may find that you get more choice and better access to rarer crystals by purchasing in this way.

Many specialist online crystal retailers are passionate about their job, going the extra mile with providing exact photographs of the crystals you're buying, rather than just a general image of ones you might receive. This can help considerably with giving you a clear idea of what you're purchasing. It's also worth looking out for websites that use videos to share their crystals, or who sell via social media, such as Instagram or Facebook live events, as these experiences provide a more personal shopping style.

If you're unsure which crystals to purchase, why not try using your pendulum to dowse? Use it in front of, or over, a picture of the crystal and be guided by its response as to whether it's right for you or not. Sometimes the results may be surprising, but you may later discover why that crystal was right at that particular time.

Many specialist crystal retailers and jewelers are passionate about their craft and will support you to choose the crystal that's right for you.

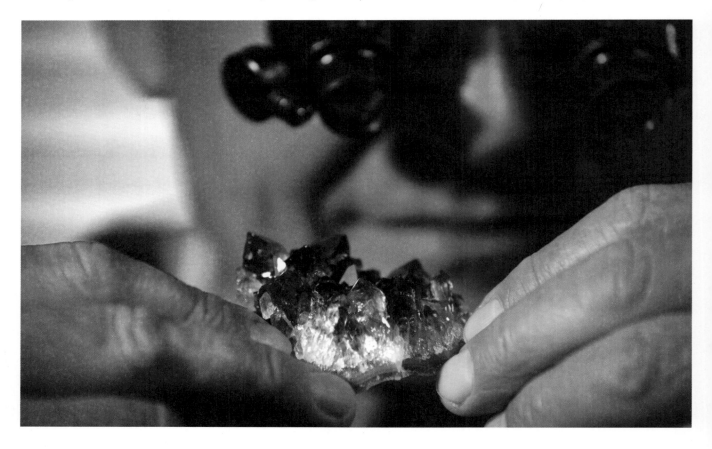

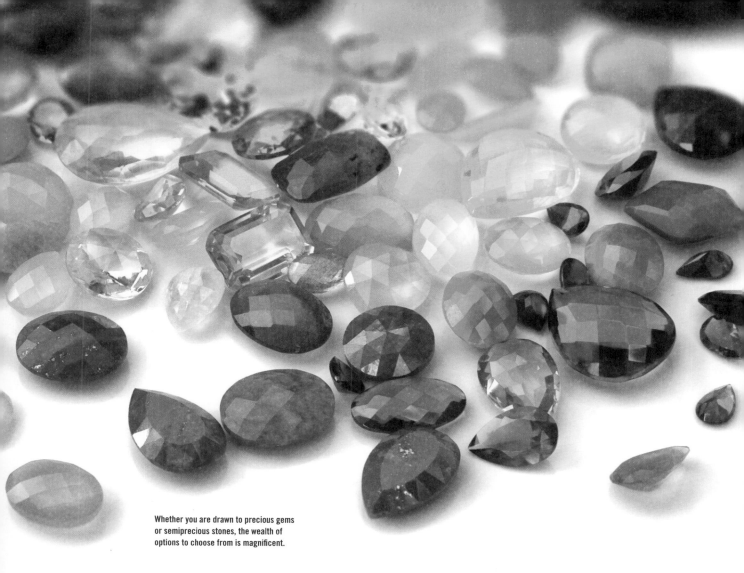

Whether you are drawn to precious gems or semiprecious stones, the wealth of options to choose from is magnificent.

CRYSTAL BIRTHSTONES AS GIFTS

Certain crystals are traditionally associated with months of the year, with a different crystal representing each one. The idea is that the crystal associated with your month of birth can bring a protective energy to your aura, and carrying or wearing that stone acts as a form of talisman. Buying a piece of jewelry or other crystal items that links to a month of birth has become a popular gift idea.

The notion of crystal birthstones has a long history and is believed to date back to at least Biblical times. One example of 12 stones representing the 12 months of the year was found in the Breastplate of Aaron, a sacred object worn by the High Priest of the Israelites (Aaron, the elder brother of Moses)

to communicate with God. (If you want to read more about this, a description can be found in the Book of Exodus in the Bible.)

Over the years, there have been a lot of variations on crystal birthstones, relating to different traditions and beliefs. For example, some people go by specific zodiac sun signs rather than the months of the year, or choose gems relating to planets.

It can be confusing to know which crystal is the right one to gift, which is why the association the Jewelers of America created their modern birthstone list in 1912. It's since become widely accepted as a standard guide to crystal birthstones.

According to the list, the birthstones are as follows:

January—Garnet
February—Amethyst
March—Aquamarine
April—Diamond
May—Emerald
June—Alexandrite, Cultured Pearl, and Moonstone
July—Ruby
August—Peridot
September—Sapphire
October—Opal, Tourmaline
November—Citrine, Yellow Topaz
December—Turquoise, Blue Zircon, Tanzanite

PROGRAMMING YOUR CRYSTALS

Once your crystals are purified and cleansed, it's time to program them.

The idea of programming your crystals is that you're getting them ready for the special purpose you want them to serve. Each crystal has its own individual strengths and abilities, and some can have more than one benefit.

By programming a crystal, you clearly set your intention for the specific purpose for which you want to use the stone. Programming helps the crystal energies to focus on specific intentions, goals, or desires, which is said to enhance its vibrations, ability, and power.

STEP-BY-STEP GUIDE TO PROGRAMMING CRYSTALS

—

First, spend a few quiet moments holding each crystal and connecting to its energy. Look at its color and appearance, touch it, and notice how it feels in your hands. You can do this as part of a mindfulness or meditation exercise if you wish.

Next, set your positive intention for how you want to use the crystal. Choose one specific intention or purpose for your crystal. For example, if you want to use a crystal to help attract prosperity into your life, state that. If you're seeking help with dealing with a health condition, be specific about the exact condition or symptoms.

Form the intention into a single sentence—you may find it helpful to write this down. Once you have your sentence, say it out loud while holding the crystal.

For example, a quartz crystal can be beneficial for dispersing negativity and helping you feel more energized. So, you could program a quartz crystal with the words, "I program this crystal to boost my energy and disperse negativity from my life."

In the case of a citrine crystal, which is associated with manifesting abundance, you could program it with the words, "I program this crystal to manifest more money into my life."

Repeat the process and reprogram your crystals frequently, especially before and after using them.

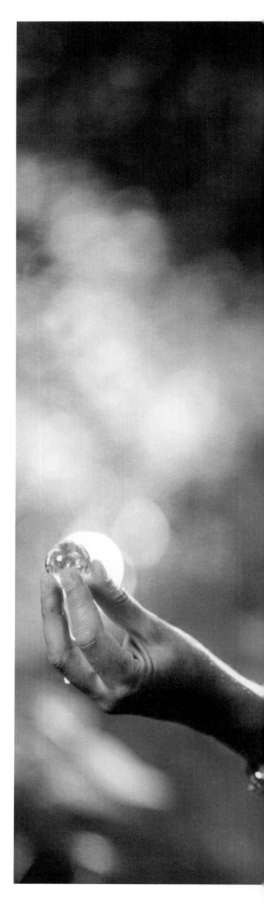

RIGHT: Charge your crystals with sunlight and nature before programming them for your set intention.

NEXT PAGE:
There are many ways to get the best from your crystals, including charging plates, crystal grids, crystal altars, and more. Discover which methods work best for you.

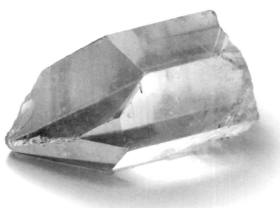

Quartz crystals can be a good choice for boosting energy and expelling negativity.

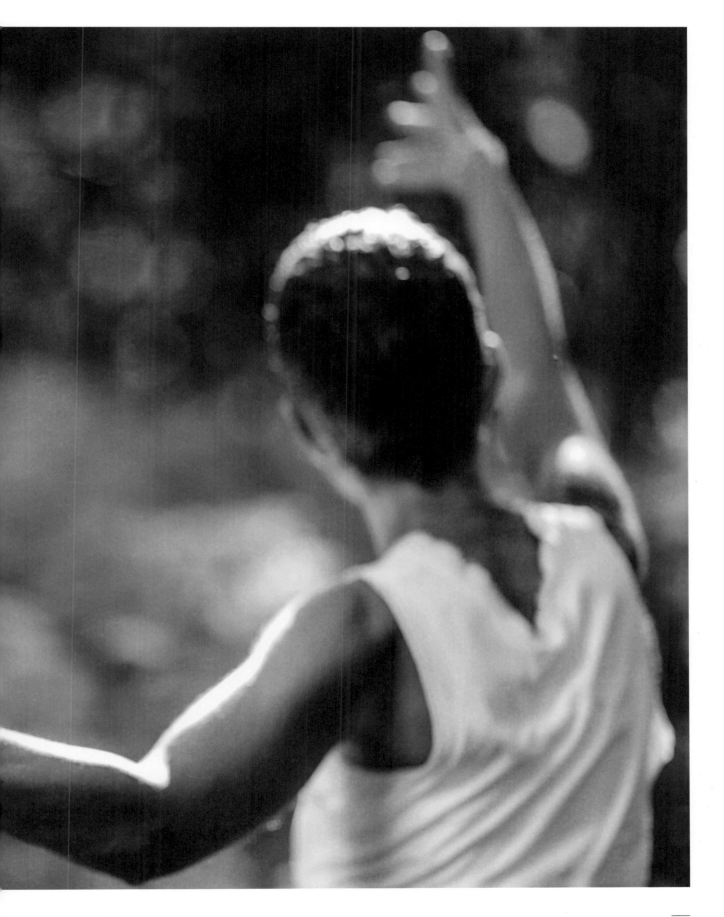

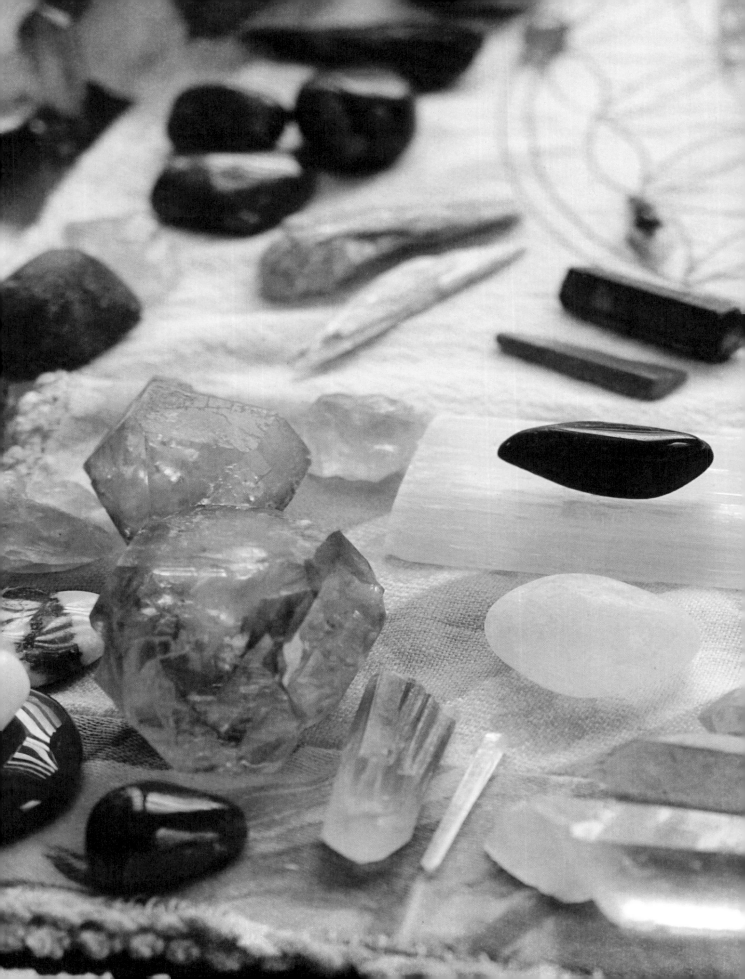

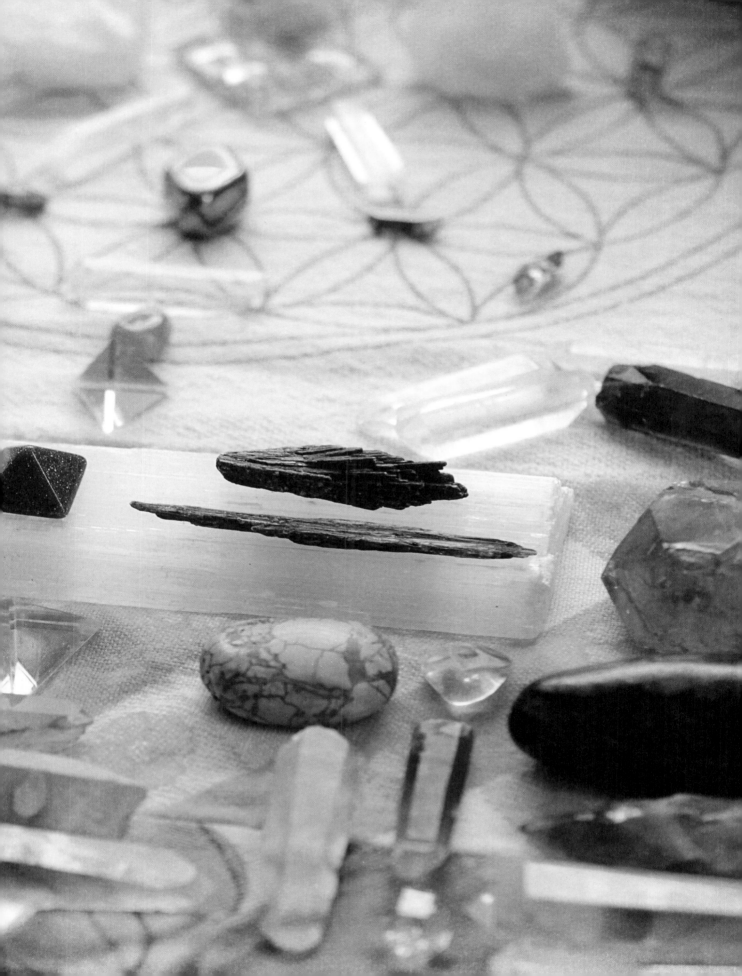

PURIFYING YOUR CRYSTALS

In order for your crystals to be in prime condition for use, you'll need to purify and cleanse them first.

This is especially important when you first buy crystals, or after you've been using them. Purifying crystals helps rejuvenate their energy and remove negativity, as well as revive their color, sparkle, and shine.

There are several methods you can use to purify crystals:

Many crystals can be purified in a bowl or jug of clear, clean water. Avoid placing water-soluble stones, or those that contain minerals, in water and instead use a method such as sunlight, moonlight, incense, or earth.

Running water—hold your crystals under running water for a few minutes, then leave them to dry naturally or pat dry with a towel.

Still water—place your crystals in a bowl of still water. As an optional extra, add a teaspoon of salt. Leave them to cleanse for up to an hour.

Sunlight—place your crystals in sunlight to purify them. Be aware that some crystals, such as quartz, could be a fire risk if left in direct sunlight, even on a windowsill, so avoid leaving them unattended.

Moonlight—place your crystals outside or on a windowsill to charge them by moonlight. This is especially good in the light of a full or new Moon.

Incense—burn incense sticks, such as sandalwood, or a traditional sage smudge stick, and let the smoke waft over your crystals to purify them.

Earth—bury your crystals overnight in soil (outside in your garden or inside in a plant pot) to help them reconnect with the earth.

CAUTION

Some crystals, such as selenite, fluorite, calcite, and azurite, are water soluble, so are not suitable for water cleansing. As a general rule, any crystals that are rated five or below on the Mohs' hardness scale should not come into contact with water. Plus, crystals that contain minerals, such as hematite and magnetite, should not be purified with water as they contain iron ore and iron oxide, which will rust when in contact with water.

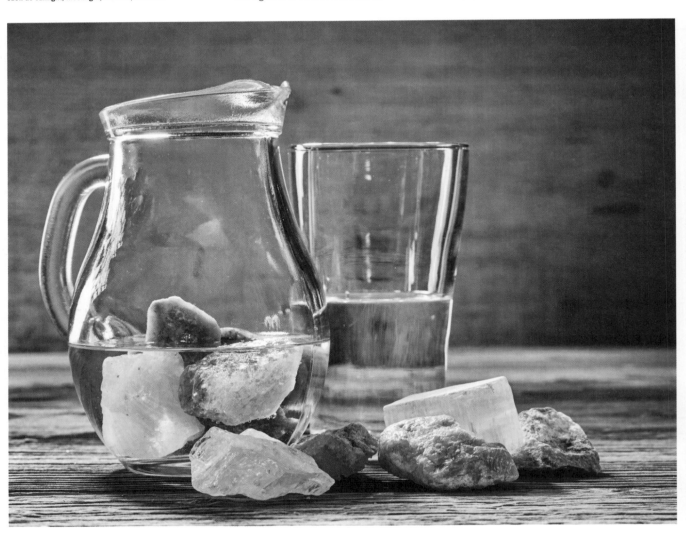

USING OTHER CRYSTALS TO CLEANSE AND PURIFY

Some crystals have a unique ability to purify other crystals.

For example, crystals can be placed onto selenite to become purified. Look for selenite carved in the form of round plates, long bars, or bowls, as these are designed so that you simply place your crystals onto or into them and leave them to purify.

If you have a crystal geode or a crystal cluster, such as quartz, you can place your crystals on or inside them for cleansing.

Carnelian is also a good purifying crystal. Keep a piece of carnelian in a bag of tumbled gemstones to keep them cleansed and purified, ready for use.

CREATE YOUR OWN CRYSTAL PURIFIER

—

One nice idea that is not only practical but also looks really attractive as a decorative accessory in your home is to create your own crystal-purifying station.

Find a suitable empty, clean, glass container to use, such as a round bowl or an empty terrarium (normally used for plants) and fill the base with Himalayan pink salt. Himalayan salt is a form of fossilized sea salt, which has traces of minerals in it that gives it a delicate pink color. Salt is traditionally used for purification purposes and it can work as a means of cleansing crystals, too.

Once you have a good layer of salt in the base of your container, place your chosen crystals inside, onto the salt, to purify and recharge. Position your charging station where you can see it and where you can access your crystals easily when you need to.

Take care not to place your purifying station in direct sunlight, though, as the crystals could catch the sun's rays and become a fire risk.

CRYSTAL CLEANING AND OTHER CARE

Crystals that are out on display in your home or regularly in use will inevitably get dusty. In addition to your crystal-purifying practices, it's a good idea to clean crystals in other ways to help keep them in good condition.

For example, dust is drawn to collect on the surface of crystal clusters and geodes, such as quartz, citrine, or amethyst, and can get between the points. If the dust is left there, over time you'll notice the color and shine of the crystal has dulled, plus it won't be as powerful for healing purposes. Crystals can also pick up sticky residues—for example, from sprays or perfumes.

Crystal points and tumblestones can easily be cleaned with a duster—simply wipe clean the surface. For crystal clusters, use a small brush, such as a toothbrush, paintbrush, or makeup brush to remove excess dirt and dust. Any sticky residue can be wiped off with a damp cloth.

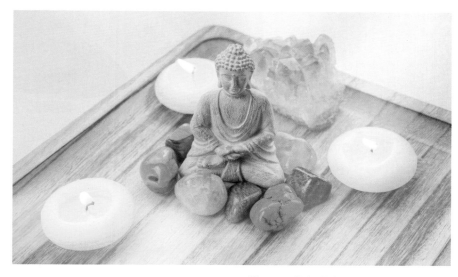

When not on display, it's important to store your crystals safely and securely, where they won't damage each other.

STORING YOUR CRYSTALS

—

It's lovely to keep some crystals out where you can see and admire their beauty, whether at home or work. But if you're building up a large collection of different crystals for healing purposes, you're likely to need to think about storage options, too.

Crystals can be delicate, so it's important not to put them all together loose in one bag or box, where they could knock against each other. You don't want your treasured stones becoming cracked, broken, or damaged.

As a rule of thumb, crystals that are rated hard on the Mohs' scale shouldn't be stored loose with softer stones.

Look for storage boxes that are split into compartments or consider wrapping your delicate crystals in tissue paper, Bubble Wrap, or fabric.

You could arrange your crystals alphabetically, by color, by shape, or by purpose—the choice is yours.

CRYSTAL DIRECTORY

PART TWO

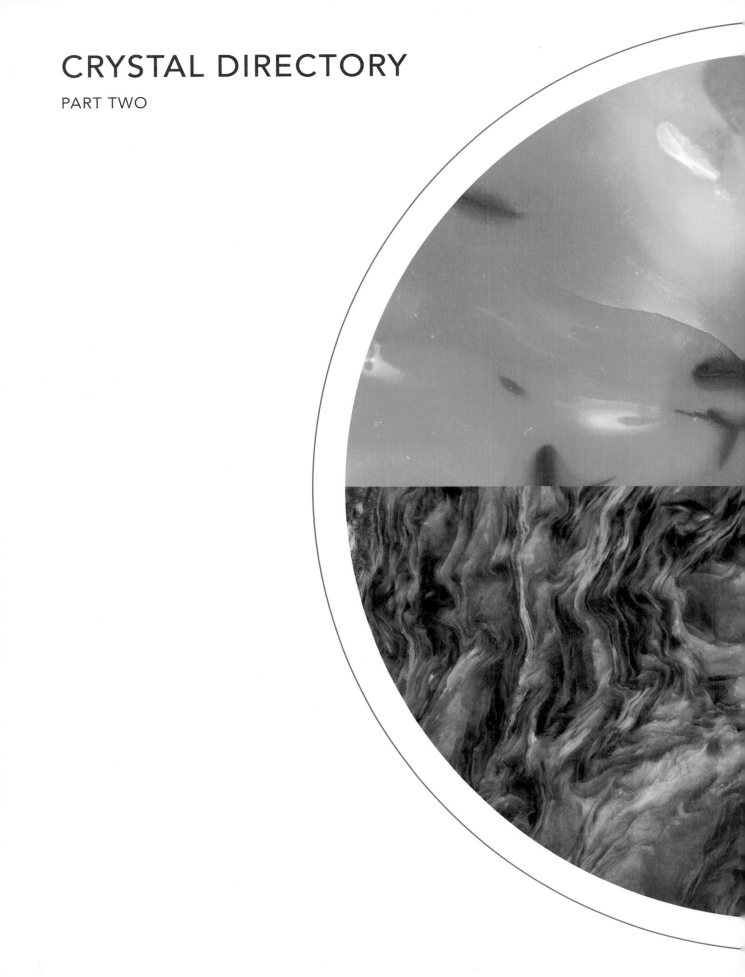

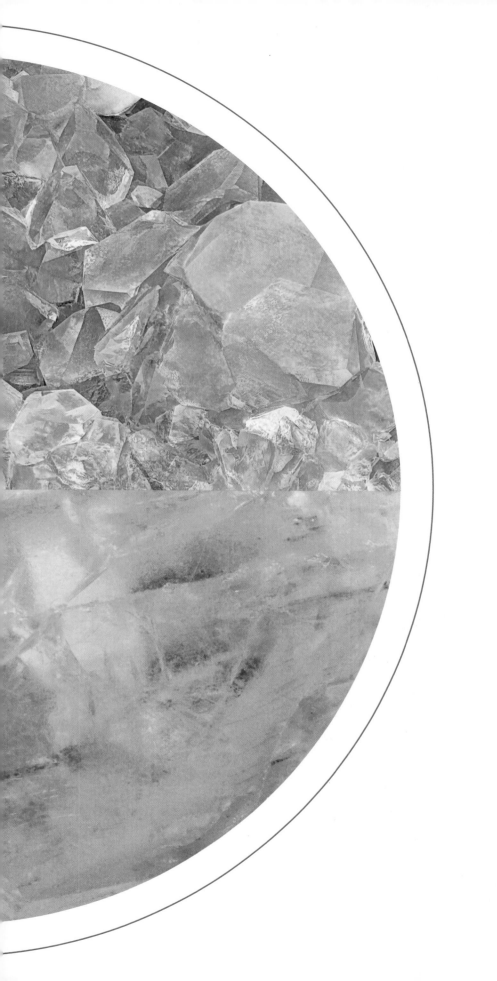

BLACK, GRAY, AND BROWN

These crystals of earth and darkness find particular resonance with the root and earth chakras. Many also connect with the third eye, allowing us to look clearly at what we most fear. Working with black, gray, and brown crystals can enable us to ground ourselves, both emotionally and practically. If we are in need of protection, dark crystals can offer it. Yet when we connect fully with their power, they are freeing, allowing us to see endless possibilities.

From humanity's earliest days, black—the color of the night sky—has represented the unknown. The goddess Kali, of Hinduism and Buddhism, is often depicted with black skin. She is the bringer of both life and death, knowledge and formlessness. In ancient Egypt, black was associated with the dark, rich soil of the Nile River's seasonal floods, bringing new life after death and stasis. Black crystals offer the chance of rebirth. They offer the possibility of facing our fears of darkness and loss, gaining the power of knowledge and courage. Brown and gray crystals are gentler than black; while connecting strongly with the earth, they provide stability and comfort. They allow us to open more fully to the needs of others and of our planet itself.

BLACK TOURMALINE

APPEARANCE
—

A translucent to opaque crystal, black tourmaline is often found in columnar, radiating, or needle-shaped forms that are triangular in cross section.

RARITY
—

This semiprecious stone is widely available in specialist stores. Crystals are often mined in Africa, the United States, and Brazil.

FORMATION
—

Tourmaline is a boron silicate mineral. Brownish-black to black tourmaline is often known as schorl, while dravite (named for the Drava district of Austria) is dark yellow to brown. Both varieties are rich in iron and sodium. Schorl forms in the igneous rock granite, while Dravite is more common in metamorphic rocks such as marble and schist.

ATTRIBUTES
—

Black tourmaline offers both spiritual grounding and protection. It frees from fear and allows us to look deep inside ourselves, for the negative emotions and motivations that we find difficult to confront. Due to its iron content, opaque black schorl has high magnetic susceptibility. This makes it a powerful crystal to work with when clearing blockages and dispersing negative energy. It is also said to expel toxins and reduce bloating.

HEALING ACTION
—

A black tourmaline wand can help when seeking a solution to a seemingly impossible problem. Gardeners may find that black tourmaline wind chimes help their plants to flourish. Place a black tourmaline paperweight on your desk to balance the left and right brains.

COMBINATIONS
—

Use with clear quartz for a powerful boost in emotional strength. While meditating, combine with lepidolite to help with repetitive or self-harming behaviors.

CARE
—

Tourmaline rates 7–7.5 on the Mohs' scale. Clean in warm, soapy water with a soft cloth. Do not inhale tourmaline dust, which can cause silicosis.

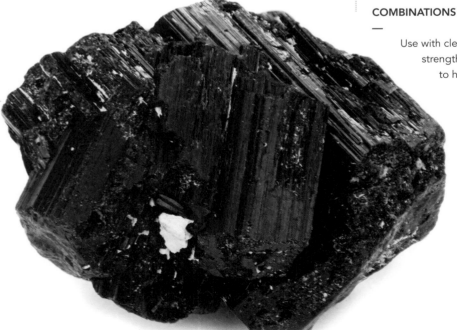

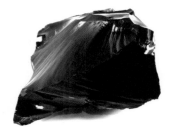

BLACK OBSIDIAN

APPEARANCE
—

A smooth, translucent, volcanic glass, black obsidian is a mineraloid rather than a mineral. It is often found as sharp-edged chunks.

RARITY
—

Obsidian is widely available from stores and may also be collected in areas of rhyolitic eruptions, particularly Argentina, the Canary Islands, Chile, Greece, Iceland, Italy, and the United States.

FORMATION
—

Obsidian forms when lava rich in lighter elements—such as silicon, oxygen, aluminum, sodium, and potassium—cools rapidly, giving no time for crystal growth. This accounts for obsidian's glass-like texture.

ATTRIBUTES
—

Ancient peoples used obsidian for cutting tools and weapons. For a modern user, obsidian aids emotional and mental clarity. If you are well supported by friends and professionals, it is a powerful tool for the examination of past trauma. Jet-black obsidian is not a gentle stone, so should be handled with care and wisdom. Crystal therapists advise that obsidian can speed healing after an injury or surgery.

HEALING ACTION
—

An obsidian pendant may open the door to success in exams or further studies. Placing an obsidian knife on your desk will encourage creativity. Used during meditation, obsidian encourages truth-seeking and clearness of vision. Avoid placing obsidian in the bedroom if you are troubled by repetitive night thoughts.

COMBINATIONS
—

To free yourself from a negative attachment while soothing the pain of an emotional break, combine with amber.

CARE
—

Obsidian is brittle and amorphous, so is prone to fracturing. It scores 5–6 on the Mohs' scale. Do not breathe in obsidian dust, as it contains silicon, so can cause silicosis. Clean in lukewarm, soapy water with a soft cloth.

SHUNGITE

APPEARANCE
—

Shungite is black, matte, and opaque. However, when polished it can take on an almost metallic luster.

RARITY
—

This is a rare mineraloid. Most genuine specimens are found in Russia, usually near the village of Shunga, in Karelia.

FORMATION
—

Shungite is almost pure carbon, around 98 percent, although the term "shungite" is sometimes used for shungite-bearing rocks with lower proportions of carbon. The mineraloid forms from organic-rich sediments deposited in brackish, shallow-water settings.

ATTRIBUTES
—

In the early 1700s, Russia's Peter the Great followed the example of folk medicine and ordered his army to use shungite for purifying water. He also founded a spa in Karelia to benefit from shungite-cleansed water. Today, shungite is still often used for water purification. On the emotional plane, shungite frees the mind of troubling thoughts and helps us to focus on what is truly important. On the physical plane, it is said to cleanse the body of toxins.

HEALING ACTION
—

Hold the crystal over the root chakra to ground yourself in the earth and all the lives that have been lived before your own. Place carvings or bowls made of shungite in a room that often plays host to family arguments, so this mineraloid can help to dispel negativity and focus positivity instead.

COMBINATIONS
—

In combination with sardonyx, shungite can encourage us to make the right choices in difficult times, to be honest about past mistakes, and to turn our backs on bad habits.

CARE
—

With a score of just 3.5–4 on the Mohs' scale, shungite can be damaged by drops and bangs. Clean in warm, soapy water.

BLACK ONYX

APPEARANCE

—

Onyx is translucent to opaque. It may be pure black or display parallel white bands. Traditionally layered white and black, onyx was intricately carved into cameos so that the white layer formed a raised image against the black base layer.

RARITY

—

Black onyx is a fairly common rock. The term "onyx" is sometimes used in a descriptive rather than scientific sense to describe parallel-banded alabaster or obsidian, so ensure you are buying genuine onyx. Some black onyx specimens are artificially colored.

FORMATION

—

Onyx is a form of chalcedony, a cryptocrystalline (with microscopically small crystals) blend of the silicate minerals quartz and moganite.

ATTRIBUTES

—

This rock offers strength and courage. When we feel we lack the willpower to carry on, black onyx can bolster us. It also offers the wisdom to know what is best said and left unsaid, revealed, or kept secret. It is said to protect and nourish the digestive system, pancreas, and gallbladder.

HEALING ACTION

—

If training for a marathon or studying for exams, wear black onyx on your body for willpower and the belief that you will triumph through hard work. If you suffer from bad dreams or night terrors, place black onyx under your pillow.

COMBINATIONS

—

If you are working through grief, meditate with black onyx and rhodochrosite for the strength to continue when the loss feels unbearable.

CARE

—

Onyx is durable, with a hardness of 6.5–7 on the Mohs' scale. Do not inhale onyx dust, which can cause silicosis. Clean in warm, soapy water with a soft cloth.

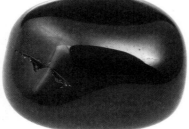

ANDRADITE

APPEARANCE

—

This mineral often forms clearly defined dodecahedrons and trapezohedrons. Andradite is usually black or brown, but is on rare occasions yellow-green or bright green. It ranges from transparent through translucent to opaque.

RARITY

—

Crystals of andradite are fairly common in the United States, Italy, Russia, and Ukraine.

FORMATION

—

Andradite is a member of the garnet group of minerals. It contains the elements calcium, iron, silicon, and oxygen. It forms in metamorphic rocks, particularly those that have been altered by contact with magma or hydrothermal fluid.

ATTRIBUTES

—

The garnet group is known for its powerfully revitalizing crystals. Andradite is no exception, awakening both creativity and inspiration. It encourages us to reach out to others to form new relationships and reawaken old ones.

HEALING ACTION

—

When entering a challenging social situation, such as a new job, flatshare, or course of study, wear andradite close to the body for the self-confidence to build new bonds. Meditate with andradite when you are in need of inspiration in your working or home life. Place andradite by your computer if you are experiencing trouble with problem-solving. Some crystal therapists use andradite externally for easing stomach complaints such as irritable bowel syndrome, but medical advice should always be sought.

COMBINATIONS

—

When seeking contact with the spirit realm, place angelite at the third eye or crown chakra, with andradite at the root chakra. In combination with blue sapphire, andradite will enhance learning, both academic and spiritual.

CARE

—

Andradite may be cleaned in warm, soapy water with a soft cloth. It scores 6.5–7 on the Mohs scale.

PYROLUSITE

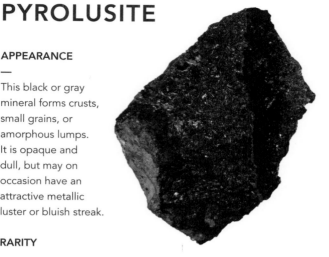

APPEARANCE
—

This black or gray mineral forms crusts, small grains, or amorphous lumps. It is opaque and dull, but may on occasion have an attractive metallic luster or bluish streak.

RARITY
—

Pyrolusite is readily available from specialist stores, both as tumbled stones and in combination with other crystals and rocks.

FORMATION
—

Pyrolusite is manganese dioxide, making it an important ore of manganese. It forms in bogs and hydrothermal deposits.

ATTRIBUTES
—

Pyrolusite was used as a pigment for cave painting from the Stone Age. It has often been found at Neanderthal sites. The mineral's name comes from the Greek words for "fire wash," as it was used to remove the green or brown tints from glass during glassmaking. In terms of healing, this mineral has the power to transform, turning negative thoughts to positive, fear to courage, and anger to renewed love. Some crystal therapists use pyrolusite externally for balancing the metabolism.

HEALING ACTION
—

Pyrolusite soils the fingers and is heavy, so it is not suitable for wearing or excessive handling. Turn conflict to agreement by placing pyrolusite in a meeting room or office that sees frequent turmoil.

COMBINATIONS
—

Place pyrolusite and variscite in the bedroom of someone who is recovering from illness or mild depression to help rebuild their physical and emotional strength. Team pyrolusite with sodalite during meditation if you are searching for higher truths.

CARE
—

Keep pyrolusite away from babies and children. Do not inhale the dust from pyrolusite, which is toxic. Wash hands after touching. It scores 6–6.5 on the Mohs scale, but may be softer in large chunks. It can be cleaned in warm water with a soft cloth.

JET

APPEARANCE
—

A semiprecious mineraloid, jet is black or dark brown, occasionally with sparkling pyrite inclusions. It is opaque and may be polished to a high shine.

RARITY
—

Jet is found in a few locations, including Whitby, in England, the southwestern United States, northern Spain, and eastern Turkey. True jet is warm to the touch, unlike imitation black glass, which feels cool.

FORMATION
—

Jet is a type of coal, formed from ancient wood—usually araucarian coniferous trees—that has been subjected to intense pressure in a watery environment. Jet is around 75 percent carbon, plus oxygen, hydrogen, and sulfur.

ATTRIBUTES
—

Jet pendants have been worn as protective talismans since ancient times. This is a powerfully protective and cleansing stone. It also strengthens the links between past and present; and between present hopes and future fulfillment. It is said to both strengthen the immune system and expel toxins.

HEALING ACTION
—

Wear as a pendant, earrings, bracelet, or ring to awaken the protection of ancestors or lost loved ones. When working toward a goal, from passing exams to saving for a vacation, place a jet stone or carving in a prominent position. Jet can awaken memories of past lives and, during meditation, aids awareness of nature's natural cycles.

COMBINATIONS
—

When accessing past lives or scrying, combine with variscite and muscovite for powerful visualizations, as well as the ability to learn from them.

CARE
—

Jet is soft, only 2.5–4 on the Mohs' scale. When placed in a flame, jet burns like coal. Do not ingest or use in gem elixirs.

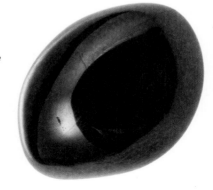

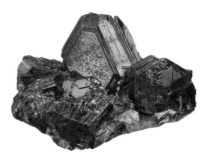

SPHALERITE

APPEARANCE
—
Gray-black, gray, brown, or yellow, sphalerite forms clearly defined cubic or tetrahedral crystals. Some specimens are shiny or metallic.

RARITY
—
A common mineral worldwide, sphalerite is the most important ore of zinc.

FORMATION
—
Sphalerite contains zinc and sulfur, with varying quantities of iron. The higher the iron content, the blacker the crystal. The mineral forms in hydrothermal veins and contact metamorphic zones, often in association with galena.

ATTRIBUTES
—
This mineral is warming, soothing, and comforting. The paler, more translucent varieties of sphalerite connect with the earth and with home. The darker, more metallic varieties, which may be called marmatite, have the same quality, along with a rejuvenating and uplifting effect. It is said to speed recovery from mild viruses such as colds.

HEALING ACTION
—
When placed at the root chakra, sphalerite soothes feelings of rootlessness and homesickness. If placed at the throat chakra, it helps us to comfort those who need kind words. Sphalerite is the ideal mineral for imbuing a family room with positive energy.

COMBINATIONS
—
If you are prone to hatching plans that never come to fruition, meditate with sphalerite together with blue sapphire and black onyx for the practicality, clear sight, and willpower that will help you see everything through.

CARE
—
Scoring 3.5–4 on the Mohs' scale, sphalerite is soft and fragile, so handle with care. Do not use in gem elixirs. Clean in warm, soapy water with a soft cloth.

AEGIRINE

APPEARANCE
—
Aegirine forms greenish-black or dark green crystals that grow as tall, rectangular prisms, sometimes side by side or fanning from a central point. It ranges from translucent to opaque.

RARITY
—
When aegirine was discovered in Norway in the 1800s, it was named after Aegir, the Norse god of the sea. Today, the mineral is mined from locations in Norway, Greenland, Russia, Canada, Scotland, Kenya, and the United States.

FORMATION
—
A silicate mineral, aegirine also contains sodium and iron. It forms in sedimentary, igneous, and metamorphic rocks that are rich in silicon.

ATTRIBUTES
—
Aegirine is the crystal of integrity. When our honesty and decency are most under threat, aegirine gives strength. It also helps to free us from negative attachments and habits. Some crystal therapists say that it helps to heal the lungs and sinuses after infection.

HEALING ACTION
—
Use an aegirine wand during scrying to signal the way forward. Meditate with aegirine if you are facing a difficult choice, where financial or social gain points in the opposite direction from truth or fairness. If you are able to purchase a "nest" of aegirine, featuring crystals clustered together as in a blackbird's nest of twigs, place it in the family corner of the home (to the left and midway through the house if you enter by the front door) to encourage honest conversation between the generations.

COMBINATIONS
—
Meditate with obsidian and aegirine if you need to call on both clarity and integrity to make a difficult decision. Use with shungite for help with ending bad habits, from nail-biting to excessive snacking.

CARE
—
This crystal scores 6 on the Mohs' scale. Do not inhale aegirine dust. Do not use in gem elixirs. It can be cleaned in warm, soapy water with a soft cloth.

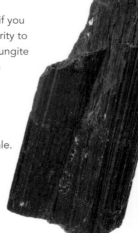

BLACK SPINEL

APPEARANCE
—

Spinel takes its name from the Latin word for "spine," due to its pointed crystals. It is often found in eight-sided shapes or flat, triangular plates. Specimens range from transparent to opaque.

RARITY
—

Transparent spinel is priced as a semiprecious gemstone, but tumbled opaque stones are far more common.

FORMATION
—

Crystals of spinel grow in igneous and metamorphic rocks. Spinel is formed from atoms of magnesium, aluminum, and oxygen. Spinel and ruby are often found together, with ruby formed mainly from aluminum and oxygen.

ATTRIBUTES
—

All varieties of spinel offer hope in times of difficulty, with black spinel having particular resonance with material concerns, such as financial problems, house moves, and legal issues. It opens the door to fresh energy and ideas when they are needed the most. On a physical level, it is also said to be highly reenergizing, particularly after periods of overwork.

HEALING ACTION
—

While lying down, place spinel on the root chakra to open the door to hope. If positioned on the third eye, spinel can help with problem-solving. Sleep with tumbled spinel under your pillow to awake refreshed and to be able to find new routes around old obstacles.

COMBINATIONS
—

For a powerful boost at times of despair, meditate with black spinel, sugilite, and sunstone.

CARE
—

This strong crystal scores 7.5–8 on the Mohs' scale. It can be cleaned with warm, soapy water and a soft cloth.

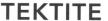

TEKTITE

APPEARANCE
—

Tektites are natural glass pieces that may be black, gray, brown, or green. Taking the shape of raindrops, balls, shards, or plates, tektites are usually gravel-sized.

RARITY
—

Most tektites come from one of four meteorite-strewn fields: North American (34 million years old), Central European (15 million years old), Ivory Coast (1 million years old), and Australasian (0.8 million years old). Usually, Australasian and Ivory Coast tektites are black, Central European tektites are green (see Moldavite), and North American tektites are green, brown, or black.

FORMATION
—

Tektites formed when the earth's rocks and soil were melted and ejected during massive meteorite impacts. Many tektites fell back to the earth thousands of miles from the site of the impact.

ATTRIBUTES
—

Tektites have the power to open our hearts and minds to necessary changes, new ideas, or challenging journeys. These are ideal stones for those interested in dream work or conversing with the spirit realm. They are also said to ease headaches caused by staring at a screen.

HEALING ACTION
—

Place on the third eye to open your mind to ideas or voices. Placed on any chakra, tektite helps with blockages and the balancing of energy flow. Meditate with tektite to take your consciousness beyond its usual limits, or place under your pillow to aid lucid dreaming.

COMBINATIONS
—

To facilitate contact with the angelic realm, combine with angelite. Use tektite together with moonstone for powerful lucid dreams.

CARE
—

Tektite scores 5.5 on the Mohs' scale. Store carefully to prevent accidental breakage. Do not inhale tektite dust, which can cause silicosis. Clean in lukewarm, soapy water with a soft cloth.

GRAY KYANITE

APPEARANCE
—
Kyanite forms columnar, striated crystals. It ranges from transparent to opaque.

RARITY
—
Kyanite is a common mineral, available from most specialist stores. Crystals are more usually blue than gray: the crystal's name comes from the ancient Greek *cyanos*, meaning "dark blue."

FORMATION
—
Kyanite contains the elements aluminum, silicon, and oxygen. Its crystals grow during the metamorphism of fine-grained sedimentary rocks. It is commonly found in aluminum-rich gneiss and schist.

ATTRIBUTES
—
Gray kyanite dispels formless fears, illusions, and irrational anxieties. It is also a great healer of rifts, bringing together families, friendship groups, and workforces so that they can strive together for a common purpose. Some crystal therapists say that gray kyanite supports the body's automatic nervous system.

HEALING ACTION
—
Kyanite wands are useful for dispelling negative energy. Position near your pillow if you are troubled by night terrors or anxiety-induced insomnia. Place on your desk or position at the crown chakra if you are beset by self-doubt.

COMBINATIONS
—
To see your way through a quandary, meditate with kyanite and pietersite.

CARE
—
Kyanite crystals are much stronger (6.5–7 on the Mohs' scale) if pressed or banged at right angles to their direction of growth, than if struck parallel to their striations (4.5–5 on the Mohs' scale). Clean with warm, soapy water and a soft cloth. Do not soak. Do not use in gem elixirs.

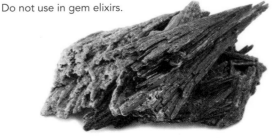

ZOISITE

APPEARANCE
—
Brown zoisite may be pleochroic, exhibiting different colors from different angles and in different lights. It is transparent to translucent. Zoisite is found as chunks, striated prisms, and columns. Different shades of zoisite are known as tanzanite (blue to violet), thulite (pink), and anyolite (green zoisite combined with ruby).

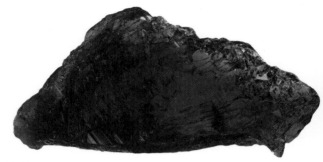

RARITY
—
Translucent zoisite is fairly common. High-quality transparent zoisite is priced as a semiprecious stone.

FORMATION
—
Zoisite is found in metamorphic rocks or igneous rocks that formed at high temperature and pressure deep underground. It contains atoms of silicon, aluminum, calcium, oxygen, and hydrogen.

ATTRIBUTES
—
Zoisite can help the user turn sadness to hope, anger to acceptance, and anxiety to calm. It is an ideal crystal for those looking for a fresh start, either practically or emotionally. Where relationships have gone astray, it may help with rebuilding trust. It is said to strengthen the joints, particularly the hips, although medical advice should always be sought.

HEALING ACTION
—
For those suffering from writer's block or anxiety about a new creative project, place zoisite on your desk as a paperweight. Meditate with zoisite to help find your way toward positive change.

COMBINATIONS
—
For those experiencing the physical and emotional changes of menopause, meditate with zoisite and moonstone.

CARE
—
Zoisite scores 6–7 on the Mohs' scale. Do not use in gem elixirs. Clean in warm, soapy water with a soft cloth.

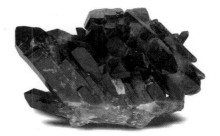

SMOKY QUARTZ

APPEARANCE
—

Smoky quartz is gray to black, sometimes with yellowish tints, and ranges from transparent to almost opaque. Quartz crystals often grow as six-sided prisms ending in pyramids.

RARITY
—

Smoky quartz is common worldwide. Ensure that you buy from a reputable source that does not sell quartz that has been artificially irradiated.

FORMATION
—

Pure quartz is made of silicon and oxygen atoms. Smoky quartz gets its appearance from natural irradiation of traces of aluminum in the crystal structure. Quartz is a common rock-forming mineral, found in felsic rocks such as granite.

ATTRIBUTES
—

Smoky quartz offers strength in the face of difficulty, as well as practical solutions to nebulous problems and fears. This crystal helps us to accept ourselves as we truly are, both physically and mentally. Some crystal therapists say this variety of quartz helps with ailments of the legs, including nighttime cramps.

HEALING ACTION
—

Positioned at the earth or root chakra, smoky quartz is grounding, helping us to turn ideas and dreams into workable reality. This crystal is an ideal gift for anyone who struggles with body image or is overly self-critical. A wand of smoky quartz is particularly effective at dispelling negative energy.

COMBINATIONS
—

Meditate with golden topaz, ametrine, and smoky quartz to overcome low self-worth and lack of confidence.

CARE
—

Quartz, which is named for the old Germanic word for "hard," scores 7 on the Mohs' scale. Do not inhale quartz dust, which can cause silicosis. Clean in warm, soapy water with a soft cloth.

LORENZENITE

APPEARANCE
—

Usually brown to black in hue, lorenzenite forms needles or rectangular prisms. It ranges from dull to glassy, opaque to transparent.

RARITY
—

This is a rare mineral that may be most easily purchased when interlocked with other crystals, such as aegirine.

FORMATION
—

Lorenzenite, named for the Danish mineralogist Johannes Lorenzen, contains the elements sodium, titanium, silicon, and oxygen. It is most often found in pegmatites, which are igneous rocks containing enlarged crystals.

ATTRIBUTES
—

This crystal engenders stability, balance, and rootedness. In times of anxiety or change, it offers calm and comfort. It helps to combat worries about the future by encouraging us to see the patterns of life and death, endings and renewal, that maintain our planet's natural cycles. Some crystal therapists say that lorenzenite can be helpful while experiencing the transition of menopause.

HEALING ACTION
—

If you are suffering from home sickness, place lorenzenite under your pillow or in a corner of your hotel room. Wear as a pendant if you are prone to episodes of anxiety. If you have difficulty existing in the moment during meditation, position lorenzenite at your root chakra.

COMBINATIONS
—

When aegirine and lorenzenite crystals grow side by side, they form a powerful combination, encouraging both stability and integrity.

CARE
—

Scoring 6 on the Mohs' scale, lorenzenite is strong enough to withstand frequent handling. Do not inhale lorenzenite dust, which can cause silicosis. Do not use in gem elixirs. It can be cleaned in warm, soapy water with a soft cloth.

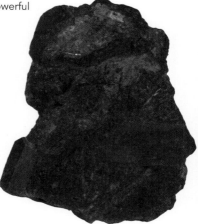

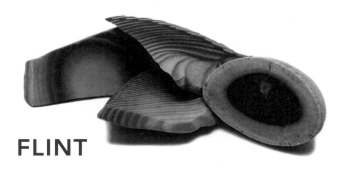

FLINT

APPEARANCE
—
Usually gray, brown, black, green, or white, flint has a glassy appearance. It is translucent to opaque. The flint is often surrounded by an outer layer of rough white rock. Flint chips and breaks into sharp-edged pieces.

RARITY
—
This extremely common mineral can be found on beaches and beside rivers and lakes. It is commercially quarried in countries such as Belgium, Germany, Poland, Romania, and the United States.

FORMATION
—
Flint forms as nodules, often in the burrows of long-dead worms and echinoids, in sedimentary rocks such as chalk and limestone. Flint is a tiny-crystalled variety of the mineral quartz, which is composed of silicon and oxygen.

ATTRIBUTES
—
Flint is a fire-starter. In practical terms, it produces a spark when struck against steel. In emotional terms, it awakens love, passion, and inspiration. For millennia, flint was used for cutting tools and weapons. Today, it encourages perception, incisive thought, and decision-making. Some crystal therapists say that flint reenergizes after illness.

HEALING ACTION
—
Meditate with flint at times when you feel emotionally adrift and disconnected. To keep love and passion alive, place flint in the love and marriage corner of the home, which is at the back right if you enter by the front door.

COMBINATIONS
—
When involved in complex or emotionally draining decision-making, meditate with flint and black obsidian.

CARE
—
Flint scores 6.5–7 on the Mohs' scale. Do not breathe in flint dust, which could cause silicosis. Clean in warm, soapy water with a soft cloth.

BROWN ZIRCON

APPEARANCE
—
Many zircons are golden brown, earning the mineral its name, which comes from the Persian word *zargun*, meaning "gold-hued." Some crystals are colorless, yellow, red, blue, or green. Specimens range from gem-quality transparent crystals to opaque stones. Zircon forms as plates, prisms, or chunks.

RARITY
—
Transparent, colorless zircons are priced as semiprecious stones and are often used as diamond substitutes in jewelry. Brown, lower-quality crystals take a lower price tag. Many zircons are mined in Australia or South Africa.

FORMATION
—
Zircon, which is zirconium silicate, forms in magma that is high in silicon. It is often found in granite.

ATTRIBUTES
—
Zircon enhances self-worth and dignity. It offers direction when we are listless or forced into inactivity by not knowing what to do for the best. It teaches us to trust our best instincts while rising above our basest desires. It is said to benefit the liver, kidneys, gallbladder, and pancreas.

HEALING ACTION
—
Zircon jewelry is an ideal gift for someone who is searching for a path in life or struggling with low self-worth and negative body image. When you need to find direction at times of doubt and ambivalence, position at the earth or root chakra.

COMBINATIONS
—
To improve self-confidence, build a grid with zircon, citrine, and lapis lazuli.

CARE
—
Zircon is hard, ranking 7.5 on the Mohs' scale. Do not use in gem elixirs, as zirconium may be toxic. It is soluble in acids, so may react dangerously with stomach acid. Clean only in warm water with a mild soap.

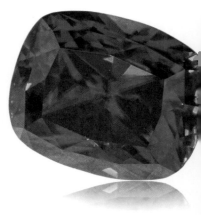

MOQUI MARBLE

APPEARANCE
—

Moqui marbles are brown-black balls, ranging from pea-sized to grapefruit-sized. Some balls are conjoined, while other forms are buttons, plates, and flying saucers.

RARITY
—

True moqui marbles are found in Utah and Arizona, particularly in State and National Parks and Reservations, where collecting is absolutely prohibited. Ensure that you buy from a reputable store. Moqui marbles may also be called Hopi marbles, Navajo berries, or shaman stones.

FORMATION
—

Known to geologists as iron concretions, moqui marbles are balls of iron oxide and sandstone that crystalized in groundwater flowing through Jurassic Navajo sandstone. After the overlying sandstone was eroded, the hard, weather-resistant iron concretions were exposed, often in large groups.

ATTRIBUTES
—

According to legend, the ancestor spirits of the Hopi People return to the earth at night to play marbles with these balls, leaving them behind to remind their descendants they are safe and well. Moqui marbles bring joy and light to the everyday. They help us to see the dawn just when the night is darkest. Moqui marbles are said to enhance memory.

HEALING ACTION
—

Moqui marbles are best used in pairs. Some say that flatter marbles are male, while spheres are female. Hold a marble in each hand during meditation to free yourself from anxiety and darkness. Place a marble at either end of your desk or dinner table to balance energies and surround yourself with loving kindness. Marbles can also be rubbed gently as a stress reliever.

COMBINATIONS
—

Combine with ruby and other warming, healing stones, such as red jasper, to help with depression, hopelessness, or even grief.

CARE
—

Moqui marbles score around 5.5–6.5 on the Mohs' scale. Do not submerge your marbles in water when cleaning, as their sandstone centers may dissolve over time. Wipe clean with a damp cloth, then dry thoroughly. Do not use in gem elixirs.

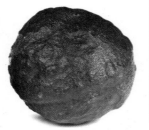

STAUROLITE

APPEARANCE
—

Staurolite is a reddish-brown to black opaque crystal. Crystals are often twinned at right angles to each other, forming a cross. Fittingly, this mineral's name comes from the ancient Greek for "cross" (*stauros*) and "stone" (*lithos*).

RARITY
—

Staurolite is rare, but can be found in Switzerland, Norway, and the United States, where it is the state mineral of Georgia. Fairy Stone State Park, in Virginia, is named for staurolite and the folk beliefs connected with it. This cross-shaped mineral is said to have formed when the fairies heard of Christ's death. Staurolite is often bought in its matrix (the rock in which it grew).

FORMATION
—

This mineral grows where regional metamorphism has occurred, as when mountains have been forced upward by the convergence of tectonic plates, putting rock under extreme heat and pressure.

ATTRIBUTES
—

Staurolite is a good luck charm, warding off harm and negativity. It finds hope and the possibility of renewal in the midst of sorrow and darkness. This mineral can be a beacon to those dealing with addiction. It is also said to strengthen the immune system.

HEALING ACTION
—

Position staurolite near the entrance to your home, to welcome kindly visitors and keep negativity at bay. Meditate with staurolite to give rise to feelings of lightness and hope. Practitioners of white magic use staurolite to strengthen spells and elixirs.

COMBINATIONS
—

Combined with motivating amber and cleansing peridot, staurolite is a comforting guide for those battling addiction, as long as they are also supported by professionals.

CARE
—

With a hardness of 7–7.5 on the Mohs' scale, staurolite is durable. Clean in warm, soapy water with a soft cloth.

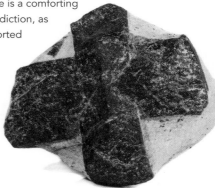

RED

Red crystals resonate with the root chakra, where our primal needs and desires are centered. Red crystals speak to our will to survive, to our passions, and our drive for love, success, and fulfillment. These crystals can aid motivation and stamina. Although they are empowering, they are also wholly practical and realistic. They help us to put plans into action, not to daydream our time away.

Red, the color of blood, has always been linked with our most primitive needs and self-preservation. From around 40,000 years ago, artists used red iron-oxide minerals to paint depictions of wild animals and hunters on cave walls. In the safety of these firelit caves, these artists conjured up images of fear, danger, heroism, and survival. By drawing conquest, they made it real. Through the millennia, from depictions of martyred saints on the walls of Venetian churches to children's scribbled drawings, red has been the color of the heart, of flesh, and of love, both sensual and self-sacrificing. These crystals are for those who desire to live fully, seriously, and passionately

RUBY

APPEARANCE
—

This variety of the mineral corundum is named for the Latin for red (*ruber*). Rubies range from orange-red to purple-red. Gem-quality corundums of other shades are known as sapphires. Rubies are translucent to transparent. When crystals have enough materials, space, and time to grow, they form hexagonal prisms.

RARITY
—

Rare and desirable, rubies are considered to be precious stones. Along with diamonds, sapphires, emeralds, and amethysts, they are among the traditional cardinal stones, priced above all others. Today, however, other high-quality gems, such as alexandrite, may take larger price tags. Rubies are priced by their color, cut, clarity, and carat weight. Uncut, cloudy rubies are distinctly more affordable than high-quality, faceted gems.

FORMATION
—

Corundum is composed of aluminum and oxygen. Traces of chromium tint the mineral red. Rubies form underground under extreme heat and pressure.

ATTRIBUTES
—

Ruby encourages us to be extrovert, sociable, loving, and passionate. It supports dynamic leadership and go-getting. Ruby should be used with wisdom, so that the raw power of this stone does not encourage selfishness or blinkered thinking in the pursuit of goals. Some say that ruby is beneficial for the heart and cardiovascular system.

HEALING ACTION
—

To boost confidence in social or professional situations, wear a ruby pendant. Place at the root chakra during meditation to encourage positive and loving feelings. Position ruby in the bedroom to keep sensuality alive.

COMBINATIONS
—

While working toward a professional goal, team with crystals of empathy and circumspection, such as moldavite, to encourage teamwork.

CARE
—

Ruby is extremely hard, scoring 9 on the Mohs' scale. Clean only with warm, soapy water and a soft cloth. Take fine jewelry to a professional jeweler for cleaning.

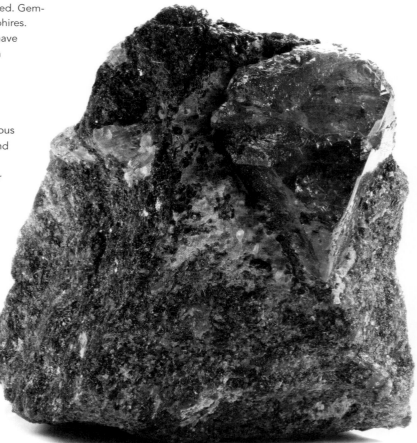

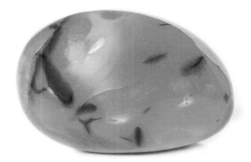

CARNELIAN

APPEARANCE
—
Carnelian, also called cornelian or sard, ranges from orange-brown to brown-red. It is translucent and may have a waxy appearance.

RARITY
—
Most carnelian is mined from India, Indonesia, Russia, Germany, or Brazil. High-quality crystals are priced as semiprecious gems.

FORMATION
—
Carnelian is a form of chalcedony, which is composed of fine intergrowths of the silicon dioxide minerals quartz and moganite, the two forms differentiated by their crystal structures at the microscopic level. Carnelian is tinted red by traces of iron oxide.

ATTRIBUTES
—
This mineral promotes energy and effort, both physical and emotional. It has particular resonance with business pursuits, allowing us to see the right course of action and giving the courage and conviction to pursue it. Carnelian discourages the will to fail. It is also said to improve stamina and muscle strength.

HEALING ACTION
—
When energy is at a low ebb in midwinter, wear carnelian close to the skin for a much-needed boost. To aid success in business, position in the wealth corner of the house, which is at the far left if you come in by the main entrance. Place carnelian under your pillow if you are kept awake by imagining failure.

COMBINATIONS
—
When constructing a grid for a favorable outcome in a business venture, team carnelian with aventurine and citrine.

CARE
—
Carnelian scores 6–7 on the Mohs' scale. Saltwater can cause carnelian to fracture. Clean with warm, soapy water and a soft cloth. Do not inhale carnelian dust, which can cause silicosis.

PYROPE

APPEARANCE
—
Pyrope is in the garnet family of minerals. It is frequently referred to only as "red garnet." It ranges from pink to purple-red. It often forms dodecahedral crystals with distinct, sharp-edged faces.

RARITY
—
Pyrope is less common than most minerals in the garnet family. High-quality pyropes are often used as "garnets" in jewelry. Pyrope is hard to distinguish from the similar garnet mineral, almandine.

FORMATION
—
Most pyrope forms in rocks such as peridotite deep in the earth's mantle. It contains magnesium, silicon, aluminum, and oxygen.

ATTRIBUTES
—
This crystal encourages love, from romance to devotion to family and friends. It reminds us that through loving, we become loveable. Pyrope also exhorts us to seize the moment, living passionately and sensuously in the here and now. It is said to be an aphrodisiac.

HEALING ACTION
—
Wear pyrope in jewelry to encourage new relationships, whether you are looking for love or friendship. Meditate with pyrope if you find it difficult to exist in the moment. Place in the love and relationships corner of the house, which is at the far right if you enter by the front door.

COMBINATIONS
—
If you are embarking on a new relationship, combine the passion of pyrope with the wisdom of black onyx to ensure you commit yourself only to those who are worthy.

CARE
—
Pyrope scores 7–7.5 on the Mohs' scale. Clean only with warm, not hot, soapy water.

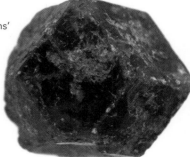

RHODOCHROSITE

APPEARANCE
—

Ranging from cherry red to pale pink, rhodochrosite forms columns, blades, and rhombohedrons. Its name comes from the ancient Greek for "rose-colored." Rhodochrosite is transparent to translucent.

RARITY
—

Easily obtained, rhodochrosite is a key ore of manganese. However, faceted stones are rarely available due to this mineral's softness. Attractive, banded rhodochrosite is mined from Argentina.

FORMATION
—

This mineral grows in hydrothermal veins, where it is often found in association with silver.

ATTRIBUTES
—

While many red stones inspire personal and particular love, rhodochrosite inspires a selfless love—for humankind, for other species, and for our planet itself. It allows us to balance our own needs and self-respect with the desire to help others.

HEALING ACTION
—

Those who devote their time to caring, whether for young children or adults, may find it useful to meditate with rhodochrosite. When placed at the root chakra, rhodochrosite helps us find balance between selfless love and self-care. Place this mineral at the higher heart chakra if your goal is to raise money for charity or to maintain planet-friendly resolutions, such as cycling to work or planting seedlings.

COMBINATIONS
—

If you are burying your own needs and desires to avoid failure or change, combine rhodochrosite with courageous aquamarine as well as moonstone or diamond, which are both stones of new beginnings.

CARE
—

This mineral is very soft, just 3.5–4 on the Mohs' scale. Always remove jewelry before exercise or chores. Do not wipe or rub when dry, as even household dust could scratch. Clean only with warm, soapy water and a soft cloth. It is soluble in acids, so may react dangerously with stomach acid. Do not use in gem elixirs as it contains manganese.

BROOKITE

APPEARANCE
—

Brookite crystals may be flat, pyramidal, or hexagonal. They range from deep red to brown, from opaque to transparent.

RARITY
—

This mineral is found in locations including the United States, Russia, Wales, and Pakistan. Although brookite is not extremely rare, it usually occurs as flat, plate-like crystals that cannot be cut, so faceted gems are collector's items.

FORMATION
—

A form of titanium dioxide, this mineral grows in veins in metamorphic rocks such as gneiss and schist.

ATTRIBUTES
—

Brookite has high, positive energy. It helps us to understand ourselves, what drives us and what terrifies us. It encourages perception, insight, and, finally, acceptance. It is said to help with healing of the tissues after surgery.

HEALING ACTION
—

Position brookite on any chakra that is blocked or imbalanced for a suffusion of healing, warming energy. While positioning brookite on the root chakra allows us to understand our own desires, placing on the third eye encourages us to see and accept others as they truly are.

COMBINATIONS
—

To fully understand the reasons for our own damaging habits or mistakes, meditate with brookite and iolite. If you struggle with body image, combine brookite with kind and accepting rose quartz.

CARE
—

Fairly brittle, brookite scores 5.5–6 on the Mohs' scale. Store jewelry away from harder gems. Clean with warm, soapy water.

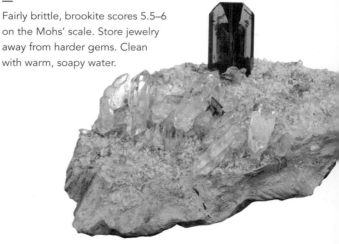

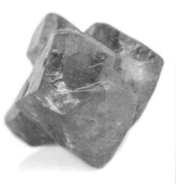

RED SPINEL

APPEARANCE
—

Red spinel ranges from transparent to opaque. It takes its name from the Latin word for "spine," due to its pointed crystals. It is often found in eight-sided polyhedrons or flat, triangular plates.

RARITY
—

Transparent spinel is priced as a semiprecious gemstone. Famous red spinels, once mistaken for rubies, include the British Crown Jewels' Timur Ruby and Black Prince's Ruby. Poorer-quality or opaque stones are much lower priced.

FORMATION
—

Spinel and ruby are often found together, with ruby formed mainly from aluminum and oxygen, while spinel also contains magnesium. Spinel grows in the intense heat of igneous and metamorphic rocks.

ATTRIBUTES
—

Spinel is an invigorating crystal that improves mental and physical strength. It offers hope and comfort when we are in need. It allows us to express the best of ourselves while holding back our flaws and hostilities. It can also help us to see past the imperfections of others to the vulnerable person inside.

HEALING ACTION
—

If convalescing from a long illness, place spinel by the bed or under the pillow to improve strength. If you are training for a marathon or revising for exams, wear spinel jewelry for a boost in stamina. Place spinel in a meeting room to aid positive and respectful communication.

COMBINATIONS
—

When physical strength is at its lowest ebb, a combination of red spinel and hematite may offer the necessary boost in energy. Combine with black tourmaline when facing emotional attack from challenging personalities.

CARE
—

Spinel is strong and durable, with a rating of 7.5–8 on the Mohs' scale. Light-colored stones may fade in intense heat. Clean with warm, soapy water and a soft cloth.

RED JADE

APPEARANCE
—

The decorative stone known as jade is one of two minerals with similar properties and appearance, jadeite and nephrite. Red specimens are jadeite. They range from translucent to opaque.

RARITY
—

Natural red jadeite is extremely rare. Many specimens of "red jade" have been dyed. Some stones marketed as jade may be jasper or other substitutes.

FORMATION
—

Jadeite forms during metamorphism, where two tectonic plates are converging. Much jadeite is found around the rim of the Pacific Ocean, in the Ring of Fire. The mineral is often found as pebbles and boulders in stream valleys, with a dark, weathered rind covering its beauty.

ATTRIBUTES
—

All colors of jade bring harmony. Jade helps to balance the chakras, as well as finding equilibrium between the conflicting demands of body and mind. Red jade has particular resonance with the emotions, helping to reduce mood swings, irritability, and angry outbursts. It is said to regulate the hormones and the metabolism.

HEALING ACTION
—

Hold red jade over any chakra that is blocked or overstimulated. If you are experiencing mood swings, use this mineral for meditation. If you feel that justified anger is building inside you, position red jade over the throat chakra so that you can voice your feelings calmly and kindly.

COMBINATIONS
—

If you suffer from hormonally influenced mood swings, build a grid containing red jade, turquoise, and moonstone.

CARE
—

Jadeite scores 6.5–7 on the Mohs' scale. Wipe jadeite clean with a soft, soapy cloth, then rinse with clean water and dry carefully. Jadeite should not be soaked. Keep out of direct sunlight.

RED JASPER

APPEARANCE

—

Jasper is an opaque stone, with red its most common color. It breaks with a smooth surface and takes a high polish.

RARITY

—

Red jasper is common worldwide. Note that "jasper" is sometimes used as a descriptive term for a colorful, shiny stone rather than as a scientific term.

FORMATION

—

Jasper is an opaque variety of quartz, usually combined with chalcedony, which is itself composed of very fine intergrowths of quartz and moganite. Both these minerals are composed of silicon and oxygen atoms, but have different molecular structures. Jasper often forms where fine, soft sediments are cemented together by silicon dioxide. It is the included particles of sediment that make jasper both opaque and colorful. Red jasper is tinted by iron inclusions.

ATTRIBUTES

—

All varieties of jasper are supportive and protective. Red jasper also helps us bring to light intangible truths: the meanings of dreams, the genuine nature of our own desires, and the best path to take at times of indecision. It is said to strengthen bones, joints, and ligaments.

HEALING ACTION

—

Place red jasper under your pillow to access the spiritual truths of your dreams. Wear a red jasper pendant or bracelet as a guide through difficult decisions, from home-buying to business negotiations.

COMBINATIONS

—

To experience lucid and revealing dreams, place danburite and red jasper under your pillow.

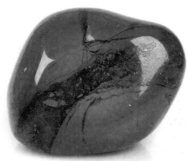

CARE

—

Jasper is fairly hard, scoring 6.5–7 on the Mohs' scale. Clean with warm, soapy water and a soft cloth. Do not inhale quartz dust, which can cause silicosis.

RED CALCITE

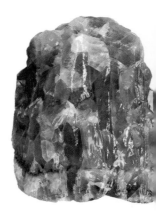

APPEARANCE

—

Calcite often grows in pyramid-shaped crystals, as well as in countless other forms that range from simple grains to complex, radiating "flowers." This mineral is transparent to translucent.

RARITY

—

Red calcite is far less common than white or colorless. However, calcite is a ubiquitous crystal worldwide, so this shade is readily available from specialist stores.

FORMATION

—

Calcite is calcium carbonate, which is colorless. It is the presence of impurities, such as iron, that tint it red. Calcite is an essential component of sedimentary rocks including limestone and chalk, as it formed the shells and skeletons of the sea creatures of which these rocks are composed. Magnificent calcite crystals can be found in limestone caves.

ATTRIBUTES

—

All varieties of calcite stimulate the intellect and insights. Red calcite is particularly useful for giving us insight into the deep-seated reasons behind our own fears. At the same time, this energetic and comforting crystal gives us the willpower to confront those fears. It is said to clear constipation and blockages, although medical advice should always be sought.

HEALING ACTION

—

If feeling anxious or irrationally fearful, meditate with red calcite. Place at the third eye for a window into your worries, but hold at the root chakra for the courage to face them.

COMBINATIONS

—

If you are already working with professionals to combat your phobias, you may find it helpful to build a grid with red calcite, motivating chrysocolla, and courageous black onyx and pyrolusite.

CARE

—

Calcite is brittle and soft, scoring just 3 on the Mohs' scale. It should not be handled excessively. Calcite is not soluble in pure water but is soluble in rainwater, which is slightly acidic. It may react dangerously with stomach acid. If cleaning is necessary, wipe very gently with a soft cloth.

RED BERYL

APPEARANCE
—
Sometimes called bixbite, red beryl is pinkish-red and translucent to transparent. It grows in hexagonal crystals, but may also be found as plates, grains, and chunks.

RARITY
—
Genuine red beryl is the rarest form of beryl, found only in the Wah Wah Mountains and Juab County in Utah, as well as Paramount Canyon and Round Mountain, New Mexico. Good-quality stones are very highly priced.

FORMATION
—
Red beryl crystals grow in cavities and along fractures in rhyolitic rocks. Beryl is composed of beryllium, aluminum, silicon, and oxygen. Pure crystals are colorless. Red beryl is tinted by traces of manganese.

ATTRIBUTES
—
All varieties of beryl help us to meet our potential. Red beryl has particular resonance with our emotional and sexual lives, helping us to find fulfillment in our closest relationships. It gives us the self-confidence to love and be loved. Some say that it has powerful aphrodisiac properties.

HEALING ACTION
—
Place red beryl at the root chakra to stimulate passionate love, either new or long-standing. Meditate with this beryl when you are searching for what you truly feel, as opposed to what others tell you to feel. Wear red beryl jewelry to gain emotional self-confidence and stability.

COMBINATIONS
—
If you are embarking on a new romantic relationship, build a grid containing red beryl, loving sugilite, and optimistic golden topaz.

CARE
—
Red beryl scores 7.5–8 on the Mohs' scale, making it highly suitable for jewelry. Clean with warm, soapy water and a soft cloth. Red beryl contains beryllium, a known carcinogen, so do not inhale its dust.

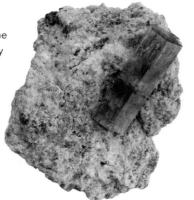

MAHOGANY OBSIDIAN

APPEARANCE
—
Streaked or speckled in red-brown and black, this variety of obsidian often displays a pattern like the grain of rich mahogany wood. Its texture is smooth and glass-like.

RARITY
—
This shade of obsidian is less common than the jet-black variety. Much commercially available mahogany obsidian comes from Mexico.

FORMATION
—
Obsidian forms when lava rich in lighter elements—such as silicon, oxygen, aluminum, sodium, and potassium—cools quickly, giving little time for crystal growth. Mahogany obisidian's reddish shade is caused by traces of elements such as iron.

ATTRIBUTES
—
Mahogany obsidian is gentler than its jet-black sister. While it aids searchers for emotional and mental clarity, it also offers the support and nurturing that discovering the truth often requires. It allows us to balance acknowledgment of the past with future growth. It is said to ease headaches.

HEALING ACTION
—
Worn as a pendant or bracelet, mahogany obsidian offers direction, as well as nurturing the courage to pursue those goals. Meditate with mahogany obsidian to sow the seeds of resourcefulness. Place on the root chakra to encourage honest but forgiving self-confidence.

COMBINATIONS
—
Wear with golden topaz to shed light on the way forward and offer support as you take the first difficult steps toward a new goal or departure.

CARE
—
With a score of 5–6 on the Mohs' scale, obsidian is relatively easy to fracture and scratch. Clean only with warm, soapy water and a soft cloth. Do not breathe in obsidian dust.

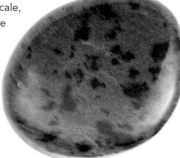

CUPRITE

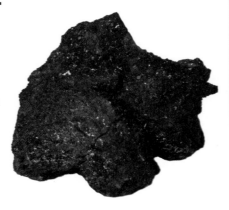

APPEARANCE
—

This blood-red to deep-burgundy mineral is transparent or translucent. It is found as crusts, needles, cubes, and octahedrons.

RARITY
—

Although cuprite is fairly widespread, crystals large enough to be faceted are extremely rare, making them valuable collector's items. Any seller should advise about cuprite's toxicity, as it contains copper.

FORMATION
—

Containing only atoms of copper and oxygen, cuprite is an important ore of copper. Cuprite forms where copper lodes are oxidized (react with oxygen).

ATTRIBUTES
—

Cuprite calms anger, turning destructive energy into creative release. It soothes anxiety, making us feel calm and supported when we are most challenged. Cuprite's warming, healing powers can quicken the flow of energy through any sluggish chakra.

HEALING ACTION
—

Before using cuprite, consult with a qualified crystal therapist, as cuprite dust is toxic. When your own feelings of anger or bitterness are overwhelming, meditate with cuprite. Place this mineral on the root chakra to direct energy away from recrimination and toward forgiveness.

COMBINATIONS
—

To dispel repetitive angry thoughts, cuprite can be combined with peridot, magnetite, and lapis lazuli.

CARE
—

Scoring only 3.5–4 on the Mohs' scale, cuprite is too soft to be widely used as a gemstone. Care should also be taken to avoid knocks and scratches. Cuprite dust, which contains copper, is highly toxic. Do not use in gem elixirs. Cuprite is soluble in acids, so may react dangerously with stomach acid. Clean gently with warm, soapy water and a soft cloth. Extended exposure to light could cause fading.

PINK

Pink crystals and stones are well placed at the higher heart chakra, where they promote positivity, generosity, and empathy. While red crystals are fiery and may encourage hardheadedness, pink crystals imbue passion and drive with thoughtfulness and awareness of others. They encourage gentle, tender, love and kindness. That love is also for ourselves, in self-acceptance and calm self-worth. Pink crystals soothe overpowering emotions.

Pink has difficult connotations in our society, which too often bases its judgements on false binaries. We fear that pink furnishings, pink dresses, and pink dolls will undermine a little girl's seriousness and ambition. It takes a self-confident man to wear pink. Our fear of this nurturing color not only reveals its power but belies its cultural history. Before the mid-1900s, pink was as likely to be worn by boys as girls. Pink crystals teach us that, far from being opposites, gentleness and strength must always be blended. "Male" and "female" qualities are nothing more than culturally constructed myth. Pink crystals are for those searching for a better and more honest life, a life filled with love, kindness, and connection with others.

RHODONITE

APPEARANCE
—

Rhodonite is usually fuchsia to rose-pink. It is commonly found as grains and irregular chunks, but may also form plate-shaped crystals. It is transparent to translucent.

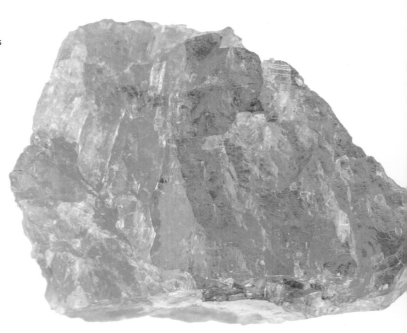

RARITY
—

This relatively rare mineral is sourced in Argentina, Australia, Brazil, Canada, India, Russia, and the United States. Large, well-formed crystals are highly sought after.

FORMATION
—

Alongside other minerals rich in manganese, rhodonite forms in rocks that are altered by contact metamorphism (baking by nearby magma) and hydrothermal fluids.

ATTRIBUTES
—

Rhodonite is a crystal that brings balance, between the heart and head, between jealousy and coldness, between generosity and self-denial. It soothes and harmonizes energy flow between the chakras. Rhodonite is also said to balance the metabolism and the action of the body's glands.

HEALING ACTION
—

Meditate with rhodonite if you are prone to extremes of emotion or find yourself alternating between acting out and guilt. Place on the higher heart chakra to encourage a love that is suffused with kindness, friendship, and respect. To encourage supportive, nurturing relationships, position a rhodonite crystal in the love corner of the home, which is in the back right if you enter by the front door.

COMBINATIONS
—

If you are prone to stormy relationships, meditating with rhodonite and calming aquamarine—along with talking therapies—may help you break the pattern.

CARE
—

Rhodonite scores 5.5–6.5 on the Mohs' scale. Do not expose rhodonite to dramatic changes in temperature. Clean with lukewarm, soapy water and a soft cloth. Do not use in gem elixirs as it contains manganese and is soluble in acids, so may also react dangerously with stomach acid.

THULITE

APPEARANCE
—

This variety of the mineral zoisite is cherry pink. It may be pleochroic, exhibiting different colors from different angles and in different lights. It is usually found as chunks.

RARITY
—

First identified in Norway, thulite was named after the mythical, far-northern island of Thule of the ancient Greeks and Romans. Specimens may also be found in North America, Austria, and New Zealand. This fairly rare semiprecious stone is often carved into jewelry and artworks.

FORMATION
—

Thulite is found in metamorphic or igneous rocks that formed at high temperature and pressure deep underground. In addition to zoisite's silicon, aluminum, calcium, oxygen, and hydrogen, thulite contains manganese, which bestows its beautiful pink shade.

ATTRIBUTES
—

Thulite awakens positive feelings and abilities that have been dampened or forced into dormancy. It stirs love, generosity, and creativity. Like other forms of zoisite, it is a perfect crystal for those looking for a fresh start, either practically or emotionally. It is said to help reenergize the body after shock or illness.

HEALING ACTION
—

Wear thulite jewelry if you suffer from lack of self-confidence or fear of voicing your feelings and ideas. Position it in the workplace to encourage positive discussion and the conception of creative ideas. When friendships or love affairs have cooled, meditate with thulite to bring fresh energy and connection.

COMBINATIONS
—

To rekindle a relationship, create a grid with other pink stones of love and warmth, including rose quartz and kunzite.

CARE
—

Thulite is fairly brittle, scoring 6.5 on the Mohs' scale. Clean with warm, soapy water and a soft cloth.

COBALTOAN CALCITE

APPEARANCE
—

This variety of calcite ranges from petal-pink to purple. It is found as crusts and pyramid-shaped crystals, as well as complex forms such as "flowers." It is transparent to translucent.

RARITY
—

Cobaltoan calcite is a relatively rare form of the common mineral calcite. Specimens are often sourced from Spain, Morocco, the Democratic Republic of the Congo, and Australia.

FORMATION
—

Pure calcite is calcium carbonate. In cobaltoan calcite, the calcium has been partially replaced by cobalt, which is responsible for this mineral's pink shade. It is found in hydrothermal veins.

ATTRIBUTES
—

All forms of calcite stimulate the intellect and insights. This extrovert variety of the mineral particularly empowers our empathy for others. It also heightens our insights into the true natures of those we meet. It is said to benefit eyesight.

HEALING ACTION
—

Meditate while facing cobaltoan calcite to awaken empathy for anyone with whom you experience conflict or disagreement. If you are running out of patience with a teenager, place this mineral in the children corner of the house, which is in the middle of the right side if you enter by the front door.

COMBINATIONS
—

If you work in a caring profession such as teaching, nursing, or volunteering, combine empathy with generosity by working with this crystal alongside any shade of topaz.

CARE
—

Cobalt is toxic, so do not ingest, do not use in gem elixirs, do not breathe in dust, and do not handle excessively. Cobaltoan calcite scores just 3–4 on the Mohs' scale. Calcite will dissolve in rainwater or other acids, such as vinegar. It may also react dangerously with stomach acid. If cleaning is necessary, wipe with a soft cloth.

KUNZITE

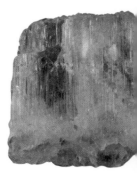

APPEARANCE
—

This transparent to translucent crystal is usually pink to purple. It exhibits an effect called pleochroism, or appearing different colors in changing lights and from different angles. Kunzite is striated, which means that many parallel hairline grooves can be seen.

RARITY
—

Discovered in 1902, kunzite was named after George Kunz, Tiffany & Co.'s chief jeweller. This crystal is more widely available than in the past. It is now mined in the United States, Canada, Mexico, Brazil, Myanmar, Afghanistan, and Pakistan.

FORMATION
—

Kunzite is a form of the mineral spodumene, which grows in intrusive igneous rocks, such as granite, that are rich in lithium. It is a lithium aluminum silicate. The pink to purple tint is given by the presence of small quantities of manganese.

ATTRIBUTES
—

Kunzite activates the heart chakras, helping to bring them into balance and cooperation with the other chakras, particularly those of the throat and third eye. In this way, kunzite awakens love and chases away negativity, but also encourages the expression of creativity and frees intuition. It is said to strengthen the cardiovascular system.

HEALING ACTION
—

Place over the higher heart or heart chakra to boost mood and alleviate mild depression. Wear as a pendant to heal heartache, particularly the pain caused by intrusive memories of past events. Some call kunzite the "mother's stone" because, when placed under the pillow, it can help new mothers to get a good night's sleep while calming and rejuvenating the heart—ready to start the new day with compassion and unconditional love.

COMBINATIONS
—

Use with rose quartz for a powerful boost, particularly for those suffering with self-doubt or low self-esteem. While meditating, combine with lapis lazuli or azurite to encourage spiritual growth.

CARE
—

Keep out of sunlight, which causes fading. Clean only in warm, soapy water. Do not use in gem elixirs as it contains lithium. Kunzite scores 6.5–7 on the Mohs' scale.

PINK LEPIDOLITE

APPEARANCE
—

An opaque to translucent crystal, lepidolite is pink to purple with plate-like layers or mottled grains. It is often found as masses, scaly aggregates, and pseudohexagonal crystals.

RARITY
—

Lepidolite is straightforward to source, with plentiful occurrences in the United States, Canada, Brazil, Russia, and Zimbabwe. However, buy from a reputable source as there are many fakes on the market.

FORMATION
—

Like kunzite, lepidolite grows in granite that is rich in lithium. Lepidolite is the most abundant lithium-bearing mineral, making it a valuable ore.

ATTRIBUTES
—

Lepidolite opens and clears the heart, throat, third eye, and crown chakras. It dispels negative and obsessive thoughts, helps to combat addiction, and boosts mood. This crystal can also be of benefit during decision-making, as it filters out distractions and nagging thoughts while encouraging objectivity and perception.

HEALING ACTION
—

Position lepidolite on your desk to ward off negativity and stress in the workplace. Place under the pillow for a good night's sleep and so that you awake feeling positive. Try using this crystal as a pendulum when seeking an answer to spiritual questions.

COMBINATIONS
—

When facing intense negativity, in yourself or others, combine with powerful dark-colored stones such as obsidian, black onyx, and pyrolusite.

CARE
—

Lepidolite is very soft, scoring just 2.5–3 on the Mohs' scale, so be careful with knocks to pendants. Avoid contact with chemicals, particularly acids, which will dissolve this mineral. It may react dangerously with stomach acids, so do not ingest. Do not immerse in water. If necessary, wipe clean with a soft cloth.

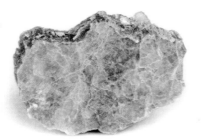

PINK SAPPHIRE

APPEARANCE
—

Small stones may be brightly transparent (and extremely costly), but larger uncut and unpolished blocks will be cloudy.

RARITY
—

Pink sapphires are a precious gemstone, with high-quality stones at least as rare and valuable as their blue counterparts. Less-good-quality, uncut stones are, however, easy to source. Large sapphire deposits are found in Kashmir, Myanmar, Thailand, Sri Lanka, Madagascar, and China.

FORMATION
—

Like all sapphires and rubies, pink sapphires are a variety of the mineral corundum, an aluminum oxide. The pink shade is given by the presence of chromium.

ATTRIBUTES
—

All sapphires bestow wisdom, but pink stones focus particularly on emotional wisdom. They encourage true intuition and perception, helping with decision-making in matters that involve (or should involve) the heart. In addition, pink sapphires encourage the integration of conscious and unconscious thought. It is said to speed the healing of wounds.

HEALING ACTION
—

Wear as a ring, earrings, brooch, or pendant to encourage insightful decision-making in business or while making complex life decisions where head and heart must work together, such as house-buying.

COMBINATIONS
—

For help when reaching a decision seems impossible, use alongside brown stones, such as brown jasper, pietersite, and brown jade, which are deeply grounding and help to overcome uncertainty and instability.

CARE
—

Scoring 9 on the Mohs' scale, pink sapphires are strong and durable, often being passed down through the generations of a family, along with their wisdom. Take to a jeweler for cleaning, or use warm, soapy water and a soft cloth. However, cavity-filled, fracture-filled, or dyed gems should be cleaned only with a damp cloth. Do not use them in gem elixirs.

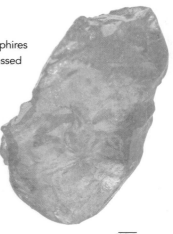

POUDRETTEITE

APPEARANCE
—

This pale-pink gemstone grows in barrel-shaped prismatic crystals. It is transparent and pleochroic, appearing pink-violet or colorless from different angles.

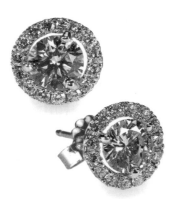

RARITY
—

An exceptionally rare, precious gemstone, poudretteite is named after the Poudrette family, who originally owned the quarry where it was first found, in Mont St. Hilaire, Quebec, Canada. Poudretteite gems should be bought only from reputable jewelers.

FORMATION
—

Poudretteite is composed of potassium, sodium, boron, silicon, and oxygen atoms. It forms in the metamorphic rock marble.

ATTRIBUTES
—

Poudretteite enhances happiness, helping us to laugh and to find pleasure in the moment. This gemstone helps us to find love, to build long-lasting relationships, and to show affection open-heartedly. It also soothes stress and alleviates low mood. Some say that poudretteite energizes the immune system.

HEALING ACTION
—

Wear poudretteite jewelry to feel joyful, loving, and full of zest for life. Meditate with poudretteite to lift mood and awaken love. Place at the higher heart chakra to feel a surge of comforting energy.

COMBINATIONS
—

Poudretteite and amber make a strong partnership against mild depression.

CARE
—

Scoring just 5 on the Mohs' scale, poudretteite should be treated with extreme care because of its value. It is too soft for rings or bracelets, but can be worn as earrings or a brooch. It may be washed in warm, soapy water with a soft cloth, but valuable gems should be taken to a reputable jeweler for cleaning.

ROSE QUARTZ

APPEARANCE
—

This variety of quartz ranges from pale pink to rose red. Quartz crystals often grow as six-sided prisms ending in pyramids. Rose quartz may display diasterism, a star-shaped pattern of light when lit from behind.

RARITY
—

Rose quartz is common worldwide. Sources include the United States, Brazil, and India.

FORMATION
—

Quartz is a ubiquitous rock-forming mineral, often found in felsic rocks such as granite. Colorless quartz is made of silicon and oxygen atoms, but traces of manganese, titanium, or iron can tint it pink.

ATTRIBUTES
—

Rose quartz is a crystal of love, kindness, and forgiveness. It is the ideal stone for someone who has loved and lost, and is now finding it hard to move forward and welcome new relationships. Rose quartz also helps us to truly understand others, opening the door to selfless nurturing. It is said to aid the regeneration of the body's cells.

HEALING ACTION
—

To welcome love into your life, wear a rose quartz pendant close to the heart. To nurture your existing relationships, both romantic and familial, place a rose quartz twin (two conjoined crystals) or cluster in the relationship corner of your home, which is in the back right if you enter by the main door.

COMBINATIONS
—

To forgive, heal, and move on together in a relationship that has foundered, or to move forward from one that has irretrievably broken down, meditate with chrysoprase and rose quartz.

CARE
—

Quartz scores 7 on the Mohs' scale. Clean using warm, soapy water and a soft cloth. Do not inhale quartz dust, which can cause silicosis.

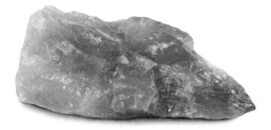

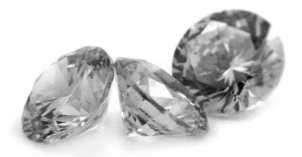

MORGANITE

APPEARANCE
—

Morganite is a pink variety of the mineral beryl. It grows in pale-pink to salmon-colored crystals that are transparent to translucent. It often forms hexagonal columns, but may also be found as plates, grains, and chunks.

RARITY
—

Morganite is a fairly rare, semiprecious stone. Sources include Brazil, the United States, Madagascar, and Myanmar.

FORMATION
—

Pure, colorless beryl is composed of beryllium, aluminum, silicon, and oxygen. Pink beryl is tinted by traces of manganese. It is often found in granitic pegmatites, which are igneous rocks studded with enlarged crystals. This variety of beryl was named after the American banker J.P. Morgan.

ATTRIBUTES
—

All varieties of beryl help us to meet our potential. Pink beryl is particularly useful for freeing ourselves from the negative feelings that hold us back from achieving our goals. With its warm, encouraging energy, beryl removes the will to fail. It is also said to strengthen the bones and joints.

HEALING ACTION
—

Place morganite at the higher heart chakra to truly know you are worthy of achieving success. Meditate with this beryl when you fear failure. To feel constantly encouraged and supported, wear a morganite pendant close to the heart.

COMBINATIONS
—

Use with smoky quartz if you are paralysed by fear of failure.

CARE
—

Morganite scores 7.5–8 on the Mohs' scale. Use warm, soapy water and a soft cloth for cleaning. Beryl contains beryllium, a known carcinogen, so do not inhale its dust.

PINK TOURMALINE

APPEARANCE
—

Pink to red tourmaline is sometimes called rubellite. A translucent to opaque crystal, pink tourmaline is often found in columnar, radiating, or needle-shaped forms that are triangular in cross-section.

RARITY
—

This semiprecious gem is available from jewelers and specialist stores. Some specimens may have been artificially irradiated to deepen their color.

FORMATION
—

Tourmaline is one of the most complicated silicate minerals, containing elements such as aluminum, iron, lithium, magnesium, potassium, and sodium, among others. Pink tourmaline is usually rich in lithium and manganese. Prolonged natural irradiation deepens the pink to red. Pink tourmaline is found in metamorphic rocks such as schist and marble.

ATTRIBUTES
—

Like all tourmalines, this variety offers spiritual protection. It is a powerful crystal for clearing blockages and dispersing negative energy. Pink tourmaline also encourages trust and generosity in our close relationships. It teaches us to love so that we can be loveable. This tourmaline is also said to treat the endocrine system.

HEALING ACTION
—

Wear a pink tourmaline pendant to open your heart to loving and being loved. Meditate with pink tourmaline when you find it hard to trust yourself and others. Position a pink tourmaline crystal on the higher heart chakra when you know you are guilty of not feeding relationships with your loved ones.

COMBINATIONS
—

Use with clear quartz to stimulate and warm the chakras. For enhanced spiritual protection, combine with fluorite, particularly green.

CARE
—

Tourmaline rates 7–7.5 on the Mohs' scale. Clean with warm, soapy water and a soft cloth.

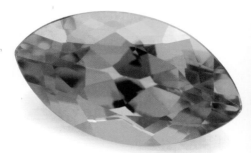

PINK PETALITE

APPEARANCE
—
Petalite, also known as castorite, is transparent to translucent. Pink specimens are usually the color of sugared almonds. Crystals may be in the form of columns or plates.

RARITY
—
Transparent, faceted gems are highly priced. Cloudier, smaller specimens are easier to source and may be cut into cabochons. Petalite is often mined in Brazil or Madagascar.

FORMATION
—
Petalite contains aluminum, lithium, silicon, and oxygen. It is found in granite pegmatites, which are coarse-grained igneous rocks.

ATTRIBUTES
—
Pink petalite encourages us to be strong yet flexible, outgoing yet able to listen, alert yet calm. Its soothing tranquility is of particular benefit during meditation. It encourages us to open our minds to new ideas and our hearts to new relationships. It is said to ease muscle aches and pains, particularly after overexertion.

HEALING ACTION
—
When an overly busy mind makes meditation difficult, turn to pink petalite. Position it on your desk to encourage yourself to listen well to colleagues and to be receptive to new approaches. If you are facing conflict with a teenager's strong will, position pink petalite at the higher heart chakra to enable yourself to compromise at the right times and in the right way.

COMBINATIONS
—
An excellent combination for enhancing meditation is pink petalite, larimar, and apophyllite.

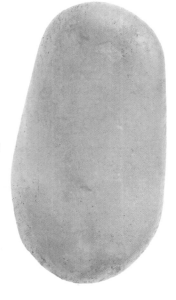

CARE
—
Scoring 6–6.5 on the Mohs' scale, petalite should be stored away from other crystals and jewelry to avoid scratches. Clean only with warm, soapy water and a soft cloth.

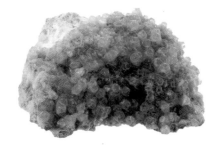

PINK SMITHSONITE

APPEARANCE
—
Rarely found as well-formed crystals, smithsonite is most often seen as globular masses resembling a foam of bubbles. This translucent mineral is found in a range of pastel shades.

RARITY
—
Smithsonite is widely available from specialist mineral stockists.

FORMATION
—
Smithsonite was identified in 1802 by English mineralogist James Smithson, whose bequest established the Smithsonian Institutation. The mineral, composed of zinc, carbon, and oxygen, forms where zinc ores are weathered.

ATTRIBUTES
—
Smithsonite encourages us to be warm, outgoing, and charming. It facilitates good communication and idea-sharing. It is the crystal of collaboration and partnerships, whether those relate to business, study, friendship, or marriage. Some say that smithsonite can strengthen the immune system.

HEALING ACTION
—
To encourage teamwork, position smithsonite in the center of the workplace, or in the love and marriage corner of the home, which is in the back right if you enter by the front door. Meditate with smithsonite to find resolution in disputes with romantic or working partners.

COMBINATIONS
—
If you suffer from shyness, meditate with tiger's eye and smithsonite.

CARE
—
Smithsonite scores just 4.5 on the Mohs' scale, so should be handled with care. Do not use in gem elixirs as it contains zinc and is soluble in acids, so may react dangerously with stomach acid. Clean with warm, soapy water and a soft cloth, removing any water and soap residue before storage. Do not soak.

PINK COMMON OPAL

APPEARANCE

—

Unlike precious opals (see page 137), common opals are not iridescent, but they do display adularescence, a milky sheen of light that originates from inside the stone. This effect is caused by light interacting with the mineraloid's molecular structure.

RARITY

—

Common opal is found worldwide and costs significantly less than precious opal.

FORMATION

—

Opal, whether common or precious, is a mineraloid, a mineral-like substance without a regular crystal structure. Up to 20 percent of an opal is water, with the mineraloid's silicon dioxide containing clusters of water molecules. Opal forms as water trickles through rocks such as sandstone and claystone, collecting particles of silicon dioxide. Over time, the solution forms opal in cracks and holes.

ATTRIBUTES

—

Common opal is both less powerful and less fickle than precious opal. It encourages us to feel centered and rooted in our love for others. While common opal can be a transformative stone, its changes are wrought slowly and incrementally, supporting us to be gentler, kinder, and more nurturing day by day. It may help with regaining strength after illness or surgery.

HEALING ACTION

—

For support in the daily care of elderly or young loved ones, position pink common opal in the health and family corner of the home, which is on the left and midway through the house if you enter by the front door. Meditate with this opal to find joy in bestowing small kindnesses.

COMBINATIONS

—

Build a kindness grid using pink common opal, rose quartz, green tourmaline, and sunstone.

CARE

—

Opal scores 5.5–6 on the Mohs' scale, so care must be taken to avoid chips and breaks. Do not expose to extremes of temperature. Do not immerse in water. Do not use in gem elixirs. Wipe clean with a lukewarm, soapy cloth, then dry quickly.

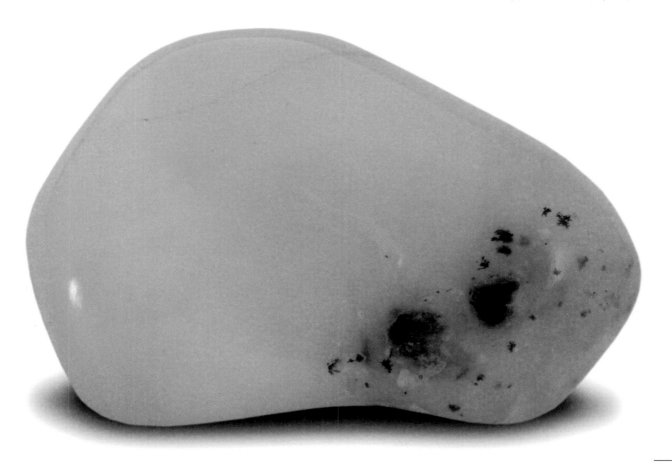

ORANGE

The sacral chakra—center of emotions, creativity, and sexual pleasure—chimes with orange crystals. These crystals offer the passionate energy of red crystals, but with a more creative and cooperative bent. They encourage us to find joy by realizing what truly matters in our lives; by enjoying the company of others, whatever their flaws. Orange crystals encourage us to strengthen our relationships, build bonds with others, and focus on being a better partner. At the same time, these crystals help us to face abandonment and separation, by building true self-esteem and self-reliance.

Orange is the colour of both the harvest and falling leaves; of ripeness and change. In Confucianism, orange is the color of both transformation and balance. While yellow was the colour of perfection and spirituality, red was the colour of happiness and sensuality. By balancing and combining the two, orange brought the power of change. In English, orange was known as "yellow-red" until the early 1500s, after the arrival of the orange fruit via Spain. Orange remains associated with partnerships, innovation, and the ability to adapt to change.

AMBER

APPEARANCE
—
Amber is usually golden-yellow to red-brown, smooth, and translucent. It sometimes contains plant or animal material, such as ancient insects.

RARITY
—
Common sources of amber include Kaliningrad, Russia; Kachin, Myanmar; and the Dominican Republic.

FORMATION
—
Amber is not a mineral: it is fossilized tree resin. Millions of years ago, resin-coated logs—sometimes with insects trapped in the sticky resin—were carried by rivers to coastal deltas, where they were buried by sediment. Over time, the amber and the surrounding sediment hardened.

ATTRIBUTES
—
Amber's warming, brightening energy helps us to find joy in the everyday. It encourages loyalty and partnership, strengthening our bonds with the people who are most important to us, whether they are friends, children, or life partners. For those who feel prickly or insecure in social situations, it encourages friendliness and affability. Some say that amber eases problems of the bladder and kidneys.

HEALING ACTION
—
If you are suffering from low mood, meditate with amber regularly. Wear amber jewelry to feel open and at ease in the company of others. To strengthen your bond with a life partner, place in the love and marriage corner of the house, which is at the back right if you enter by the front door.

COMBINATIONS
—
If your mood needs lifting, work with amber, sunstone, and staurolite. To relieve shyness, combine amber with ruby or red beryl.

CARE
—
Amber has a hardness of just 2–2.5 on the Mohs' scale, so it should be protected from scratches. Avoid extremes of heat and prolonged exposure to sunlight. Wipe clean with a damp, soft cloth. Do not soak. Do not use in gem elixirs.

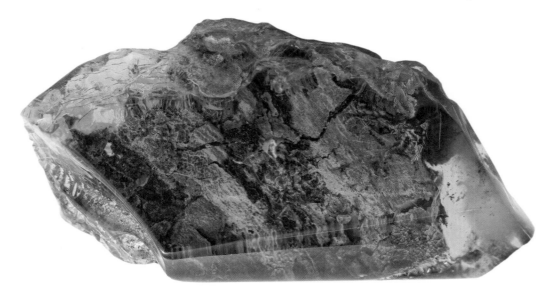

SUNSTONE

APPEARANCE
—

This transparent to translucent mineral is often found in shades of yellow, orange, and red. It has a spangled appearance, as if it contains glitter, caused by light reflecting from small copper or hematite inclusions.

RARITY
—

Sunstone is found in the United States, Australia, Norway, and Sweden. Gem-quality specimens are often Norwegian.

FORMATION
—

Sunstone is a form of oligoclase, a member of the feldspar group of rock-forming minerals. Oligoclase is found in igneous and metamorphic rocks.

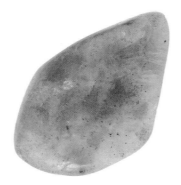

ATTRIBUTES
—

Sunstone helps us to offer those small acts of human kindness that make everyday life joyful. It also encourages us to recognize and accept the kindness of others. This stone brings happiness, not through great change or drama, but through pleasure in the ordinary, from a walk in the park to a cake shared with a friend. Sunstone is said to regulate the metabolism and ease aches and pains.

HEALING ACTION
—

Meditate with sunstone to experience joy in the moment, to focus on the here and now, not the troubled past or the doubtful future. If you find your workplace fraught or stressful, carry sunstone or place it on your desk. Place sunstone on the sacral chakra to combat feelings of dissatisfaction and irritability with others.

COMBINATIONS
—

Build a friendship grid with sunstone, gray kyanite, pink smithsonite, and thulite.

CARE
—

This mineral scores 6–6.5 on the Mohs' scale. Remove sunstone jewelry before exercise or chores. Clean with warm, soapy water and a soft cloth. Do not use in gem elixirs as its inclusions may be toxic.

ZINCITE

APPEARANCE
—

Zincite is often found as small grains within a rocky matrix, but when crystals form they are blade-like. This mineral usually takes flame-like colors, ranging from yellow through orange to red. It is translucent to transparent.

RARITY
—

Natural, well-formed zincite crystals are extremely rare, found only in Franklin Mine and Sterling Hill Mine, in New Jersey. Most commercially available crystals are grown artificially or formed through zinc smelting.

FORMATION
—

Pure zincite is colorless zinc oxide, but an orange shade is provided by traces of iron and manganese.

ATTRIBUTES
—

Zincite is the crystal for communal creative endeavors, from art clubs to choirs, orchestras, and theaters. While encouraging each person to fulfill their own creative potential, zincite draws everyone together for a common goal. Zincite encourages mutual support, collaboration, and idea-sharing. Used externally, zincite is said to be beneficial to the hair and skin.

HEALING ACTION
—

Place zincite in communal spaces, where everyone can be boosted by its positive energy. Position at the sacral chakra to feel confident enough in your own ideas to accept constructive criticism from others. If you are worn down by negative comment on social media, meditate with zincite to be able to discern helpful from unhelpful posts.

COMBINATIONS
—

For the success of any spoken or sung performance, meditate with zincite, aquamarine, and blue calcite.

CARE
—

Zincite is soluble in acids, so it may react dangerously with stomach acid. Do not use in gem elixirs. It scores just 4 on the Mohs' scale. If cleaning is necessary, dust carefully with a soft cloth.

ORANGE ARAGONITE

APPEARANCE
—

Orange aragonite ranges from brown-red to sunshine-yellow. Aragonite crystals form hexagonal prisms, stalactites, needles, fibers, and branching forms known as *flos ferri*, meaning flowers of iron. Aragonite is transparent to opaque.

RARITY
—

Aragonite is a very common mineral, but *flos ferri* and other delicately shaped crystals are collector's items.

FORMATION
—

Pure aragonite is white, but it can be tinted orange by impurities such as iron or inclusions of sand. A type of calcium carbonate, aragonite forms through biological and geological processes. It is made naturally in most mollusk shells. Crystals precipitate from saltwater and freshwater, often around hot springs and in caves.

ATTRIBUTES
—

This variety of aragonite gives us patience in our dealings with others, while also helping us to think creatively about how to work around conflicts. Crystal therapists say that this warming variety of aragonite is particularly helpful with problems of the circulatory system.

HEALING ACTION
—

If struggling through conflict with a teenager, meditate with orange aragonite to feel both calmed and able to view the conflict from a fresh perspective. Place orange aragonite on your desk to find resolutions to office discord.

COMBINATIONS
—

Orange aragonite and blue zircon are a soothing combination when dealing with family friction.

CARE
—

Scoring just 3.5–4 on the Mohs' scale, aragonite is extremely fragile and must be handled with care. Aragonite is soluble in acids and in water. Do not use in gem elixirs as it may react dangerously with stomach acid. If cleaning is necessary, dip briefly in lukewarm soapy water.

SYLVITE

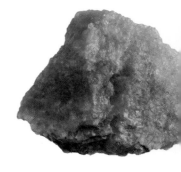

APPEARANCE
—

This mineral is usually found as chunks and crusts, but may form cubes and octahedrons. It is transparent to translucent.

RARITY
—

Sylvite is economically important as a potassium fertilizer, but it is rarely represented in mineral and crystal collections. A seasoned mineral collector could source their own specimen from evaporite deposits in places such as the southwestern United States and Saskatchewan, Canada.

FORMATION
—

This mineral is potassium halide. The orange shade is provided by hematite inclusions. Sylvite is an evaporite mineral (formed as water evaporates from mineral-rich solutions) that is found in dry saline lakes, salt beds, and volcanic fumaroles such as those around Italy's Mount Vesuvius.

ATTRIBUTES
—

This earthy, practical, realistic crystal helps us to see what is truly important and what is merely distraction or evasion. It encourages us to sow seeds for future plans and then to work patiently and assiduously to bring those plans to fruition in their own time. It is said to aid physical stamina when training for a marathon or other sporting goal.

HEALING ACTION
—

Meditate with sylvite to focus on what is meaningful, forgetting the concerns about appearances, petty comments, and social wrangling that so often occupy our minds.

COMBINATIONS
—

To rid yourself of irrational worries and to focus on what is truly important, carefully build a grid with sylvite, lorenzite, and gray kyanite.

CARE
—

Sylvite rates just 2 on the Mohs' scale, so avoid frequent handling or placing on the body. It is soluble in water, so wipe clean very gently with a dry, soft cloth if necessary. Do not use in gem elixirs. Store in a closed box as moisture in the air can degrade its appearance.

SPESSARTINE

APPEARANCE
—

A member of the garnet family, spessartine ranges from yellow-orange to burgundy. Yellow-orange specimens are sometimes called mandarin garnets. Transparent to translucent, spessartine may form roughly cubic crystals or formless chunks.

RARITY
—

Spessartine often grows as a blend with other garnets, such as almandine (a red to purple garnet). Specimens are found in many locations around the world, including in Madagascar, Australia, Tanzania, and the United States.

FORMATION
—

Composed of manganese, aluminum, silicon, and oxygen, spessartine is often found in granite pegmatites, which grew large crystals at high temperature and pressure deep inside the crust.

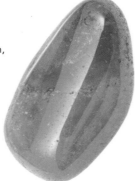

ATTRIBUTES
—

Spessartine encourages us to work practically when we help others, rather than offering nebulous support or good wishes. It also engages our rational minds when we are making decisions involving love and family. It helps us to be realistic about our relationships so that we can work constructively. It is said to treat problems of the lungs and cardiovascular system, although there is no scientific proof of this claim.

HEALING ACTION
—

Position spessartine at the sacral chakra when emotion is overpowering decision-making. Wear spessartine jewelry to build strong, lasting relationships based on honesty and mutual understanding. Place spessartine in the helpful people corner of the home, which is to the right as you enter, if you want to focus on nourishing your longstanding friendships.

COMBINATIONS
—

For insight into how to help a troubled friend, meditate with spessartine and black obsidian.

CARE
—

Spessartine scores 6.5–7.5 on the Mohs' scale. Clean in warm, soapy water with a soft cloth. Do not breathe in garnet dust, which can cause silicosis.

HONEY CALCITE

APPEARANCE
—

As its name suggests, this variety of calcite is the color of honey. Calcite often forms pyramid-shaped crystals or grains, as well as complex forms such as "flowers." It is transparent to translucent.

RARITY
—

Much of the world's honey calcite is sourced from Mexico. It may also be called golden or amber calcite.

FORMATION
—

Calcite is calcium carbonate, which is colorless. It is the presence of impurities including iron that give it a golden tint. Calcite is a major ingredient of sedimentary rocks such as limestone and chalk, as it formed the shells and skeletons of the tiny sea creatures from which these rocks formed.

ATTRIBUTES
—

All varieties of calcite stimulate the mind. This kindly stone teaches us to use our intellectual gifts wisely, never to score points against others. It also encourages us to use our skills for more than pure financial gain, whether that means finding a better balance between work and home life or devising a complete career change. Some say that honey calcite improves dexterity and hand–eye coordination.

HEALING ACTION
—

Place honey calcite in the career area of the home, which is immediately as you enter the front door. Meditate with this mineral if you are feeling burned out from overwork.

COMBINATIONS
—

If you are considering retraining for a new job, build a grid containing honey calcite, clear-sighted obsidian, and motivating ruby or carnelian.

CARE
—

Calcite is brittle and soft, scoring just 3 on the Mohs' scale. It should not be handled excessively. Calcite is not soluble in pure water but is soluble in rainwater, which is slightly acidic. Do not use in gem elixirs. If cleaning is necessary, wipe with a soft cloth.

HESSONITE

APPEARANCE

—

Also called cinnamon stone, hessonite is an orange variety of the mineral grossular, a member of the garnet family. The crystals form cubes, dodecahedrons, and masses.

RARITY

—

Hessonite is a semiprecious stone often used in jewelry. It is sourced mainly from Sri Lanka and India.

FORMATION

—

Composed of atoms of calcium, aluminum, silicon, and oxygen, hessonite grows in metamorphic rocks. It is often found in streambed deposits.

ATTRIBUTES

—

This crystal allows us to view our relationships both clearly and kindly. It encourages us to see where we are needy, where we feel inferior, and where we could be more supportive. While bestowing this insight, hessonite also bolsters our forgiveness of ourselves and others, so we can mend or build where necessary. Hessonite is said to speed the mending of broken bones.

HEALING ACTION

—

When troubled by imbalances in a friendship or romantic relationship, meditate with hessonite. Place hessonite on the sacral chakra to build emotional self-confidence. To focus on relationships with good friends, place hessonite in the helpful people corner of the home, which is at the near right if you enter by the front door.

COMBINATIONS

—

If you frequently feel unloved or unwanted, even if you know that is far from the case, meditate with hessonite, red spinel, red beryl, and brown zircon.

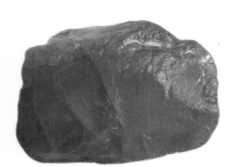

CARE

—

Hessonite scores 7 on the Mohs' scale. Clean in warm soapy water with an untreated cloth. Do not breathe in garnet dust, which can cause silicosis.

TANGERINE QUARTZ

APPEARANCE

—

This orange, transparent, or translucent variety of quartz is often found as six-sided prisms ending in pyramids, arranged as single wands, pairs, or clusters.

RARITY

—

Most tangerine quartz crystals are sourced from Brazil.

FORMATION

—

Pure quartz is made of silicon and oxygen atoms. This variety of the crystal has inclusions of—or is coated with—iron oxide (commonly known as rust), which gives it its orange hue. Quartz is a common rock-forming mineral, found in felsic rocks such as granite.

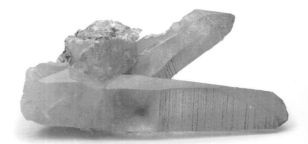

ATTRIBUTES

—

Tangerine quartz offers the possibility of moving on from guilt, of freeing ourselves from past mistakes and failures. This crystal also helps with change and transition, whether that is moving out of the parental home, a relationship breakup, or retirement. Some say that it eases premenstrual tension and the hormonal changes of menopause.

HEALING ACTION

—

Position a wand's point toward the third eye to open your mind to different belief systems or opportunities. When positioned at the sacral chakra, a cluster of tangerine quartz can give us the self-esteem and self-forgiveness to move forward from trauma. Meditating with a long, slender crystal of tangerine quartz will help point the way forward at times of transition.

COMBINATIONS

—

Combine with hematite if fear of new challenges is preventing you from taking the plunge with a relocation, change of career, or new relationship.

CARE

—

Avoid acid cleaning or polishing, which can remove the iron oxide film. Do not immerse in water or use in gem elixirs. Wipe clean with a dry, soft cloth if necessary. Do not inhale quartz dust.

DESERT ROSE SELENITE

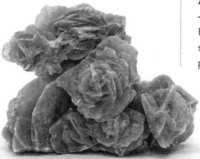

APPEARANCE
—

This variety of the mineral selenite has a coating of sand or contains sand throughout its structure. Its rose-like form is composed of rosettes of blade-like crystals.

RARITY
—

This crystal may sometimes be called Sahara rose, rock rose, or sand rose. Specimens are found in locations such as North Africa, the Middle East, Australia, Spain, Mexico, and Arizona and Texas.

FORMATION
—

An evaporite mineral, selenite is calcium sulfate dihydrate, which means it contains molecules of water. Selenite tends to form rosettes when it grows in dry, sandy conditions, such as when water is evaporating from a desert salt basin. The crystals take the color of the sand that encrusts them, with iron oxides giving a rusty shade.

ATTRIBUTES
—

Like other forms of selenite, desert rose enhances our insights. Desert rose is particularly useful for shining a light on how we can find joy or relief in a difficult situation. It shows us what we need to do to make positive changes in our life. It is said to ease headaches caused by eyestrain.

HEALING ACTION
—

When struggling with low mood, use this crystal as a focus for meditation to open your eyes to all the goodness that is in your life. To increase your family's optimism and resourcefulness, place in the knowledge corner of the home, which is to the left of the main entrance.

COMBINATIONS
—

When a project, large or small, has taken a wrong turn, meditate with black obsidian and desert rose to find a life-enhancing solution.

CARE
—

Selenite dissolves in water, so wipe clean if necessary with a dry, untreated cloth. Do not use in gem elixirs. It scores just 2 on the Mohs' scale, which makes it soft enough to be scratched by a fingernail.

APRICOT AGATE

APPEARANCE
—

Ranging from dusty pink to peach, this variety of agate has bands showing subtle color variations. It is translucent and can be polished to a high shine.

RARITY
—

Natural apricot agate is quite rare. Specimens sold in stores may be heat-treated gray agate.

FORMATION
—

Agate is a translucent form of quartz and chalcedony, which is itself composed of fine intergrowths of quartz and moganite. Both these minerals are composed of silicon and oxygen atoms, but have different molecular structures. Agate is often found as nodules within extrusive igneous rock. Cavities in the lava are filled with silica-rich fluid, which forms solid layers as it crystallizes on the walls then slowly works its way inwards. Variations in the solution or the conditions create bands of different shades and crystal structures.

ATTRIBUTES
—

All forms of agate heighten vision, concentration, and memory. Apricot agate has particular resonance with the family, allowing us to see relationships with children or parents with greater clarity so that we do not repeat mistakes from generation to generation—or oversteer in our attempts to avoid those mistakes.

HEALING ACTION
—

If you face frequent conflict with toddlers or teens, meditate with apricot agate to see deeper into those struggles and what lies behind them. Place in the children corner of the home, which is on the right and midway through the house if you enter by the front door.

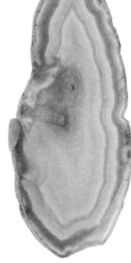

COMBINATIONS
—

To free yourself from lingering memories and bitterness caused by your own childhood conflicts, meditate with apricot agate and pyrolusite.

CARE
—

With a rating of 6.5–7 on the Mohs' scale, agate is suitable for jewelry. However, store it separately to avoid scratches from harder gems. Clean with warm, soapy water and a soft cloth. Do not inhale quartz dust.

YELLOW

Yellow crystals are well placed at the solar plexus chakra, home to our sense of self. These crystals nurture self-confidence, willpower, and belief in our own powers. They also benefit emotional stability and strong emotional communication. If your search is to find your truest self, a more authentic life, or broader enlightenment, yellow crystals act as a guide.

We associate the color yellow with the Sun. When children paint a yellow sun in the corner of their picture, they are expressing warmth and happiness. Indeed, sunlight does have a yellowish shade when the Sun is near the horizon, thanks to the scattering of shorter wavelengths of light. Just as the Sun rises every day, yellow is associated with new beginnings and fresh starts. The legendary first emperor of China was known as the Yellow Emperor. Throughout Asia, the color is associated with power and harmony. The Maya glyph for yellow, k'an, also meant ripe. Yellow is the color of ripe corn, of fulfillment, and of hope for a bright future.

YELLOW JASPER

APPEARANCE
—

Jasper is an opaque stone that is often found as tumbled pebbles. It can be polished to a high shine and is frequently used for carvings.

RARITY
—

Although less common than red jasper, yellow jasper is widely available to purchase. Be aware that the term "jasper" is sometimes used to describe colorful stones with a different mineral makeup than true jasper.

FORMATION
—

Jasper is a mix of quartz and chalcedony, which is composed of microscopically small intergrowths of quartz and moganite. Both these minerals are composed of silicon and oxygen atoms, but have different molecular structures. Jasper often forms where fine sediments are cemented by silicon dioxide. It is the included particles, such as hematite and pyrolusite, that create different shades of jasper.

ATTRIBUTES
—

Like other varieties of jasper, yellow jasper is supportive and protective. It has particular resonance when we are on a physical or mental journey, ranging from pregnancy to a road trip. It prevents us from feeling overcome by anxiety, trepidation, and self-doubt. Yellow jasper is said to benefit the immune system.

HEALING ACTION
—

Place yellow jasper under your pillow when you are traveling far from home. For a feeling of centered calm, meditate with jasper during emotional journeys, such as studying for exams or returning to the parental home after a long absence.

COMBINATIONS
—

When attempting to journey into past lives, combine with variscite. If an emotional journey is fraught and distressing, use with healing amber.

CARE
—

Jasper scores 6.5–7 on the Mohs' scale. Clean with warm, soapy water and a soft cloth. Do not inhale quartz dust, which can cause silicosis.

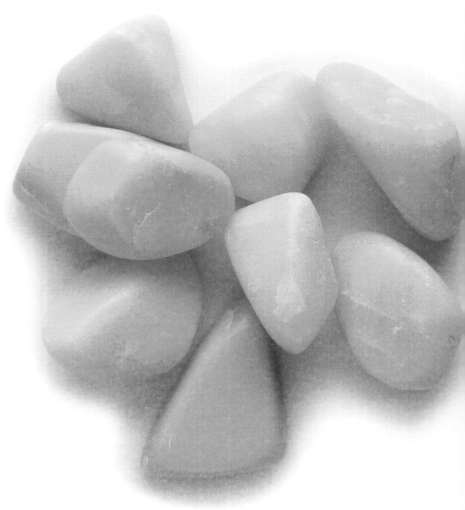

CITRINE

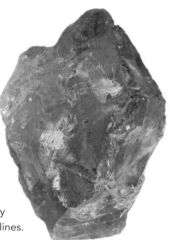

APPEARANCE
—

This variety of quartz ranges from yellow to orange to brown. It grows as six-sided prisms ending in six-sided pyramids, as well as in clusters inside geodes, which are hollow spherical rocks. A natural citrine has a cloudy appearance, while a heat-treated amethyst or smoky quartz may display faint internal lines.

RARITY
—

Natural citrines are rare, with most specimens sourced from southern Brazil. Many citrines on the market are artificially heat-treated amethysts.

FORMATION
—

Citrine contains silicon and oxygen, with traces of iron causing its yellow tint. Citrine geodes form when cavities in volcanic rock are filled with hydrothermal fluid rich in silica.

ATTRIBUTES
—

Traditionally, citrine is called the "money stone," due to the belief that it will bring wealth. Although no crystal has that power, citrine does enhance the forward-planning and self-belief that aid success in business. Citrine helps with concentration and clears the mind, helping us to overcome self-doubt, confusion, anxiety, and phobias.

HEALING ACTION
—

To dispel anxiety that is causing difficulties with eating, place at the solar plexus chakra, Meditate with citrine if money worries are disturbing your peace of mind. To help with planning and book balancing, place a citrine geode in the wealth corner of the house or office, which is at the rear left if you come in by the main entrance.

COMBINATIONS
—

To help with financial planning, place paperweights of tree agate and citrine in your office.

CARE
—

Citrine scores 7 on the Mohs' scale. Wash in warm, soapy water with a soft cloth. Do not inhale citrine dust, which can cause silicosis.

YELLOW FLUORITE

APPEARANCE
—

This transparent to translucent crystal grows in cubes, octahedrons, columns, and fibers. Many crystals fluoresce (a phenomenon named after the mineral) in ultraviolet light.

RARITY
—

Fluorite is a common mineral worldwide, with many practical uses from smelting to pharmaceuticals. Fine specimens are used for decorative purposes, although the mineral's softness usually precludes being used in most jewelry.

FORMATION
—

Fluorite commonly forms in felsic igneous rocks, which are rich in lighter elements. It is composed of calcium and fluorine. Pure fluorite is colorless, but impurities, natural irradiation, and structural defects (called "color centers") can tint it any shade.

ATTRIBUTES
—

All varieties of fluorite help us to make positive changes in our lives. Yellow fluorite has particular resonance with the emotions. When we are struggling with repetitive patterns of feeling, thought, and behavior, fluorite can give us the strength to move forward. It helps us to recognize why we return to the same place again and again, then gives us the self-belief to break the cycle. Some say that yellow fluorite releases toxins and cleanses the liver.

HEALING ACTION
—

If you would like to break free from a negative pattern of emotions, whether that is a self-fulfilling will to fail or frequent jealousy, place at the solar plexus chakra. To cleanse repetitive thoughts or compulsions, place at the crown chakra. Meditate with yellow fluorite for the insight to know why we behave as we do.

COMBINATIONS
—

To ease repetitive thoughts, meditate with yellow fluorite, citrine, and pink topaz.

CARE
—

Fluorite scores just 4 on the Mohs' scale, so it is best to avoid knocks and scratches. Fluorite is not water safe, so clean with a dry cloth if necessary. It is toxic, so do not use in gem elixirs and do not ingest. Do not expose to acids.

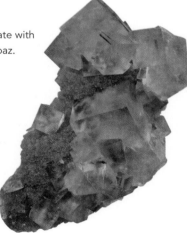

YELLOW APATITE

APPEARANCE
—

Yellow apatite may be one of two minerals in the apatite group, known to mineralogists as hydroxyapatite or chlorapatite. Both minerals form hexagonal plates, nodules, and crusts.

RARITY
—

These crystals are usually sourced from Mexico, although some specimens may be from Japan. Transparent, brightly colored specimens are occasionally used as gems.

FORMATION
—

Apatite is a calcium phosphate, with chlorine-rich chlorapatite and water-rich hydroxyapatite. It forms in many rock types. In the human body, hydroxyapatite is a component of tooth enamel and bone. However, it should not be ingested.

ATTRIBUTES
—

This shade of apatite encourages creativity and spontaneity. It spurs us to find joy in the moment, whether that is whiling away a train journey with a book or getting through chores. It encourages us to focus on what is good in ourselves and our lives.

HEALING ACTION
—

If you have a creative job, place yellow apatite in your office. If you would like to be more creative with your spare time, whether through artistic hobbies or imaginative outings, place this mineral before you during meditation. Put in the creativity corner of the house, which is in the center right if you enter by the front door.

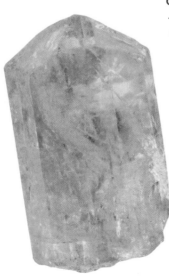

COMBINATIONS
—

For mild depression or low mood, combine with uplifting sunstone.

CARE
—

Yellow apatite scores 5 on the Mohs' scale so should be treated with care. Apatite is toxic, so do not use in gem elixirs and wash your hands after handling. Do not immerse in water. If necessary, wipe clean with a damp cloth.

CHRYSOBERYL

APPEARANCE
—

Most commonly, chrysoberyl is greenish-yellow and transparent to translucent. Its crystals often grow as plates or short prisms. When yellow chrysoberyl exhibits chatoyancy, caused by numerous tiny inclusions, it is called cat's eye.

RARITY
—

Chrysoberyl is one of the rarest, hardest, and most brilliant gemstones. However, there is little demand for it so it does not command the highest prices. It is often mined in Madagascar, Myanmar, Pakistan, Brazil, and the United States.

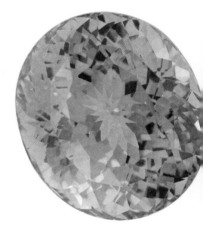

FORMATION
—

Chrysoberyl is composed of beryllium, aluminum, and oxygen atoms. It forms in igneous rocks called pegmatites, which formed by slow crystallization at high temperatures. Despite its name, chrysoberyl is not a form of beryl, although both contain beryllium.

ATTRIBUTES
—

This is an uplifting crystal that encourages us to feel optimistic. It helps us to feel pride in our achievements, families, and abilities. It discourages us from confusing self-worth with possessions or social media feeds. Some crystal therapists say that chrysoberyl enhances lung function and supports healing of the lungs after infection, but there is no scientific basis for these claims.

HEALING ACTION
—

Place chrysoberyl on the solar plexus to enhance feelings of true self-worth. When placed on the crown chakra, chrysoberyl works against materialism. Wear chrysoberyl jewelry to be self-confident without egoism.

COMBINATIONS
—

To wean yourself or a loved one away from social media, build a grid with chrysoberyl, smoky quartz, andradite, and aegirine.

CARE
—

Chrysoberyl is extremely hard, scoring 8.5 on the Mohs' scale. Clean in warm, soapy water with a soft cloth.

YELLOW PREHNITE

APPEARANCE
—
This lemon-colored mineral is often found as rounded, bubbly, or stalactitic forms. Shapes popular with collectors include "fingers," "Roman helmets," and "snakeheads." This mineral is usually translucent.

RARITY
—
Crystals are easily bought from specialist suppliers. Much gem-quality prehnite is mined in South Africa and Australia.

FORMATION
—
This mineral contains calcium, aluminum, silicon, and oxygen, with traces of iron. It is often found in basalt and gneiss. Crystals may be found with a brown ferrous coating, which is chemically removed.

ATTRIBUTES
—
Prehnite is a stone of trust, in oneself, in other people, and in the Universe's overarching patterns. This crystal replaces doubt with belief, anxiety with acceptance, and pessimism with optimism. When we fear change, it brings optimism. Used externally, prehnite is said to treat arthritis, including gout, although there is no scientific proof of that claim.

HEALING ACTION
—
Place on the solar plexus chakra to engender a warming, strengthening self-belief. If placed at the universal mind chakra, it connects us with the ebb and flow of this world and beyond. If you are feeling trepidation about a new chapter in your life, meditate with yellow prehnite to feel ready to grasp new opportunities.

COMBINATIONS
—
To encourage team-building in an office, club, or cooperative, build an orange-yellow grid with yellow prehnite, amber, zincite, and spessartine.

CARE
—
Prehnite may react dangerously to stomach acid, so do not use in gem elixirs. It scores 6–6.5 on the Mohs' scale. Wipe clean with a soft cloth and warm, soapy water. Never use acidic cleaning products as they will dissolve this mineral. Prehnite will fade gradually over time if on display.

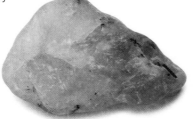

GOLDEN BERYL

APPEARANCE
—
Golden beryl ranges from lemon to gold. Greenish-yellow shades of beryl are known as heliodor (from the ancient Greek for "gift of the Sun"). Beryl often forms hexagonal columns, but may be found as plates or grains.

RARITY
—
Both golden beryl and heliodor are priced as semiprecious gems. The stones with the most golden shade take the highest prices. Crystals are sourced from Sri Lanka, Namibia, Brazil, and Madagascar.

FORMATION
—
Pure, colorless beryl contains beryllium, aluminum, silicon, and oxygen. Golden beryl is tinted by traces of iron. It is found in igneous rocks.

ATTRIBUTES
—
All varieties of beryl help us to meet our potential. Golden beryl helps us to keep our emotions under control as we strive for success, and then to meet that success with calm and magnanimity. It helps us communicate calmly what we feel and to respect the feelings of others. It is said to speed up a slow digestive system.

HEALING ACTION
—
Position golden beryl at the solar plexus chakra when you feel overwhelmed by your own emotions. At the crown chakra, this beryl can help to balance emotion and intellect when it comes to decision-making. Meditate with golden beryl when you are experiencing mood swings.

COMBINATIONS
—
If you are involved in complex negotiations or trying to balance conflicting demands in the workplace, meditate with golden beryl and aegirine, the crystal of integrity.

CARE
—
With a score of 7.5–8 on the Moh's scale, golden beryl is strong and easy to facet, making it ideal for jewelry. It contains beryllium, a known carcinogen, so do not inhale its dust. Clean with warm, soapy water.

DANBURITE

APPEARANCE
—

Often straw-yellow, danburite specimens may also be colorless, white, cream, or gray. This mineral is translucent to transparent. Crystals form tall prisms and radiating masses. Most crystals fluoresce sky blue in ultraviolet light.

RARITY
—

Although this mineral is not rare, large crystals are harder to source. Transparent, faceted specimens are priced as semiprecious stones, but cloudier tumbled stones are lower priced.

FORMATION
—

This mineral was first identified in Danbury, Connecticut. It is a calcium boron silicate that forms while rocks metamorphose as they are baked by magma.

ATTRIBUTES
—

This kind and healing stone helps us to overcome past trauma and to make peace with the past. It calms nervous energy and soothes repetitive or circular thoughts, particularly those that dwell on events we cannot change. Used externally, it is said to speed recovery from stomach upsets caused by food poisoning.

HEALING ACTION
—

Danburite's warm but cleansing energy is useful for unblocked chakras. If you suffer from stress-related insomnia, place a tumbled piece of danburite under the pillow to awaken refreshed and free from worry. If anxiety is causing butterflies or stomach upset, place on the stomach while practicing breathing exercises.

COMBINATIONS
—

To move forward with optimism from loss, mistake, or disappointment, build a grid with danburite, red spinel, jet, and amplifying clear quartz.

CARE
—

Danburite scores 7–7.5 on the Mohs' scale, making it suitable for jewelry. Since danburite is mildly heat-sensitive, avoid steam cleaning. Use warm, soapy water and a soft cloth. Do not expose to acids and do not use in gem elixirs, as it may react dangerously to stomach acid.

YELLOW SAPPHIRE

APPEARANCE
—

Sapphire is the name for any gem-quality corundum crystal that is not red, with those crystals named "rubies." While sapphires are typically blue, those of other colors, known as "fancy" sapphires, do occur. A gem-quality yellow sapphire is transparent and may range from lemon to saffron in shade. Uncut crystals tend to be chunky.

RARITY
—

Sources of yellow sapphires include Sri Lanka, Myanmar, Thailand, Madagascar, Australia, and the United States. Good-quality stones are highly priced, but not as expensive as sapphires of other shades. Always buy any gem-quality stone from a reputable jeweler.

FORMATION
—

Corundum forms deep underground under intense heat and pressure. Pure corundum is aluminum oxide, but traces of iron tint it yellow.

ATTRIBUTES
—

Sapphires are powerful crystals, known for their ability to bring wisdom. Yellow sapphires encourage us to understand ourselves, to see ourselves with both honesty and kindness. They give us insight into our own motivations, gifts, and mistakes. Yellow sapphires help us to know when to trust our own instincts and when to listen to others. On a physical level, some say that these sapphires can help with ear problems, but medical advice should always be sought.

HEALING ACTION
—

If the solar plexus chakra is blocked or stuck, resulting in emotional instability or overwhelming mood swings, position this highly resonant gem on the chakra. If you frequently find yourself doubting your own judgement, wear a yellow sapphire pendant or earrings. Meditate with yellow sapphire when facing a decision that is tugging at your emotional resilience.

COMBINATIONS
—

If you struggle to find sensitive responses when interacting with a challenging parent, teenager, or work colleague, combine yellow sapphire with blue kyanite.

CARE
—

Sapphires are exceptionally hard, scoring 9 on the Mohs' scale. Clean with warm, soapy water and a soft cloth. However, cavity-filled, fracture-filled, or dyed gems should be cleaned only with a damp cloth. Do not use them in gem elixirs.

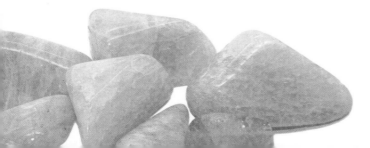

GOLDEN TOPAZ

APPEARANCE
—

Ranging from yellow to golden-brown, gem-quality topaz is transparent. It commonly forms prisms that terminate in pyramids.

RARITY
—

Relatively common but popular for jewelry, topaz is priced as a semiprecious stone. Much yellow topaz comes from Brazil, Mexico, Russia, or Germany.

FORMATION
—

Topaz is a neosilicate mineral that forms in silicon-rich igneous rocks, particularly granite and rhyolite. The presence of iron results in golden-yellow crystals.

ATTRIBUTES
—

Golden topaz enhances motivation. Whether we are training for a race, studying for exams, or trying to maintain a healthy diet, topaz bolsters willpower as well as the self-belief that tells us we can and will meet our goals. This crystal encourages us to listen for the voices that empower us rather than to focus on negative words. It is also said to strengthen the muscles, ligaments, and tendons.

HEALING ACTION
—

If your goal is a healthier lifestyle, place golden topaz at the solar plexus chakra for the strength, energy, and confidence to keep working. Wear golden topaz jewelry to foster self-assurance and fortitude. If you are working towards a career goal, place golden topaz in the career area of the home, which is just inside the front door.

COMBINATIONS
—

If you are trying to improve your lifestyle and health, combine with tree agate and green tourmaline.

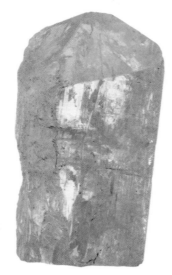

CARE
—

Although topaz scores 8 on the Mohs' scale, making it very hard, its crystals have a weakness in their atomic bonding along a certain plane, where it has a tendency to break if struck with enough force. Clean in warm, soapy water with a soft cloth.

YELLOW JADE

APPEARANCE
—

The beautiful stone we know as jade is one of two minerals with similar properties and appearance, jadeite and nephrite. Yellow specimens are jadeite, although nephrite may take a creamy shade. Yellow jade ranges from translucent to opaque.

RARITY
—

Natural yellow jade is rare. Some specimens may have been dyed or may actually be rocks, such as jasper, that seem similar in appearance to anyone who is not a mineralogist.

FORMATION
—

Both jadeite and nephrite form during the metamorphism of rocks, where two tectonic plates are converging and one plate is subducting, or moving under the other. A great deal of the world's jade is found around the rim of the Pacific Ocean, in the Ring of Fire. Jade is most often collected as pebbles and boulders in stream valleys.

ATTRIBUTES
—

Jade brings harmony, but yellow jade is less calming than other colors: it also energizes. Yellow jade brings joyfulness and a fresh appreciation of all the world has to offer. It is particularly useful for invigorating a stuck or sluggish chakra. It is said to strengthen the body after surgery.

HEALING ACTION
—

If you are suffering from mild depression or listlessness, meditate with yellow jade or wear as a pendant. Yellow jade is an ideal gift for an overworked carer or anyone who is low in energy and has lost their joy in life.

COMBINATIONS
—

If you suffer from seasonal affective disorder (SAD), meditate with yellow jade and sunstone, while also seeking advice from your physician.

CARE
—

Jadeite and nephrite score 6–7 on the Mohs' scale. Wipe jade clean with a soft, soapy cloth, then rinse with clean water and dry carefully. Jade should not be soaked. Keep jade out of direct sunlight.

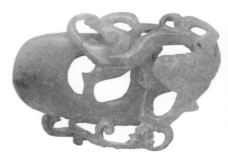

GREEN

Green crystals encourage us to love and nurture. They find particular resonance at the heart chakra. These crystals help us to express our true emotions, working against coldness, hypocriticalness, and jealousy. Yet they also rescue us when our feelings are chaotic or overwhelming, helping us to find balance—within ourselves and in our relationships.

For anyone on any continent, green is the color of nature, of life, of growth. These crystals help us connect with the natural world and to find a healthier lifestyle. Just as communing with the natural world helps us to feel at peace, these crystals renew and refresh. Since green is often the color of banknotes, these crystals are often associated with money and ambition. Yet, more truly, green crystals promote growth—whether practical, emotional, or spiritual. They also encourage us to seek freedom from restrictive rules and lifestyles, just as a plant reaches for the sky and sunlight.

PRASIOLITE

APPEARANCE
—
This pale green variety of quartz, also known as green amethyst or vermarine, is translucent to transparent. It may be found as hexagonal prisms ending in pyramids, either single, paired, or clustered. It may also be seen as tumbled pebbles.

RARITY
—
Prasiolite is rare, with most specimens mined from Brazil, Poland, or Thunder Bay in Canada. Buy from a reputable seller as some prasiolite specimens are artificially heat-treated amethyst. Dark green quartz is often the result of such heat-treating.

FORMATION
—
Quartz is made of silicon and oxygen atoms. Natural prasiolite occurs where amethyst-bearing rock has been heated by nearby lava flows.

ATTRIBUTES
—
Prasiolite offers courage, both in the ability to face up to challenges and to show love when to do so makes us vulnerable. This crystal also aids self-expression, particularly when it is hardest to say what is right and honest. Some say that prasiolite can treat problems of the cardiovascular system, although there is no scientific proof of this claim.

HEALING ACTION
—
Place at the heart chakra for the courage to love and be loved fully, whatever our faults, mistakes, and past history. When feeling fearful or doubtful, meditate with prasiolite for the strength to go forward. Place a cluster of prasiolite crystals in an office meeting room or family kitchen to encourage honest and open communication.

COMBINATIONS
—
To aid public speaking in the face of nervousness, carry prasiolite, blue agate, and blue obsidian. Meditate with ruby and prasiolite for the emotional strength to commit to a new relationship wholeheartedly.

CARE
—
Prasiolite scores 7 on the Mohs' scale, but very impure specimens may score lower. Wash in warm, soapy water with a soft cloth. Avoid extremes of temperature and chemicals. Do not inhale dust, which can cause silicosis.

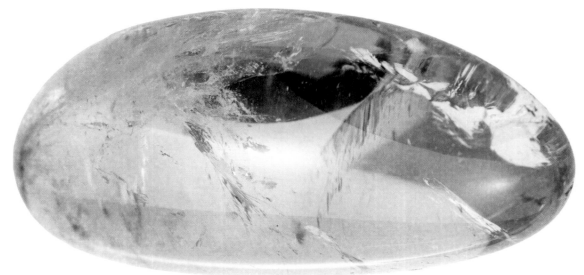

HIDDENITE

APPEARANCE
—
Grass green to emerald, hiddenite is a variety of spodumene. Its color appears to waver between these shades as it is viewed from different angles and in different lights, an effect known as pleochroism. Hiddenite often grows in striated prisms.

RARITY
—
Hiddenite is found in North Carolina (where it was first identified), Brazil, China, and Madagascar. Good-quality, transparent crystals are used as gems.

FORMATION
—
Hiddenite is a lithium aluminum silicate that is tinted green by the presence of chromium. It forms in granitic pegmatites, which are spotted with enlarged crystals.

ATTRIBUTES
—
Hiddenite helps us to focus on our ambitions. While these ambitions may be financial or career-focused, hiddenite also helps us to visualize more emotional ambitions, from spending more time with family to replanting the garden. Hiddenite encourages us to set ourselves goals, then to map out practical steps for how they can be achieved. This mineral is said to help flush out toxins from the body.

HEALING ACTION
—
During times of aimlessness and listlessness, meditate with hiddenite to find direction. If your goal is to live a healthier lifestyle, position hiddenite in the middle left of the home.

COMBINATIONS
—
If you have creative ambitions, such as writing a novel or mastering pottery, work with hiddenite and bloodstone to help put together a plan and the determination to follow it.

CARE
—
Wash in warm, soapy water with a soft cloth. Hiddenite scores 6.5–7 on the Mohs' scale. Do not store with harder gemstones in case of scratching. Hiddenite can fade with exposure to sunlight. Do not use in gem elixirs as it contains lithium.

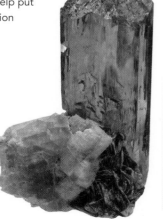

VESUVIANITE

APPEARANCE
—
Also known as idocrase, vesuvianite is found in many shades of green, as well as yellow, brown, blue, red, pink, and black. Usually translucent to opaque, it forms pyramids, prisms, columns, and masses.

RARITY
—
Fine vesuvianite crystals are found around Mount Vesuvius, Italy, as well as in the United States, Canada, and Russia. Although clear and brightly colored crystals are prized as semiprecious gems or collector's items, more opaque or tumbled specimens are low priced. A variety known as californite resembles green jade.

FORMATION
—
This common silicate mineral forms in rocks such as limestone that are baked by nearby magma. Its main ingredients are calcium, magnesium, silicon, and aluminum.

ATTRIBUTES
—
Vesuvianite is a crystal of freedom. It can free us from the social constraints and rules that inhibit true expression. It allows us to imagine different life choices, adventurous travels, and changes of career direction. Some say that vesuvianite eases muscle pain after working out.

HEALING ACTION
—
If you would like to travel, whether for weekends or for a permanent relocation, place vesuvianite in the travel corner of the home, which is at the front right as you enter through the front door. Meditate with vesuvianite to free your mind from its usual tracks. Wear vesuvianite close to the heart if you would like to speak openly and honestly.

COMBINATIONS
—
A beneficial combination for lengthy travels or relocations is vesuvianite and lorenzenite, which guards against homesickness.

CARE
—
Vesuvianite is not very hard, scoring 6.5 on the Mohs' scale. Clean in warm, soapy water with a soft cloth. Do not use in gem elixirs. It is soluble in acids, so may react dangerously to stomach acid.

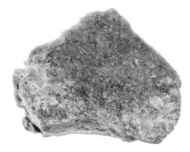

GREEN PREHNITE

APPEARANCE
—
This translucent, grass-green or dusty-green mineral is usually found as globular masses or stalactites.

RARITY
—
Crystals are easily bought from specialist suppliers, while cabochons or faceted gems can be purchased from jewelers. Most gem-quality prehnite is mined in South Africa and Australia.

FORMATION
—
This mineral, first identified by Colonel Hendrik von Prehn in South Africa, contains calcium, aluminum, silicon, and oxygen. It is often found in basalt and gneiss. Crystals often have a brown ferrous coating, which is chemically removed.

ATTRIBUTES
—
Prehnite is a crystal that frees the powers of the mind, aiding memory, intuition, and prophecy. In addition, it links our emotions with our intellect, helping decision-making and conflict resolution. Prehnite may be helpful for treating bladder infections, although there is no scientific proof.

HEALING ACTION
—
At the heart chakra, green prehnite helps us to make decisions with a combination of head and heart, reasoning, and gut feeling. If you are studying for exams or working toward a challenging goal at work, place this crystal on the crown chakra. Place on the table when undertaking tarot reading, scrying, or any form of prophecy.

COMBINATIONS
—
A beneficial crystal combination for scrying is green prehnite, apophyllite, and azurite. For a grid to help decision-making, use green prehnite, obsidian, and polyhedroid agate.

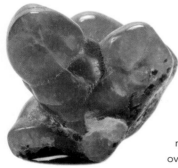

CARE
—
Prehnite may react dangerously to stomach acid, so do not use in gem elixirs. It scores 6–6.5 on the Mohs' scale. Wipe clean with a soft cloth and warm, soapy water. Never use acidic cleaning products as they will dissolve this mineral. Prehnite will fade gradually over time if it is on display.

GREEN ZIRCON

APPEARANCE
—
Green zircon, sometimes known as beccarite, may be grass-green or olive-green. Zircon crystals range from transparent to cloudy. They form as plates, prisms, or chunks.

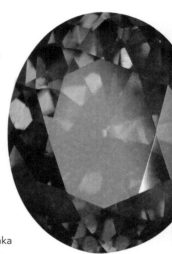

RARITY
—
Zircon is common in the earth's crust, but green is the rarest natural color. It is priced as a semiprecious stone. Green zircons are often mined in Sri Lanka or Madagascar. They are routinely heated to improve their clarity.

FORMATION
—
A zirconium silicate, zircon forms in silicon-rich magma. It is often found in felsic rocks such as granite, which are rich in lighter elements including silicon, oxygen, and aluminum.

ATTRIBUTES
—
Green zircon offers self-confidence. It helps us to overcome shyness, anxieties about public speaking, and stammering. It encourages us to trust our own intuition and instincts. It tells us that we can achieve whatever we want. Some crystal therapists say that it offers relief from menstrual cramps.

HEALING ACTION
—
Meditate with green zircon when your intuition is pulling you a different way from your reasoning. Place at the root chakra to build self-belief. Wear green zircon jewelry in situations where you need a boost of self-confidence, from interviews to sales pitches.

COMBINATIONS
—
For additional support with public speaking, combine green zircon with blue kyanite.

CARE
—
Zircon scores 7.5 on the Mohs' scale, but it can be chipped along faceted edges. Do not use in gem elixirs, as zirconium may be toxic and may react dangerously with stomach acid. Clean only in warm water wwith a mild soap.

MOLDAVITE

APPEARANCE
—
A natural glass, moldavite ranges from turquoise to dark green. Specimens are usually gravel-sized and shaped as shards, beads, raindrops, or flowers, often with internal swirls or bubbles.

RARITY
—
Moldavite is found only in Central Europe, particularly in Germany, the Czech Republic, and Moldova. The world's total amount of moldavite is believed to be around 275 tons. High-quality specimens can be relatively highly priced.

FORMATION
—
This natural glass, a form of tektite, formed 15 million years ago when a giant meteorite crashed into the earth, forming the Nördlinger Ries crater in modern-day Germany. The force of the impact melted and ejected rocks and soil, which fell back to the earth as moldavite, sometimes many hundreds of miles away.

ATTRIBUTES
—
Moldavite has an extremely high vibration that can clear chakra blockages and balance the body's energy flow. Like other forms of tektite, moldavite opens the mind to different realms, new ideas, or challenging journeys, both emotional and physical.

HEALING ACTION
—
Place on the third eye to facilitate the exploration of past lives or awaken your powers of telepathy. Meditate with moldavite to open your mind to new possibilities, whether practical, financial, or emotional.

COMBINATIONS
—
Use at the center of any grid to enhance the powers of the other crystals.

CARE
—
Store moldavite carefully to prevent accidental breakage. It ranges from 5 to 7.5 on the Mohs' scale. Do not clean with salt or toothpaste, which will scratch the surface. It can break in hot water, so clean by rinsing in lukewarm water. Do not use in gem elixirs as its ingredients could be toxic.

PERIDOT

APPEARANCE
—
Peridot is the name for gem-quality olivine. It may also be known as chrysolite. Peridot ranges from yellow, through yellow-green and olive, to lime. Crystals are orthorhombic and translucent to transparent.

RARITY
—
This popular semiprecious stone is often sourced from Afghanistan, Pakistan, Myanmar, Vietnam, China, Egypt, and the United States.

FORMATION
—
A magnesium iron silicate, olivine is found in igneous rocks, such as basalt and gabbro, which are rich in magnesium and iron. Occasionally it is found in volcanic areas in nodules called bombs. Olivine has also been discovered in meteorites, as well as on the Moon and on Mars.

ATTRIBUTES
—
Since the days of ancient Egypt, peridot has been used to ward off evil spirits and drive away nightmares. This is a crystal that guards the heart, protecting us from thoughtlessly hurtful words and deeds, while giving us the emotional strength to face loss and separation. Some say that it helps with palpitations, but medical advice should always be sought first.

HEALING ACTION
—
If you have a tendency to fall in love too easily, wear a peridot pendant so you do not give your heart away to those who do not deserve it. Sleep with peridot under the pillow if you are prone to nightmares or night terrors. When struggling with separation from a loved one, meditate with peridot.

COMBINATIONS
—
A powerful combination against nightmares is peridot and amethyst. When working through grief or loss, build a grid with peridot, black onyx, and sunstone, in addition to seeking help from family, friends, or professional counsellors.

CARE
—
Peridot scores 6.5–7 on the Mohs' scale, making it suitable for jewelry. However, peridot is sensitive to sweat, so avoid frequent wearing against the skin. Clean in warm, soapy water. Avoid dry dusting, which can cause scratches.

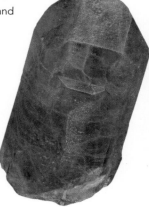

LIZARDITE

APPEARANCE
—

This member of the serpentine group of minerals is named for the Lizard Peninsula, in England's Cornwall. The group is named for the green and scaly appearance of its minerals (in contrast, the Lizard Peninsula gets its name from the Cornish words *Lys Ardh*, meaning "high court"). Although usually green, lizardite may also be white or yellow. It is translucent and generally found as chunks or grains.

RARITY
—

Although first identified in Cornwall, lizardite is found in numerous locations, including Ireland, Austria, South Africa, and India. It may be found cut into beads, cabochons, and artworks.

FORMATION
—

This magnesium silicate hydroxide forms in metamorphic rocks rich in silicate minerals.

ATTRIBUTES
—

Lizardite allows us to break with the past, shedding it as a snake sheds its skin. While ideal for those embarking in a new chapter in their life—after divorce, retirement, or illness—it must be used with wisdom. Some crystal therapists use lizardite for treating skin problems, such as acne and eczema.

HEALING ACTION
—

Meditate with lizardite to break free from old, restrictive modes of thought. Position on the heart chakra to feel ready and eager to face new people, new places, and new challenges. If you are planning a journey, either physical or spiritual, place in the travel corner of the home, which is to the right as you come through the front door.

COMBINATIONS
—

To embrace new beginnings without breaking the binds that tie us to loved ones and friends, combine with pyrope or red beryl.

CARE
—

Lizardite scores only 2.5 on the Mohs' scale. Clean gently with warm, soapy water. Do not use in gem elixirs. Note that another member of the serpentine group, chrysotile (not to be confused with chrysolite), is the most commonly encountered form of the carcinogen asbestos.

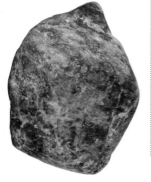

UVAROVITE

APPEARANCE
—

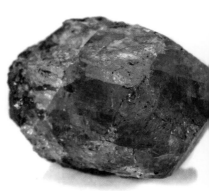

A member of the garnet group of minerals, uvarovite is emerald green and transparent to translucent. Its crystals grow as cubes, grains, coatings, and masses. Uvarovite is sometimes known as chrome garnet.

RARITY
—

Uvarovite is one of the rarest members of the garnet group. Its usual sources are Finland, Russia, and the southwestern United States. Crystals are usually too small to be faceted, but plates of crystals are sometimes used in pendants.

FORMATION
—

Composed of calcium, chromium, silicon, and oxygen, this mineral often forms through the hydrothermal alteration of chromium-rich rocks.

ATTRIBUTES
—

This crystal helps us to find harmony, both in our relationships and our own hearts and minds. If we are feeling overwhelmed by the constant buzz of modern life, it motivates us to turn to the outdoors, sport, and nature for relief. It encourages us to balance competing demands, whether those demands are our own or those of work, friends, children, or partner. Uvarovite is said to rejuvenate the body after illness or exertion.

HEALING ACTION
—

Wear uvarovite as a pendant to find relief from conflicting internal voices and circular or repetitive thoughts. When overwhelmed by work or the needs of others, meditate with this crystal. Place on the windowsill of your office to draw your heart and mind outwards.

COMBINATIONS
—

If you are suffering from overwork or feeling burned out, build a grid with uvarovite, calming blue topaz, and strengthening black onyx.

CARE
—

This mineral scores 6.5–7.5 on the Mohs' scale. Clean in warm, soapy water with a soft cloth.

GREEN TOURMALINE

APPEARANCE
—

Green tourmaline may be known by a variety of other names, including elbaite, Paraiba tourmaline, verdelite, Brazilian emerald, and chrome tourmaline. Translucent to opaque, tourmaline grows in columnar, radiating, or needle-shaped forms. Some crystals display pleochroism, or seeming to be different colors when seen from different angles.

RARITY
—

Green tourmaline is a semiprecious gem, with higher prices for the clearest and most beautifully colored stones. It is often sourced from Brazil.

FORMATION
—

Green tourmaline is commonly found in metamorphic rocks such as schist and marble. Tourmaline is a complicated silicate mineral, containing a high number of elements, including aluminum, boron, iron, lithium, magnesium, potassium, and sodium. Even small changes in the mineral structure result in a dazzling array of colors. Green tourmaline may be tinted by chromium or vanadium.

ATTRIBUTES
—

Like all tourmalines, this variety offers spiritual protection. When working with the chakras, it clears blockages and disperses negative energy. Green tourmaline encourages cooperation with others. It also opens our eyes, ears—and hearts— to the natural world.

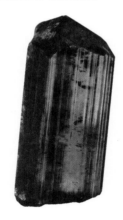

HEALING ACTION
—

Green tourmaline is an ideal gift for someone who works outdoors or is concerned about the environment. Position a green tourmaline crystal in the family room or at the center of the workplace to encourage cooperation and kindness. Meditate with this crystal if you are feeling challenged by criticism or negativity from others.

COMBINATIONS
—

If you are feeling embattled by criticism or fault-finding, combine with chlorite.

CARE
—

Tourmaline rates 7–7.5 on the Mohs' hardness scale. Clean with warm, soapy water and a soft cloth.

GREEN AVENTURINE

APPEARANCE
—

Aventurine is a form of translucent to opaque quartz that appears to sparkle or glitter. This glittering effect is known to mineralogists as aventurescence, from the Italian words meaning "by chance."

RARITY
—

Much green aventurine is sourced from India. It is often carved into beads, cabochons, and artworks.

FORMATION
—

Aventurine is a metamorphic rock composed of quartz (silicon dioxide) with flake-like inclusions of chrome-rich fuchsite, which also give its green shade.

ATTRIBUTES
—

This is an ideal stone for someone ambitious and go-getting, as it encourages us to seize the day and to spot opportunity wherever it arises. Aventurine also encourages us to nourish our relationships, finding moments to feed them and enjoy them. It is said to aid the absorption of vitamins and minerals in the intestines.

HEALING ACTION
—

If you feel you are losing touch with friends or family, wear green aventurine to encourage yourself to make time for them. Meditate with this stone to find joy in the moment. If you are striving for a career goal, place green aventurine in the career area of the home, which is immediately inside the front door.

COMBINATIONS
—

Build a grid for career success, for yourself or a loved one, using green aventurine, jet, ruby, and sylvite.

CARE
—

This rock has a hardness of around 6.5 on the Mohs' scale. Abundant inclusions can lower its hardness further. Do not inhale dust from aventurine. Clean in warm, soapy water with a soft cloth.

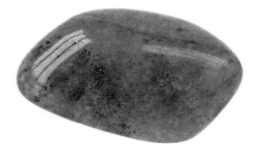

SERAPHINITE

APPEARANCE
—

Seraphinite is a variety of the mineral clinochlore, a member of the chlorite group of minerals. The group is named for the ancient Greek for green, *chloros*. Seraphinite is dark green to gray and exhibits chatoyancy (caused by light reflecting from its fibrous structure) that gives the appearance of the feathers of seraphim.

RARITY
—

This mineral is mined only in the Irkutsk Oblast of Russia's Siberia. Widely available from specialist stores and jewelers, it is priced as a semiprecious stone.

FORMATION
—

Clinochlore is composed of magnesium, iron, aluminum, silicon, hydrogen, and oxygen. It forms in metamorphic rocks. Seraphinite's feather-like chatoyancy is created by fibrous inclusions of mica.

ATTRIBUTES
—

Seraphinite helps us to access the angelic realm and to make soaring spiritual journeys. It also encourages us to take creative flight, envisioning new forms of self-expression. It encourages us to free our minds from the troubles and worries of everyday life, from bills to chores.

HEALING ACTION
—

If you are engaged in a creative project, place at the third eye chakra to gain a fresh perspective. Place at the higher chakras to make contact with the angelic realm. Leave seraphinite by the bedside to experience revelatory dreams.

COMBINATIONS
—

If attempting contact with angels and spirit guides, build a powerful grid with seraphinite, angelite, and celestite.

CARE
—

Seraphinite scores just 2–4 on the Mohs' scale, so avoid knocks and scratches. Clean in warm, soapy water with a soft cloth. Do not use in gem elixirs.

GREEN FLUORITE

APPEARANCE
—

Sometimes called fluorspar, fluorite often forms well-defined cubes and octahedrons. It is also found as columns, fibers, and chunks. Many crystals fluoresce (a phenomenon named after the mineral) in ultraviolet light. It is transparent to translucent.

RARITY
—

Fluorite is widespread worldwide, but specimens suitable for decorative rather than industrial use are less common and may be priced as a semiprecious gem. Green fluorite may be sourced from South Africa or Namibia.

FORMATION
—

This mineral forms in igneous rocks, such as granite, particularly as a result of hydrothermal activity. Pure fluorite, composed of calcium and fluorine, is colorless. Impurities, natural irradiation, and structural defects (called "color centers") can tint it any shade.

ATTRIBUTES
—

All varieties of fluorite help us to make positive changes in our lives. Green fluorite has particular resonance with our closest relationships, with partners, siblings, parents, and children. It encourages us to show and voice love, even when we are beset by self-doubt, anger, or resentment. When used externally, it is said to ease stomach upsets caused by food poisoning, although medical advice should always be sought.

HEALING ACTION
—

If you are struggling with conflict, distrust, or recrimination in a close relationship, meditate with green fluorite. Position at the heart chakra to ease negative feelings about loved ones, replacing them with empathy, compassion, and forgiveness. Place green fluorite in the family corner of the home, which is midway through the house on the left, if you enter by the front door.

COMBINATIONS
—

When a relationship with a partner is emotionally stormy, work with green fluorite, calming aquamarine, and loving thulite.

CARE
—

Fluorite scores just 4 on the Mohs' scale, so it is more suitable for display or for jewelry such as earrings than for rings or bracelets. Fluorite is not water safe, so clean with a dry cloth if necessary. It is toxic and may react dangerously with stomach acid, so do not use in gem elixirs and do not ingest. Do not expose to acids.

CHRYSOPRASE

APPEARANCE
—

Chrysoprase specimens vary from deep green to apple-green and turquoise.
It ranges from opaque to translucent. Specimens are often small and tumbled.

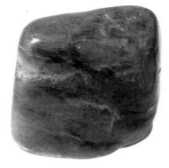

RARITY
—

This relatively common semiprecious stone is usually sourced from Tanzania or Poland, but a few specimens may be from Russia, Australia, or the United States.

FORMATION
—

Chrysoprase is a form of chalcedony, which is composed of fine intergrowths of the silicon dioxide minerals quartz and moganite, the two differentiated by their crystal structures at the microscopic level. Chrysoprase is colored green by tiny quantities of nickel. The stone is formed during the weathering of serpentinite rocks, which are usually greenish and slippery feeling.

ATTRIBUTES
—

As with other forms of chalcedony, such as carnelian, chrysoprase has resonance with business pursuits. Yet where carnelian encourages drive and ambition, chrysoprase encourages lateral thinking and creativity. It enables us to accept advice from others and to listen to other viewpoints. Chrysoprase is said to settle hormonal imbalances.

HEALING ACTION
—

Position at the heart chakras to accept the kindly advice of others and to awaken empathy even with those we find challenging. Place in the wealth corner of the house, which is at the far left if you come in by the main entrance, to encourage creative solutions to business or career issues.

COMBINATIONS
—

Combine with carnelian in grids and during meditation to encourage a holistic view of any business or scholarly venture.

CARE
—

Chrysoprase scores 6–7 on the Mohs' scale. If dropped, it may fracture into sharp-edged pieces. Since it is porous, avoid accidental contact with chemicals. Clean with warm, soapy water and a soft cloth. Do not inhale chrysoprase dust or use in gem elixirs.

EMERALD

APPEARANCE
—

This precious gemstone ranges from vivid blue-green to yellow-green. Crystals grow in hexagonal prisms.

RARITY
—

Transparent, high-quality emeralds are rare and valuable, but clouded or opaque specimens are readily available. Emeralds are mined across the world, with the two biggest producers being Colombia and Zambia. Note that only emeralds with a vivid hue earn the name: paler crystals must be known as "green beryl."

FORMATION
—

A variety of the mineral beryl, emerald grows in metamorphic rock as well as in cavities and along fractures in granite. Beryl is composed of beryllium, aluminum, silicon, and oxygen. Pure crystals are colorless. Emerald is tinted by traces of chromium and sometimes vanadium.

ATTRIBUTES
—

Emerald is a powerful nurturer of relationships. It helps us to nourish our relationships through love, good communication, and empathy. It helps us to be true to our own emotions, escaping coldness, hypocrisy, and pretence. Emerald is said to help with recovery after illness, particularly viruses.

HEALING ACTION
—

To focus on the needs and lives of those we love, meditate with emerald. Position on the heart chakra to awaken honest emotions and the ability to express them. To focus positive energy on your relationship with your spouse or partner, place an emerald crystal in the back right of the home, if you enter by the front door.

COMBINATIONS
—

To nurture your relationship with your life partner, build a grid with emerald, passionate red beryl, kind rhodonite, and communicative blue kyanite.

CARE
—

Emerald scores 7.5–8 on the Mohs' scale, but crystals usually contain a high quantity of inclusions, giving them low resistance to breakage. Clean with warm, soapy water and a soft cloth. Care must be taken with handling this mineral. Emerald contains beryllium, a known carcinogen, so do not inhale its dust.

ATACAMITE

APPEARANCE
—
Named after the Atacama Desert, where it was first described in 1801, atacamite ranges from emerald-green to black-green. Atacamite grows in slender prisms, fibers, and masses. It is transparent to translucent.

RARITY
—
Atacamite is a relatively rare mineral that is found in dry regions of Chile, Australia, Russia, and the southwestern United States. It is available from specialist mineral stockists.

FORMATION
—
This copper chloride hydroxide forms where copper minerals are oxidized in dry climates. It has been found on the weathered copper of the Statue of Liberty.

ATTRIBUTES
—
Atacamite is a crystal of long-lasting love and friendship. It helps life partnerships stand the test of time. It encourages friendships to weather changes in circumstance. Atacamite also helps us to take a long-term view of life's obstacles and difficulties, and not settle for a quick fix. Some say that it eases the discomfort of arthritis and rheumatism.

HEALING ACTION
—
Place atacamite at the heart chakra to awaken dormant feelings of love and friendship. Place in the marriage corner of the home, which is at back right if you enter at the front door. Meditate with atacamite if you feel beset by problems and stresses.

COMBINATIONS
—
Build a friendship grid containing atacamite, thulite, pink smithsonite, and amber.

CARE
—
Atacamite scores only 3–3.5 on the Mohs' scale. Its high copper content means it should not be used in gem elixirs. It is also soluble in acids, so may react dangerously to stomach acid. Do not inhale dust. Clean gently in warm, soapy water.

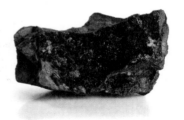

GREEN JADE

APPEARANCE
—
Green jade may be one of two minerals, jadeite and nephrite, which share a similar appearance and properties. It ranges from pale apple-green to bright emerald, from translucent to opaque.

RARITY
—
Green is the most common color of both nephrite and jadeite. Jadeite is the rarer and more highly priced of the two minerals. Both forms of jade have been used for statues and carvings for millennia, in cultures from China to New Zealand, Mexico to India.

FORMATION
—
Both nephrite and jadeite form during the metamorphism of rocks, particularly where two tectonic plates are converging. Much jade is found as pebbles and boulders in stream valleys, with a brown, weathered rind hiding its beauty.

ATTRIBUTES
—
While all colors of jade bring harmony, green jade has particular resonance with relationships. It offers insight into why conflict has arisen and how we can best move forward, without anger, blame, or denial. It is said to calm the nervous system.

HEALING ACTION
—
Green jade helps to balance the chakras, so position over any chakra that is blocked or overstimulated. If you are encountering conflict, with anyone from a teenager to a work colleague, meditate with green jade for calmness and fresh insight. Place a jade carving in the relationships corner of the house, which is at the back right if you enter by the front door.

COMBINATIONS
—
If you find yourself responding to conflict with angry thoughts or words, meditate with green jade and calming, loving amethyst.

CARE
—
Jade is durable and easy to carve. It scores 6–7 on the Mohs' scale. Wipe jade clean with a soft, soapy cloth, then rinse with clean water and dry carefully. Jade should not be soaked. Keep jade out of direct sunlight.

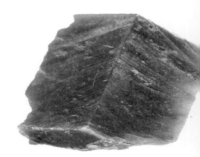

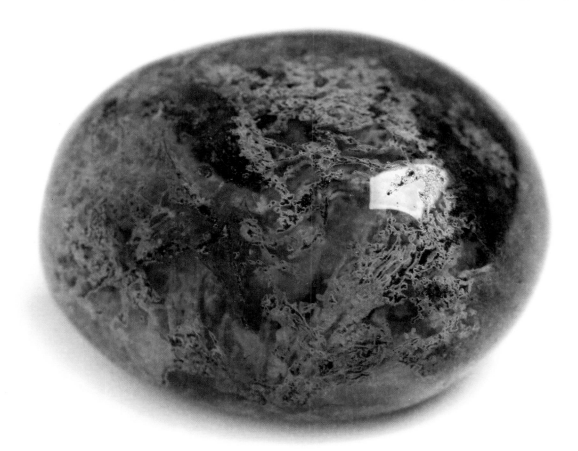

MOSS AGATE

APPEARANCE

—

This variety of agate has swirling green markings that resemble moss. The matrix is usually colorless and translucent.

RARITY

—

Moss agate is often sourced from Australia, India, or the United States.

FORMATION

—

Agate is a translucent form of quartz and chalcedony, itself composed of fine intergrowths of quartz and moganite. Both these minerals are forms of silicon dioxide, with different molecular frameworks. Agate often grows as nodules inside igneous rock. Cavities are filled with silica-rich fluid, which slowly crystallizes. The moss-like forms are inclusions of oxidized iron hornblende.

ATTRIBUTES

—

Moss agate is a nurturing crystal, encouraging us to care for our gardens, homes, families, and friends. Like other forms of agate, it heightens our vision, allowing us to see clearly how and why others need our help. It has particular resonance with the bond between parents and their children. Some say that it eases headaches caused by eyestrain or spending too long staring at a screen.

HEALING ACTION

—

Moss agate is the ideal gift for a new mother. If a loved one has recently given birth, meditate with moss agate to understand how best to show her support without overwhelming or dictating. Position moss agate in the health and family area of the home, which is on the left and midway through the house if you enter by the front door.

COMBINATIONS

—

For blessings on a new mother, build a grid holding moss agate, loving rhodochrosite, gentle pink common opal, and—most importantly—kunzite for a good night's sleep.

CARE

—

With a rating of 6.5–7 on the Mohs' scale, agate is suitable for jewelry and frequent gentle handling. Clean in warm, soapy water. Avoid extremes of temperature. Do not inhale agate dust, which can cause silicosis.

MALACHITE

APPEARANCE
—

This mineral displays bands of bright green, dark green, and blackish-green. Usually opaque, it grows as stalactites, masses, and plates. After cutting, the sawn faces exhibit the hallmark banding.

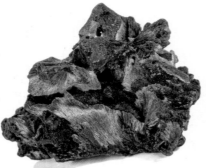

RARITY
—

Malachite is widely available from mineral stockists, who should also offer advice on its toxicity, safe storage, and care. It may also be bought as polished cabochons and beads. Gem-quality malachite is sourced from the Democratic Republic of the Congo, Australia, France, or the United States.

FORMATION
—

This copper carbonate hydroxide mineral forms underground, when carbonated water interacts with copper minerals or when a copper solution interacts with limestone.

ATTRIBUTES
—

Malachite is a crystal of empathy. It encourages us to understand and forgive the mistakes and weaknesses of others. It also allows us to journey beyond ourselves, into other lives and other worlds. While under the influence of malachite, dreamers may receive messages from spirit guides and angelic entities.

HEALING ACTION
—

This stone must be used only in its polished form and under the direction of a qualified crystal therapist.

COMBINATIONS
—

Under the care of a qualified crystal therapist, malachite can be teamed with jet to access past lives.

CARE
—

Keep malachite away from children and pets. The high copper content of malachite makes it toxic, so do not inhale its dust or use in gem elixirs. It is heat-sensitive and reacts dangerously with weak acids, including possibly stomach acid. This mineral is soft, with a Mohs' hardness of 3.5–4, so avoid excessive handling. Clean with lukewarm water and a gentle soap.

FUCHSITE

APPEARANCE
—

A green variety of the mineral muscovite, fuchsite ranges from pale green to emerald-colored. It is transparent to opaque. Its crystals are flexible and can often be cut into thin pieces with a knife. The mineral fluoresces lime green under ultraviolet light.

RARITY
—

Fuchsite can be bought from mineral stockists. Much fuchsite is sourced from Brazil.

FORMATION
—

Fuchsite is a chromium-rich variety of muscovite, which also contains potassium, aluminum, silicon, oxygen, and fluorine. It forms when clay minerals are transformed by the heat and pressure of regional metamorphism.

ATTRIBUTES
—

Fuchsite is a crystal of emotional healing. It helps us to overcome past trauma. It also helps us to find balance when we feel overwhelmed by emotion. It cleanses negative feelings, leaving the user refreshed and at peace. It is said to ease constipation, although medical advice should always be sought to find the root cause.

HEALING ACTION
—

Position at the heart chakra to modulate mood swings. Meditate with fuchsite to expel negative emotions and calm a troubled heart.

COMBINATIONS
—

Fuchsite and moonstone make a good combination for calming hormonally induced mood swings.

CARE
—

Fuchsite scores just 2–2.5 on the Mohs' scale. Do not soak in water as it may flake apart. Do not use in gem elixirs. If necessary, clean very gently with a dry, soft brush.

TURQUOISE

Turquoise crystals encourage generosity, empathy, and compassion. They are well placed at the higher heart chakra. The crystals encourage us to put effort into our relationships, to communicate freely and honestly, and to seek fellowship with others. At the same time, these crystals ease the heart by healing stress and soothing excessive emotions. They encourage temperance and serenity.

In English, the color turquoise is named for the gem turquoise, which was itself named for the French for "Turkish," as the gem was originally imported from Turkey. The color is strongly associated with the tiled domes and interiors of mosques in Samarkand and other Central Asian cities. Such domes are bridges between the earth and heaven, between material and spiritual. Turquoise crystals are also bridges, arcing between the head and heart, between ourselves and others, and between the earthly and spiritual realms.

DIOPTASE

APPEARANCE
—

Ranging from emerald green to deep blue-green, dioptase is transparent to translucent. When its crystals have ample space and materials, they form six-sided prisms terminating in rhombohedrons.

RARITY
—

Dioptase is a rare mineral. The most well-known source is Tsumeb, in Namibia. Popular with mineral collectors, crystals can be bought from specialist stores. Gem-quality specimens can be sourced from jewelers.

FORMATION
—

This mineral forms mainly in desert regions where copper sulfide mineral deposits are oxidized. It is composed of copper, silicon, oxygen, and hydrogen.

ATTRIBUTES
—

Dioptase is a powerfully optimistic crystal. It encourages us to glimpse a positive future, even when the night is darkest. It encourages us to draw strength from our happiest memories. It helps us to welcome support and kindness from family and friends.

HEALING ACTION
—

Although cut and polished dioptase specimens are considered safe to handle, this mineral is best used under the care of a qualified crystal therapist.

COMBINATIONS
—

A crystal therapist may combine dioptase with warming and uplifting ruby to help with low mood and listlessness.

CARE
—

Dioptase is fragile and brittle, scoring just 5 on the Mohs' scale. Since dioptase has a high copper content and may react dangerously with stomach acid, do not use in gem elixirs. Do not breathe in dioptase dust. This mineral is soluble in acids. If cleaning is necessary, use lukewarm, soapy water and a soft cloth.

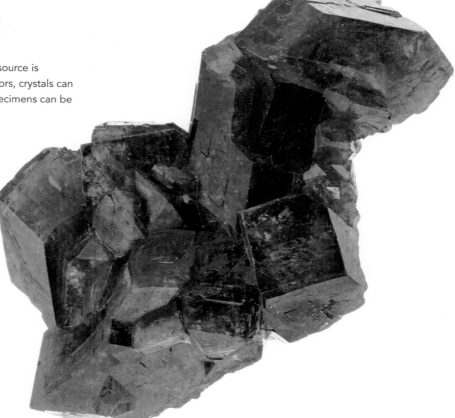

AMAZONITE

APPEARANCE

—

This green-blue or green mineral is often found as prisms, chunks, or tumbled stones. It ranges from translucent to opaque.

RARITY

—

Sources of amazonite include Russia, Mongolia, China, South Africa, and the United States. It may be bought as cabochons, carvings, and jewelry.

FORMATION

—

Amazonite is a potassium feldspar, its main ingredients being potassium, silicon, aluminum, and oxygen. Its color is formed from a complex combination of traces of other elements, including possibly lead, copper, rubidium, and iron.

ATTRIBUTES

—

Amazonite soothes the mind, spirit, and body. It eases stress, emotional turmoil, and intrusive or circular thoughts. It encourages us to find respite in our busy day, taking time to meditate, breathe, or walk in the fresh air. Amazonite also helps us to talk about our worries—and to find the right people to share them with.

HEALING ACTION

—

Amazonite is considered safe to handle, but observe the precautions below. Hold over the throat chakra to voice your fears and anxieties both calmly and freely. Meditate with amazonite to find relief from stress or a whirring, too-busy mind.

COMBINATIONS

—

To encourage a calming, spiritual connection with the natural world, build a grid with amazonite, uvarovite, and green tourmaline.

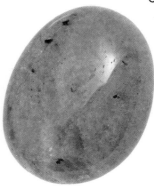

CARE

—

Keep amazonite away from children and pets. Amazonite contains traces of lead and copper, both of which are toxic. Do not use in gem elixirs or breathe in dust. Wash hands after handling. Amazonite scores 6–6.5 on the Mohs' scale. Clean in warm, soapy water with a soft cloth.

GRANDIDIERITE

APPEARANCE

—

Named after Alfred Grandidier, a French explorer of Madagascar, this gemstone is blue-green and translucent to transparent. It is trichroic, displaying three different colors—turquoise, no color, and dark green—depending on the viewing angle.

RARITY

—

Transparent, faceted grandidierite specimens are among the world's rarest and most expensive gemstones. Cloudy stones are much more affordable. Most gem-quality crystals are sourced from Madagascar or Sri Lanka, but other localities include Algeria, India, New Zealand, and the United States.

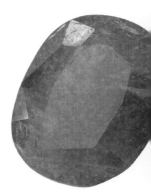

FORMATION

—

Grandidierite is composed of atoms of magnesium, iron, aluminum, boron, silicon, and oxygen. It forms in metamorphic rocks rich in aluminum and boron. The greater the quantity of iron, the bluer this gemstone becomes.

ATTRIBUTES

—

Grandidierite is a stone of forgiveness. It allows us to forgive those who have wronged us, and to forgive ourselves for mistakes. It awakens compassion and empathy. It has particular resonance with those caring for small children, helping them to turn away impatience and find kindness and love, even in exhaustion. Grandidierite is said to stimulate the thymus gland and strengthen the immune system.

HEALING ACTION

—

Place at the higher heart chakra to awaken empathy and generosity. Meditate with grandidierite while asking for forgiveness for past wrongs and bestowing forgiveness on others. Grandidierite jewelry is an ideal gift for a new parent.

COMBINATIONS

—

For the forgiveness of wrongs inflicted in past lives, combine with jet.

CARE

—

This mineral scores 7.5 on the Mohs' scale, but it can be chipped along faceted edges. Grandidierite can be cleaned in warm, soapy water with a soft cloth, but high-value gemstones should be taken to a reputable jeweler for cleaning.

VARISCITE

APPEARANCE
—

Although usually a blue-green, variscite ranges from yellow-green to emerald. Variscite is often confused with turquoise, but it is usually slightly greener. It ranges from translucent to opaque.

RARITY
—

Variscite is often used in place of turquoise in jewelry and carvings. Although rarer than turquoise, it is less well known, so it takes a lower price. Variscites from Utah are sometimes known as utahlites or lucinites. Other sources include Australia, Brazil, and central Europe.

FORMATION
—

This mineral forms as groundwater rich in phosphorus works on aluminum-heavy rocks. Variscite gets its color from traces of chromium and vanadium.

ATTRIBUTES
—

This mineral helps us to rein in excesses. When combined with professional care, it helps us to combat addictions and obsessive compulsions. It also calms mood swings and combats overpoweringly negative emotions, such as jealousy and hate. It is said to calm an overactive thyroid gland, but there is no scientific proof of this claim.

HEALING ACTION
—

Place variscite in the self-cultivation area of the home, which is to the left of the front door after entering. To support a battle against addiction, wear a variscite pendant close to the higher heart chakra.

COMBINATIONS
—

If you frequently feel overwhelmed by negative emotion, meditate with variscite in one hand and rhodonite in the other.

CARE
—

Variscite scores just 4.5 on the Mohs' scale, so protect from scratches. Clean gently in warm, soapy water with a soft cloth.

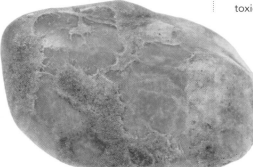

CHRYSOCOLLA

APPEARANCE
—

This blue-green to cyan mineral is most often seen as globes, nodes, and chunks. It ranges from translucent to opaque.

RARITY
—

Chrysocolla may be bought in jewelry (where it is often mistaken for turquoise) or as mineral specimens, which can be obtained from specialist stores. Pure chrysocolla is quite rare, as it has a propensity to mix with other minerals. However, this will not spoil its healing action.

FORMATION
—

This copper ore is often found in copper mines where copper compounds have been altered by water containing silica.

ATTRIBUTES
—

Chrysocolla is a deeply creative stone. It is ideal for those who work in a creative field, as well as for anyone who pursues writing, arts, crafts, or cookery as a hobby. It frees the mind to be self-confidently inventive, while gifting the hands with dexterity and deftness.

HEALING ACTION
—

Although polished chrysocolla is considered safe for jewelry and handling, this crystal is best used under the care of a qualified crystal therapist.

COMBINATIONS
—

To aid automatic or creative writing, a crystal therapist may team chrysocolla with calligraphy stone.

CARE
—

Due to its high copper and silicon content, chrysocolla dust is toxic. Do not inhale dust, do not leave it in contact with the skin, and do not ingest. Chrysocolla must not be used for gem elixirs. It scores just 2.5–3.5 on the Mohs' scale. Clean with warm, soapy water and a soft cloth.

TURQUOISE

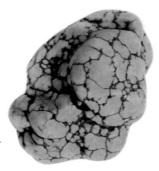

APPEARANCE
—

This blue-green, opaque mineral is found as chunks and nodes. The dark, spidery lines of limonite veining (iron ore) can often be seen.

RARITY
—

There are only a few large deposits of turquoise in the world, the best known in Iran, Egypt, Turkey, China, Mexico, and the United States. More affordable stones may be brittle and crumbly.

FORMATION
—

Turquoise is composed of copper, aluminum, phosphorus, oxygen, and hydrogen. The mineral gets its color from its copper. Typically, the mineral forms underground in a two-step process. First, hydrothermal fluid leaches copper from the host rock, filling veins and fractures with copper ore. Next, groundwater reacts with the copper ore as well as aluminum and phosphorus in the rock, slowly forming turquoise.

ATTRIBUTES
—

Turquoise has been prized as a gem since the days of ancient Egypt, when it was used for grave furnishings as well as in amulets that brought good luck and protection for the wearer. This is a stone that both heals and strengthens, helping us to overcome past trauma, to overcome emotional turmoil or anxiety, and to move forward with optimism. It is also said to speed the healing of physical wounds and injuries.

HEALING ACTION
—

When placed or worn close to the higher heart chakra, turquoise helps us to overcome anxiety, shyness, or low self-esteem. At times of emotional stress, meditate with turquoise to engender calm and hope for the future.

COMBINATIONS
—

If you are suffering from anxiety, combine turquoise with blue sapphire or gray kyanite.

CARE
—

Turquoise scores 5–6 on the Mohs' scale, so protect it from drops and knocks. If soaked, turquoise will absorb the water and any chemicals it contains. If cleaning is necessary, wipe with a soft, clean, and untreated cloth. Do not use in gem elixirs as turquoise contains copper.

HEMIMORPHITE

APPEARANCE
—

This transparent to translucent turquoise mineral is also found in white. Hemimorphite (which gets its name from the ancient Greek for "half form") is named for the unusual structure of its crystals, which have differently shaped ends, one blunt and one sharp. Typically, however, hemimorphite is found as less distinct crusts, layers, and masses.

RARITY
—

Hemimorphite is rare, particularly as a faceted gemstone, but it can be sourced from the German–Belgian border, Poland, Mexico, and the United States.

FORMATION
—

This mineral is composed of zinc, silicon, oxygen, and hydrogen. It forms in veins, vugs, and layers where zinc ores are oxidized.

ATTRIBUTES
—

Hemimorphite encourages us to be compassionate and empathetic. It also encourages us to voice our own feelings, without shame or blame. On a higher plane, hemimorphite also awakens clairvoyance, lucid dreams, and psychic visions. It is said to de-stress the nervous system.

HEALING ACTION
—

Place on the heart to awaken empathy for someone who is troubling, from a challenging work colleague to a combative teenager. Place or wear on the throat to encourage honest communication. To experience lucid dreams, sleep with hemimorphite beside the bed.

COMBINATIONS
—

To encourage frank but kindly communication with a partner or friend, combine with common pink opal. A powerful combination to stimulate clairvoyance is hemimorphite and clear selenite.

CARE
—

This mineral scores just 4.5–5 on the Mohs' scale, so protect from breaks and scratches. Hemimorphite is soluble in acids. Do not use in gem elixirs, as it may react dangerously to stomach acid. Do not breathe in its dust, which contains silicon. Clean in warm, soapy water with a soft cloth.

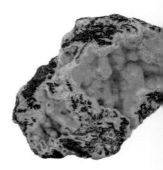

TURQUOISE SMITHSONITE

APPEARANCE
—

Sometimes called turkey fat or zinc spar, smithsonite is a translucent mineral that is found in a range of pastel shades. It forms globular masses resembling bubbles or berries.

RARITY
—

This mineral can be bought from specialist stores. Common sources are the United States, Mexico, Australia, and Greece.

FORMATION
—

Smithsonite is composed of zinc, carbon, and oxygen. It grows where zinc ores are oxidized.

ATTRIBUTES
—

Turquoise smithsonite helps us to heal our emotional wounds, as well as speeding recovery from physical wounds. It encourages us to feel whole and secure, so that we do not manifest our troubles through neediness, prickliness, or coldness.

HEALING ACTION
—

When placed at the higher heart chakra, this variety of smithsonite helps us to heal from past trauma. At the throat chakra, this smithsonite allows us to express our worries so that we can free ourselves from them and embrace life and all it offers.

COMBINATIONS
—

If you have suffered pain in this life or past lives, meditate with turquoise smithsonite and healing amber.

CARE
—

Smithsonite scores just 4.5 on the Mohs' scale, so should be handled with care. It may be toxic if ingested as it contains zinc and may react dangerously to stomach acid, so do not use in gem elixirs. Smithsonite is soluble in acids. Clean with lukewarm water and a soft cloth, but do not soak.

AQUAMARINE

APPEARANCE
—

Aquamarine is a turquoise to pale-blue variety of the mineral beryl. A deep-blue beryl may be known as maxixe. Aquamarine is transparent to translucent. It grows in hexagonal crystals, but may also be found as plates, grains, and chunks.

RARITY
—

Gem-quality aquamarine is priced as a semiprecious stone. Common sources are the United States, Brazil, Colombia, Tanzania, and Kenya.

FORMATION
—

Aquamarine crystals are often found in granitic rocks. Beryl is composed of beryllium, aluminum, silicon, and oxygen. Pure crystals are colorless, but aquamarine is tinted by traces of iron.

ATTRIBUTES
—

The ancient Romans believed that aquamarine could protect from the dangers of sea travel. Some say it truly does ease seasickness. This protective crystal gives us strength in the face of emotional and psychic attack. It helps us to see our way through stormy times, safe in the knowledge that better days will come.

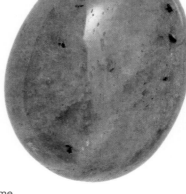

HEALING ACTION
—

For emotional and spiritual strength, wear at the heart chakra. When times are hard, meditate with aquamarine to gain strength, perspective, and optimism. A cluster of aquamarine crystals will collect positive energy and is well placed in the self-cultivation corner of the home, which is to the left of the front door.

COMBINATIONS
—

If you are in need of emotional protection, combine with jet.

CARE
—

Aquamarine scores 7.5–8 on the Mohs' scale. It contains beryllium, a known carcinogen, so do not inhale its dust. Clean with warm, soapy water and a soft cloth.

BLUE

Blue crystals resonate with the throat chakra, which is responsible for communication and the expression of personal truths. These crystals encourage wise communication, fearless speaking, and—above all—truthfulness. They work against shallowness and dishonesty. Many blue crystals also resonate at the third eye, where they help us to see truths, both physical and metaphysical. They teach us wisdom and encourage us to develop our emotional intelligence.

Blue is the color of the sky and sea, of the eternal and unchanging. Just as we are calmed by the drifting of clouds across the sky or the rhythmic breaking of waves on the seashore, so too are we soothed by blue crystals. The blue of sky and sea represent both clarity and endless depth. Blue crystals help us to focus on the detail of our daily lives while also encouraging us to see the wider picture—the truths that will remain long after we have stopped worrying about yesterday and tomorrow.

BLUE LACE AGATE

APPEARANCE
—

This variety of agate has a lace-like pattern of frills, eyes, bands, or zigzags. While most lace agate is dusty blue and white, Mexican crazy lace agate exhibits red, yellow, or white patterns.

RARITY
—

Many specimens of blue lace agate are sourced from Namibia. It is often bought as tumbled stones.

FORMATION
—

The blue lace agate found in Namibia is around 50 million years old, but it grew in fractures in igneous dolerite rock that is far older. The seams filled with silica-rich fluid, which slowly crystalized. Agate is a translucent form of quartz and chalcedony, which is itself composed of fine intergrowths of quartz and moganite. Both these minerals are composed of silicon and oxygen atoms, but have different molecular structures. Variations and inclusions in the silica create patterns and swirls of different shades and crystal structures.

ATTRIBUTES
—

When life is busy and stressful, this variety of agate helps us to find peace and inner calm. Like all forms of agate, it stimulates the mind. It encourages dreams and daydreams that shed light on our true needs and goals. Some crystal therapists say that blue lace agate relieves throat problems, as well as relaxing muscle tension of the head and neck.

HEALING ACTION
—

Meditate with blue agate at times of stress. Position on the third eye chakra to open the mind to its full potential. Place under the pillow for lucid and revealing dreams.

COMBINATIONS
—

Combine with sunstone if you are suffering from stress, overwork, or mental overload.

CARE
—

Agate rates 6.5–7 on the Mohs' scale. Do not inhale agate dust, which can cause silicosis. Clean in warm, soapy water with a soft cloth.

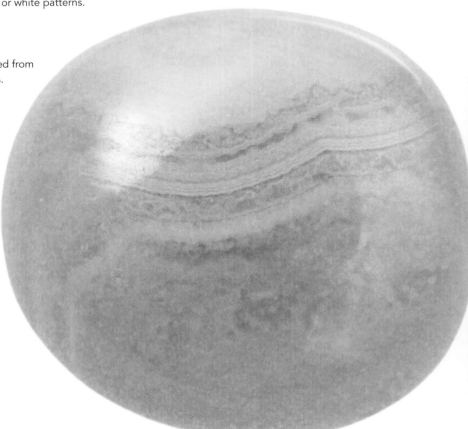

BLUE CALCITE

APPEARANCE
—

Usually a pale, dusty blue, this variety of calcite is translucent to opaque. Calcite forms pyramid-shaped crystals, grains, and crusts.

RARITY
—

The majority of blue calcite is sourced from Mexico and South Africa.

FORMATION
—

Pure calcite is colorless, but the presence of impurities can tint it a variety of colors. Limestone and chalk are largely composed of calcite, which formed the shells and skeletons of the tiny sea creatures that cemented to create these sedimentary rocks.

ATTRIBUTES
—

All varieties of calcite stimulate the intellect, but blue calcite encourages us to link our minds with our emotions. This may aid decision-making that comes from both the head and heart. It may help those engaged in creative studies or jobs, who benefit from making leaps of thought and vision. Blue calcite is said to enhance the body's circulation, although there is no scientific proof of this claim.

HEALING ACTION
—

Place at the throat chakra to give voice to your insights with self-confidence and conviction. Meditate with blue calcite if you are finding it hard to come to a decision when the head points a different way from the gut. Place blue calcite on your desk to aid problem-solving.

COMBINATIONS
—

If you are struggling with shyness or struggle with words when you are under pressure, place aquamarine and blue calcite at the throat chakra.

CARE
—

Calcite is brittle and soft, scoring just 3 on the Mohs' scale. It should not be handled excessively. Calcite is not soluble in pure water but is soluble in rainwater, which is slightly acidic. Do not use in gem elixirs, as it may react dangerously to stomach acid. If cleaning is necessary, dip in warm soapy water.

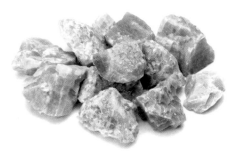

ANGELITE

APPEARANCE
—

This mineral is commonly medium-light to pale blue, but some crystals may be whitish. Flecks of red hematite are occasionally seen. When well-formed crystals are found, they are orthorhombic.

RARITY
—

This crystal is easily bought. First found in Peru in 1987, angelite is now sourced in Mexico, Egypt, Libya, UK, Germany, and Poland. Well-developed crystals are rare: the mineral is usually found as a mass.

FORMATION
—

Also known as blue anhydrite, angelite is composed of anhydrous (without water) calcium sulfate ($CaSO_4$). It is an evaporite mineral that forms as the result of gypsum losing all hydration.

ATTRIBUTES
—

As its name suggests, angelite facilitates contact with angels and spirit guides, while helping the birth of psychic gifts. It has a peaceful, soothing vibration, alleviating psychological pain, as well as tension headaches. Angelite helps the user to gain understanding of others and of the Universe itself. It encourages open communication, acceptance, and forgiveness.

HEALING ACTION
—

Placed or held at the throat chakra, angelite may have a powerful effect on communication. To aid the channeling of psychic gifts and the process of grieving, place at the third eye and crown chakras. While attempting communion with spirits, use an angelite pendulum.

COMBINATIONS
—

Use with celestite to boost its energy. To aid contact with the angelic realm, combine with seraphinite, clear quartz, and aragonite star clusters.

CARE
—

With a hardness of 3.5 on the Mohs' scale, angelite is easily damaged and must not be exposed to water. Do not use in gem elixirs as it is soluble in acids and may react dangerously to stomach acid. If necessary, wipe clean with a soft cloth.

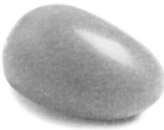

CELESTITE

APPEARANCE
—

Usually obtained as a blue crystal, celestite may also be colorless, white, yellow, or red. The transparent crystals are usually pyramidal or granular, but geodes and plates are found. Celestite may also be called celestine.

RARITY
—

This crystal is readily available as small pieces, tumbled stones, and clusters, but may be expensive. It is found in small quantities in Libya, Egypt, Madagascar, Peru, Mexico, UK, and Poland.

FORMATION
—

Composed of strontium sulfate ($SrSO_4$), celestite is often found in sedimentary rocks, with angelite and gypsum commonly nearby.

ATTRIBUTES
—

A sister stone to angelite, celestite (from the Latin *coelestis*, meaning "heavenly") also aids contact with the spiritual realm, while encouraging clairvoyance, dream recall, and artistic abilities. Its high, uplifting vibration heals the aura, promotes mental and emotional balance, disperses worries, and encourages peaceful communication. Some crystal therapists say it helps with conditions that affect the nerves, such as neuralgia.

HEALING ACTION
—

Placed or held at the throat chakra, celestite promotes communication. When placed on the crown chakra, celestite allows access to the higher chakras, particularly the soul star, to encourage psychic hearing, clairvoyance, and intuition. Leave a celestite cluster in your healing room or bedroom to aid both mental clarity and to encourage calm and positivity.

COMBINATIONS
—

Combine with other high-vibration crystals, such as blue obsidian (to stimulate intuition) and merlinite (to attract powerful magic).

CARE
—

Celestite scores only 3–3.5 on the Mohs' scale. To prevent loss of color, do not place in direct sunlight. Do not place in water, which may cause disintegration. If necessary, wipe clean with a soft cloth.

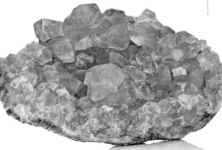

BLUE AVENTURINE

APPEARANCE
—

Translucent to opaque, aventurine is a form of quartz that sparkles and glitters. This glittering effect is known to mineralogists as aventurescence, from the Italian words meaning "by chance."

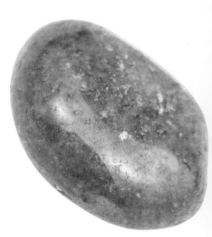

RARITY
—

Blue aventurine is sourced from India, Brazil, Tanzania, Russia, and Spain. It may be bought as tumbled stones, cabochons, and carvings.

FORMATION
—

Aventurine is a metamorphic rock composed of quartz (silicon dioxide) with inclusions of other minerals. Blue aventurine contains flakes of copper compounds, which also give its blue shade.

ATTRIBUTES
—

Blue aventurine helps us to be our best self. Morally, it encourages us to listen to the promptings of our inner angel. At work, it helps us to find inspiration and to see fresh ways around old obstacles. Socially, this rock encourages us to be extrovert, kind, and generous. Some crystal therapists say that blue aventurine benefits skin problems, although there is no scientific proof of this claim.

HEALING ACTION
—

If you are shy, nervous, or prickly in social situations, wear blue aventurine jewelry. When you are faced with a moral dilemma, meditate with blue aventurine to find the kind, decent, and generous way forward. If you are in need of creative inspiration, place this rock in the creativity area of the home, in the middle right if you enter by the front door.

COMBINATIONS
—

To escape shyness and build social confidence, team with ruby.

CARE
—

Aventurine has a hardness of around 6.5 on the Mohs' scale. Abundant inclusions can lower its hardness further. Do not inhale dust from aventurine, which can cause silicosis. Do not use in gem elixirs. Clean in warm, soapy water with a soft cloth.

BLUE APATITE

APPEARANCE
—

Crystals sold as blue apatite are often fluorapatite, a common member of the apatite group. Transparent to opaque, this variety of apatite grows as chunks and hexagonal prisms.

RARITY
—

Gem- or collector-quality blue apatite crystals are often sourced from Brazil, Russia, Madagascar, and the United States. Opaque crystals take a lower price.

FORMATION
—

Apatite is a calcium fluorophosphate. Its most important deposits are in sedimentary rocks formed in marine environments.

ATTRIBUTES
—

This shade of apatite encourages communication. It gives self-confidence during spoken and sung performances, as well as social and professional interaction. Blue apatite also frees us to speak from our hearts, with both honesty and kindness. Some believe that apatite improves problems of the throat and neck.

HEALING ACTION
—

If you work in a job where communication is key, from sales to teaching, place blue apatite in your office. If you feel there is something that must be spoken, yet you cannot find the words to say it, meditate with blue apatite placed on the floor before you.

COMBINATIONS
—

If you feel anxious in social situations, combine with confidence-boosting ruby or red beryl. If you are torn between speaking out and staying quiet, meditate with blue apatite and clear-sighted obsidian.

CARE
—

Blue apatite scores just 5 on the Mohs' scale, so it should be treated with care. Apatite is toxic so do not use in gem elixirs and wash your hands after handling. Do not immerse in water. If necessary, wipe clean with a damp cloth.

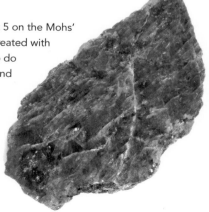

BLUE TOPAZ

APPEARANCE
—

Natural blue topaz crystals are usually a pale forget-me-not shade, but an artificially colored stone may be deeper blue. Well-formed crystals are in the shape of prisms that end in pyramids.

RARITY
—

Natural blue topaz is rare, but most gems on the market are colorless topaz that has been irradiated and heated. Blue is the most popular shade of topaz for jewelry, with dark blues often called London blue, and cornflower blues called Swiss blue. Natural blue topaz usually comes from Nigeria, Sri Lanka, or Brazil.

FORMATION
—

Topaz is a neosilicate mineral that forms in silicon-rich igneous rocks, particularly granite and rhyolite. When blue crystals form naturally, it is due to the presence of impurities such as iron and chromium.

ATTRIBUTES
—

Blue topaz enhances meditation. This is an ideal crystal for encouraging the mind to still, for filtering out unwanted thoughts, and for focusing on higher truths. Some crystal therapists say that blue topaz helps with stress-induced headaches.

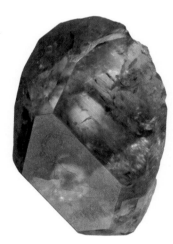

HEALING ACTION
—

If you find it difficult to relax your body and calm your mind during meditation, use blue topaz. If you are plagued by stress-related insomnia, place blue topaz by the bedside. Wear blue topaz jewelry to focus your mind on what truly matters in your life.

COMBINATIONS
—

To calm and open the mind, hold blue topaz and blue lace agate in either hand during meditation.

CARE
—

Clean blue topaz in warm, soapy water with a soft cloth. Do not inhale topaz dust. Although topaz scores 8 on the Mohs' scale, making it very hard, its crystals have a weakness in their atomic bonding along a certain plane, giving it a tendency to break along this plane if struck with enough force.

BLUE ZIRCON

APPEARANCE
—

Zircon specimens range from gem-quality transparent crystals to opaque. Zircon forms as plates, prisms, or chunks. In addition to pale blue, zircons may be golden-brown, colorless, yellow, red, or green.

RARITY
—

Many blue zircons on the market are brown zircons that have been heat-treated. Natural blue zircons are mined in Cambodia.

FORMATION
—

Often found in granite, zircon forms in silicon-rich magma. It is composed of zirconium, silicon, and oxygen.

ATTRIBUTES
—

Blue zircon helps us to resolve conflict, both interpersonal and internal. It bolsters our communication when dealing with family or workplace conflict. It also helps us to sift through our own conflicting desires, weighing and choosing judiciously. It is said to boost the immune system, particularly when jetlagged.

HEALING ACTION
—

Meditate with blue zircon if you are faced with a quandary you cannot resolve. To mitigate family discord, place this crystal in the family area of the home, which is midway along the left side.

COMBINATIONS
—

To aid the resolution of workplace conflicts, work with blue zircon and calming variscite.

CARE
—

Zircon scores 7.5 on the Mohs' scale, but it can chip along faceted edges. Do not use in gem elixirs, as zirconium may be toxic and it may react dangerously with stomach acid. Clean only in warm water with a mild soap.

LARIMAR

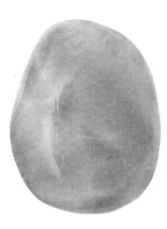

APPEARANCE
—

Larimar is a blue, turquoise, or purple variety of the mineral pectolite. The translucent to opaque crystals are found in a variety of forms, from radiating fibers to spheres, plates, and chunks.

RARITY
—

Larimar is rare, found only in the Dominican Republic. Jewelry inlaid with larimar is a local specialty. Jewelry pieces, tumbled stones, and crystals are also available worldwide.

FORMATION
—

Larimar is formed in holes, known as vugs, in volcanic rocks. It is composed of sodium, calcium, copper, silicon, oxygen, and hydrogen. It is the copper content that creates the blue coloration.

ATTRIBUTES
—

Larimar facilitates energy flow through the body and between chakras. It removes the mental blocks that prevent us expressing ourselves emotionally and creatively. In the same way, it removes the blocks that stop us from reaching out to other realms. Larimar is believed to enhance the circulatory system, although there is no scientific proof of that claim.

HEALING ACTION
—

Meditate frequently with larimar to facilitate contact with angelic beings. Position larimar at the third eye—or place on your desk—to encourage creative expression. Place on any chakra that is blocked or sluggish.

COMBINATIONS
—

Use with a wand of blue kyanite during scrying. If attempting to contact a spirit guide, combine with tektite.

CARE
—

Scoring just 4.5–5 on the Mohs' scale, larimar can be brittle. Larimar will fade over time if exposed to heat and light. Wipe clean with a damp, soapy cloth, then rinse thoroughly. Do not use in gem elixirs. Do not inhale larimar dust.

BLUE SAPPHIRE

APPEARANCE
—

Sapphire is the name for any gem-quality corundum crystal that is not red, with those crystals named "rubies." A precious stone of great beauty, a blue sapphire is vividly colored. When polished, sapphires are transparent, but they are otherwise cloudy.

RARITY
—

Blue sapphire is easily obtained as an uncut stone, but is expensive. Sapphires are mined in Myanmar, Thailand, India, Sri Lanka, Kenya, Madagascar, the Czech Republic, Brazil, Canada, and Australia. High-quality faceted sapphires are valuable.

FORMATION
—

Sapphires are a variety of the mineral corundum, an aluminum oxide. Corundum forms deep underground under intense heat and pressure. The blue coloration is caused by trace amounts of iron and titanium.

ATTRIBUTES
—

All sapphires are wisdom stones, but blue sapphires—in common with other blue crystals and stones—are particularly useful for encouraging psychic knowledge and spiritual truth. Blue sapphire encourages the user to stay on the right spiritual path, works against negative energy, and encourages self-expression. Blue sapphire is said to regulate the action of the body's glands.

HEALING ACTION
—

The throat chakra is the right position for encouraging self-expression. When placed or held on the third eye chakra, blue sapphire unlocks psychic abilities, enhances learning, and helps to heal wounds from past lives. Place under the pillow to stimulate lucid dreaming. Wearing sapphire jewelry can help mild depression and dispel anxiety.

COMBINATIONS
—

To let go of negativity, combine with citrine, ruby, or amber. To help with recognizing the truth, use alongside azurite and amazonite.

CARE
—

Sapphire scores 9 on the Mohs' scale, so is very durable. Clean with warm soapy water and a soft cloth. However, cavity-filled, fracture-filled, or dyed gems should be cleaned only with a damp cloth. Do not use them in gem elixirs.

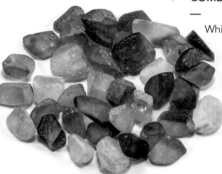

BENITOITE

APPEARANCE
—

This deep-blue, transparent gemstone is found as grains and dipyramids, or two pyramids symmetrically placed base-to-base. It fluoresces blue under ultraviolet light.

RARITY
—

Gem-quality benitoite is sourced only from California, but smaller, cloudier crystals are also found in Arkansas and Japan. This mineral is named for the place where it was first found, in 1909, near the headwaters of the San Benito River, in California. Most specimens are small, with large crystals exceptionally rare and expensive.

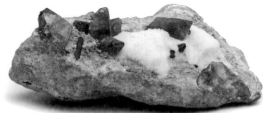

FORMATION
—

Benitoite is composed of atoms of barium, titanium, silicon, and oxygen. It forms in veins and dikes in serpentinite rock, along with other rare minerals.

ATTRIBUTES
—

An extremely high-energy crystal, benitoite is said to expand consciousness. It facilitates clairvoyance and clairsentience. For those with the gift, it is a guide through astral travel and shamanic journeying. It also invigorates the body after intense periods of overwork or exhaustion.

HEALING ACTION
—

Benitoite unlocks the door to the higher chakras, if the lower chakras are stimulated by its powerful vibrations first. Use benitoite to facilitate entering a deep and enlightening meditative state. Place on the table while scrying or channeling.

COMBINATIONS
—

While working with benitoite, keep a protective jet talisman nearby.

CARE
—

Although it looks like sapphire, benitoite is much softer, scoring just 6–6.5 on the Mohs' scale. Store in a soft bag, away from harder minerals and metals. Clean in warm, soapy water with a soft cloth.

BLUE KYANITE

APPEARANCE
—
Kyanite takes its name from the ancient Greek *cyanos*, meaning "dark blue." Kyanite forms columnar, striated crystals and ranges from transparent to opaque.

RARITY
—
Kyanite is a common mineral worldwide. When transparent and high-quality, kyanite is priced as a semiprecious gemstone.

FORMATION
—
Kyanite contains the elements aluminum, silicon, and oxygen. Its crystals grow during the metamorphism of fine-grained sedimentary rocks. It is commonly found in aluminum-rich gneiss and schist, including the Manhattan schist that underlies New York City.

ATTRIBUTES
—
Crystals of kyanite allow us to listen to our intuition and to understand our own truths, as well as those of others. This is a mineral that encourages open and honest communication, while freeing the speaker of resentment and antagonism. It is said to benefit the throat and mouth, easing sore throats and toothache, although there is no scientific proof of that claim.

HEALING ACTION
—
Kyanite wands are useful for showing the way to truth and honesty. Use a wand in meditation, scrying, or divination. Position a kyanite crystal of any shape near your pillow for healing and revelatory dreaming. Wear kyanite close to the body during public speaking, teaching, or truth-telling.

COMBINATIONS
—
If you are nervous about a presentation, performance, or speech, meditate with—or carry—crystals of kyanite and rhodochrosite, which is known for its calming properties.

CARE
—
Kyanite crystals are much stronger (6.5–7 on the Mohs' scale) if pressed or banged at right angles to their direction of growth, than if they are struck parallel to their striations (4.5–5 on the Mohs' scale). Clean with warm, soapy water and a soft cloth. Do not soak. Do not use in gem elixirs.

CAVANSITE

APPEARANCE
—
This deep-blue mineral forms crystal aggregates, or clusters, up to 1 in (2.5 cm) across. Resembling pompoms or balls, the aggregates are composed of radiating, needle-shaped crystals that usually cannot be distinguished individually by the naked eye. The crystals are transparent.

RARITY
—
Usually sourced from India, cavansite is a rare mineral. It is valued as a collector's item by mineral collectors. Cavansite aggregates are usually sold attached to their matrix.

FORMATION
—
Cavansite is named for its principal ingredients: calcium, vanadium, and silicon. It is found in extrusive igneous rocks such as basalt and andesite.

ATTRIBUTES
—
This is a crystal that encourages us to express ourselves. It enables us to speak our truths both kindly and wisely. It also facilitates creative expression, whether through painting, dance, or any other medium. Some crystal healers claim that cavansite helps problems of the ear, nose, and throat.

HEALING ACTION
—
Meditate with cavansite to focus on spiritual truths and to find the strength to move toward them. When engaged in a creative activity, place cavansite nearby. Display this mineral in the creativity area of the home, which is on the right side if you enter by the front door.

COMBINATIONS
—
Build a grid to enhance creativity using cavansite, thulite, kunzite, and bloodstone.

CARE
—
Cavansite is a brittle mineral, scoring just 3–4 on the Mohs' scale. Do not use in gem elixirs as it contains traces of copper. Do not inhale cavansite dust. Cleaning this delicate mineral should be avoided if possible, but it can be dipped in lukewarm water.

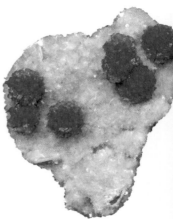

PENTAGONITE

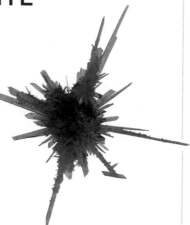

APPEARANCE
—

Pentagonite is a dimorph of cavansite, which means it has the same chemical formula but its crystals have a different structure. While cavansite forms pompoms, pentagonite clusters are spikier, with individual, bladed crystals visible to the eye.

RARITY
—

A sought-after collector's item, pentagonite is even rarer than cavansite. Be aware that cavansite may be marketed as pentagonite to justify a higher price.

FORMATION
—

Like cavansite, pentagonite forms in extrusive igneous rocks. It is composed of the same elements in the same relative quantities, but grows at a slightly different temperature. It is vanadium that gives the deep-blue shade of both dimorphs.

ATTRIBUTES
—

While cavansite facilitates self-expression, the different form of pentagonite acts as an emotional antenna. It allows us to feel the needs and pain of others, so must be used with strength and compassion. It also facilitates connection with spirits and angelic beings. Some say that pentagonite eases back and neck pain.

HEALING ACTION
—

If attempting contact with spirits, work closely with pentagonite. If you feel a lack of connection with the needs of a teenager, parent, or friend, meditate with pentagonite to open your heart to them.

COMBINATIONS
—

Pentagonite and cobaltoan calcite form a powerful empathic combination.

CARE
—

Like cavansite, pentagonite scores just 3–4 on the Mohs' scale, but its slender, bladed crystals can be even more easily snapped. Do not use in gem elixirs as it contains traces of copper. Do not inhale pentagonite dust. Avoid cleaning if possible, but pentagonite can be dipped in lukewarm water.

SHATTUCKITE

APPEARANCE
—

Ranging from dark blue to turquoise, shattuckite forms both as spherical masses and needle-like crystals. It is translucent to opaque.

RARITY
—

This relatively rare mineral is sometimes used as a gemstone. It is often found mixed with quartz. In addition to the United States, shattuckite is sourced from the Democratic Republic of the Congo, Namibia, Chile, and Australia.

FORMATION
—

This copper silicate hydroxide often forms in copper mines as copper ores are slowly oxidized. It is named after the Shattuck Mine of Arizona, where it was first described in 1915.

ATTRIBUTES
—

Shattuckite helps with developing psychic abilities, being particularly useful for channeling. This highly protective crystal also guards against dark entities and helps us to heal from the wounds inflicted during past lives. Some healers say that shattuckite helps ailments such as tonsilitis.

HEALING ACTION
—

Place at the third eye to encourage nascent psychic abilities. Keep this crystal close during channeling. Position it in the knowledge and self-cultivation corner of the home, which is to the left after entering by the front door.

COMBINATIONS
—

Combine with angelite and calligraphy stone during automatic writing.

CARE
—

Shattuckite contains copper and silicon, so do not ingest, do not use in gem elixirs, and do not breathe in its dust. It is soluble in acids, so may also react dangerously with stomach acid. It scores 3.5 on the Mohs' scale, so avoid knocks and scratches. Clean in warm, soapy water with a soft cloth.

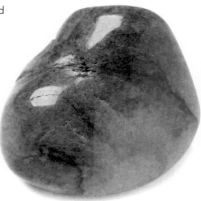

PIETERSITE

APPEARANCE

—

Featuring swirling blues, along with occasional reds, browns, and golds, pietersite may display chatoyancy (a cat's-eye effect). It is sometimes known as "tempest stone" as its swirling colors resemble stormy skies.

RARITY

—

Pietersite was identified by Sid Pieters in Namibia, in 1962, then named in his honor. Today, it is also sourced from China. When used as a gemstone, pietersite is usually cut into a cabochon. Note that jewelers who grind and cut pietersite must be aware that it contains crocidolite, a form of asbestos.

FORMATION

—

Pietersite is formed of chalcedony (a combination of the silica minerals quartz and moganite), with embedded fibers of other minerals, including crocidolite, known as blue asbestos. It is these fibers that create the cat's-eye effect as they reflect the light.

ATTRIBUTES

—

Just as tempests wreak great change, so too does the well-named tempest stone. Pietersite allows us to bring about much-needed change in our lives, freeing ourselves from habits, ingrained behaviors, and self-imposed rules. After the transformative change, pietersite brings peace and tranquility.

HEALING ACTION

—

This stone should be used under the direction of a qualified crystal therapist.

COMBINATIONS

—

Under the care of a qualified crystal therapist, pietersite may be combined with aegirine to help us break free from bad habits, addictions, or compulsions.

CARE

—

Keep pietersite away from children and animals. Pietersite contains silicon and crocidolite, or blue asbestos. Asbestos fibers cause lung cancer and asbestosis. Cut and finished cabochons of pietersite are considered low risk to display. However, do not ingest, do not use in gem elixirs, and do not breathe in pietersite dust if it shatters. Handle infrequently and wash hands afterward. Pietersite scores 6–7 on the Mohs' scale. Clean in warm, soapy water with a soft cloth.

LAPIS LAZULI

APPEARANCE

—

A rock rather than a mineral, lapis lazuli is an intense blue, flecked with white calcite or golden pyrite.

RARITY

—

Lapis lazuli is commonly available but expensive, particularly for top-quality stones. The foremost mines are in Afghanistan and Pakistan, but the rock is also sourced in Russia, Mongolia, Italy, Chile, the United States, and Canada.

FORMATION

—

Lapis lazuli is a metamorphic rock that contains large quantities of the mineral lazurite, with smaller quantities of calcite, pyrite, and sodalite, among other minerals.

ATTRIBUTES

—

As with all blue minerals and stones, lapis lazuli facilitates contact with the spirit world, enhances psychic abilities, and benefits dream work. In addition, this is a strongly protective stone that blocks psychic attack and helps the user to withstand emotional bondage. It works against repression, depression, and purposelessness, while working toward enlightenment and clarity. Lapis lazuli is also said to clear headaches caused by eyestrain and overwork.

HEALING ACTION

—

Wear or place at the throat chakra to encourage honesty and openness in communication. Wear or place at the third eye chakra to enhance psychic abilities, stimulate the mind, encourage positivity, and overcome insomnia. Wear as earrings or pendants for protection, but to avoid overstimulation do so only for short periods at first.

COMBINATIONS

—

To aid the journey to enlightenment, use with golden topaz. For clarity of thought, combine with blue lace agate or azurite.

CARE

—

Depending on its exact composition, lapis lazuli scores 5–6 on the Mohs' scale. If cleaning is necessary, briefly dip in room-temperature water with a very mild soap. Use a soft cloth to avoid scratching. Do not use in gem elixirs, as some lapis lazuli inclusions are toxic and may react dangerously with stomach acid.

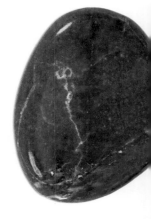

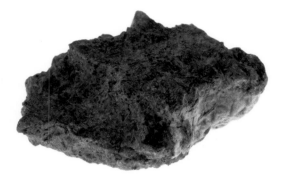

DUMORTIERITE

APPEARANCE
—

Usually blue, dumortierite is found as masses, needles, fibers, and columns. Crystals are transparent to translucent.

RARITY
—

Dumortierite is commonly sourced from France, Madagascar, Brazil, and the United States. Crystals large enough to be faceted are rare, but cabochons are easily bought in jewelry. Many specimens are impregnated with quartz.

FORMATION
—

This aluminum-boron silicate forms in aluminum-rich metamorphic rocks and in veins in boron-rich igneous rocks.

ATTRIBUTES
—

Dumortierite encourages us to be calm when under stress, and patient in the face of conflict. It allows us to not only see but to fully feel the natural order of the Universe, so that we can be at peace. Dumortierite is said to help problems of the neck and throat, although there is no scientific proof of this claim.

HEALING ACTION
—

Meditate with dumortierite to feel enlightened, peaceful, and accepting. Place at the throat chakra to encourage calm and forgiving communication. To work against stress and anxiety, wear as jewelry.

COMBINATIONS
—

If you are suffering from stress or burnout, meditate regularly with dumortierite and lepidolite.

CARE
—

Dumortierite scores 7–8 on the Mohs' scale. Since it contains silicon, do not breathe its dust. Clean in warm, soapy water with a soft cloth.

AZURITE

APPEARANCE
—

This deep-blue mineral forms plates, stalactites, prisms, and masses. It is transparent to translucent.

RARITY
—

Azurite is popular among mineral collectors, but is rarely found in jewelry due to its softness and instability (see "Care"). Sources include Namibia, Australia, Chile, and the United States.

FORMATION
—

This copper carbonate forms after carbon-dioxide-laden groundwater reacts with copper ores, dissolving some of the copper. The copper-rich water flows into fractures or pores, where precipitation slowly forms crystals of azurite.

ATTRIBUTES
—

Azurite is a crystal that facilitates scrying and channeling. It enhances telepathy and clairvoyance. On a more practical level, it aids memory and reasoning. Some crystal practitioners claim that azurite helps with stress-induced headaches.

HEALING ACTION
—

See "Care" for advice on handling. Position on the table during scrying and channeling. Meditate with azurite to allow your mind to travel freely.

COMBINATIONS
—

Azurite is particularly beneficial when scrying in smoky quartz.

CARE
—

Keep azurite away from children and pets. Avoid excessive handling and wash hands after use, particularly if a specimen is raw. Azurite scores just 3.5–4 on the Mohs' scale. It contains copper and may react dangerously with stomach acid, so do not use it in gem elixirs, do not ingest, and do not inhale its dust. Azurite lightens in color over time, as its surface weathers into malachite (see page 98). Do not expose to heat or acid. To preserve azurite's color, store in a dark, sealed box. If cleaning is necessary, dip in cold water.

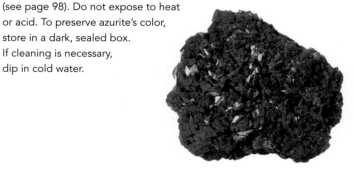

SODALITE

APPEARANCE
—

Usually royal blue, sodalite may occasionally be sourced in violet, green, or yellow. Although individual crystals are translucent, it is commonly found as opaque masses in which white veins can be seen. It fluoresces in ultraviolet light.

RARITY
—

Sodalite is a fairly rare rock-forming mineral. Royal blue sodalite is often used as cabochons and inlays in jewelry. Sources of good-quality sodalite include Canada and the United States.

FORMATION
—

Composed of sodium, aluminum, silicon, oxygen, and chlorine, sodalite forms in magma that is rich in sodium.

ATTRIBUTES
—

Sodalite is a crystal that directs us to the truth. It helps us to perceive practical, financial, emotional, and spiritual truths. It allows us to speak those truths without fear. It helps us to see the meanings and motivations of others clearly. Some crystal healers say that sodalite helps to balance the metabolism.

HEALING ACTION
—

Place on the throat chakra to allow honest and courageous speech. Meditate with sodalite if you are in need of emotional or spiritual direction. Place in the knowledge corner of the home, which is to the left if you enter by the front door.

COMBINATIONS
—

Combine wisdom with truth-telling by working with both sodalite and black onyx.

CARE
—

Sodalite scores 5.5–6 on the Mohs' scale, so is better suited to earrings and pendants than to frequently knocked rings and bracelets. Do not soak this crystal, as this could splinter a crack. Do not use in gem elixirs as it is soluble in acids and may react dangerously with stomach acid. Wipe clean with a damp, soft cloth.

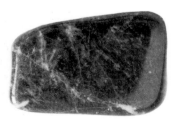

BLUE OBSIDIAN

APPEARANCE
—

This variety of the volcanic glass is deep blue, translucent, and frequently bought as jagged-edged pieces.

RARITY
—

Much blue obsidian bought online or in stores is artificially made in China. Natural stones, which are a little more expensive, may be from Morocco or Greece.

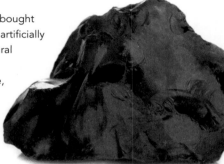

FORMATION
—

Obsidian forms when lava rich in lighter elements—such as silicon, oxygen, aluminum, sodium, and potassium—cools quickly, giving little time for crystal growth. This accounts for obsidian's glass-like texture.

ATTRIBUTES
—

Blue obsidian encourages acuity in mental processes and communication. Ancient peoples used obsidian for cutting tools and weapons. To guard against blue obsidian encouraging harshness or criticism, it should be used with care and self-knowledge. Blue obsidian is said to aid problems of the eyes, although there is no scientific proof of this claim.

HEALING ACTION
—

Place on the third eye chakra for clearness of thought and insightful reasoning. Place on the throat for the strength to speak long-withheld thoughts and needs. A blue obsidian paperweight on a desk will encourage clear-thinking, helping to cure tedious or confusing tasks.

COMBINATIONS
—

When teamed with chrysocolla, blue obsidian can encourage open communication without bitterness or destructivity. Combine with moonstone for insight hand in hand with empathy and circumspection.

CARE
—

All varieties of obsidian are brittle and easy to fracture. It scores 5–6 on the Mohs' scale. Do not breathe in dust, which can cause silicosis. Clean in lukewarm, soapy water with a soft cloth.

PURPLE AND VIOLET

These crystals resonate with the crown chakra, the seat of our spirituality, and the third eye, home to intuition. They prevent us from being overly concerned by the physical world, a concern that may manifest itself in materialism, selfishness, and obsessive or controlling behavior. Purple and violet crystals encourage us to look both deep inside ourselves and far beyond ourselves.

Purple has been associated with kings, judges, and priests for millennia. Tyrian purple dye—in ancient times obtained from *Muricidae* sea snails in the region of today's Lebanon—could be afforded only by the wealthy. During the 1960s, the color experienced a renaissance when it was adopted by the counterculture, as suggested by the band Deep Purple and Jimi Hendrix's "Purple Haze." Although these associations may seem opposing, purple crystals combine both worlds. They help us to be our best selves, focusing on the ideal qualities of kings, judges, and priests: wisdom, morality, and spirituality. They also encourage us to open our eyes, hearts, and spirits to other worlds, other experiences, and other lives.

TANZANITE

APPEARANCE
—

This variety of the mineral zoisite is blue to violet. Depending on its heat treatment, it may be trichroic or dichroic. Untreated tanzanite is trichroic, meaning that the crystal refracts and absorbs light so that an entire spectrum of shades can be seen from different angles and in different lights. After heating, tanzanite becomes dichroic, ranging from violet to blue.

RARITY
—

Mined only from a small region of Tanzania, tanzanite is rare and priced accordingly. The gem was named by Tiffany & Co. in 1968.

FORMATION
—

Tanzanite is found in metamorphic rocks or igneous rocks that formed at high temperature and pressure deep underground. It contains atoms of silicon, aluminum, calcium, oxygen, and hydrogen, with small amounts of vanadium giving its vibrant shade. Rough tanzanite may appear reddish-brown to clear, but is heat-treated to bring out the blue violet of the gem.

ATTRIBUTES
—

Tanzanite opens the conscious mind to the subconscious, allowing us to search our own motivations, needs, and desires. It also facilitates journeys beyond the physical world, into the angelic realm and our own past lives. Crystal therapists use tanzanite to work with headaches and ailments of the throat.

HEALING ACTION
—

Place on the crown chakra to free yourself from materialism and open your mind to truer and more long-lasting goals. Place on é&&éthe throat chakra to give expression to your own creativity. Wear tanzanite jewelry to form a constant bridge between the physical and metaphysical worlds.

COMBINATIONS
—

Work with tanzanite and variscite if your goal is to open your mind and heart to past lives.

CARE
—

Protect your tanzanite from blows and rough treatment, as it scores just 6.5 on the Mohs' scale. Clean only with warm, soapy water and a soft cloth.

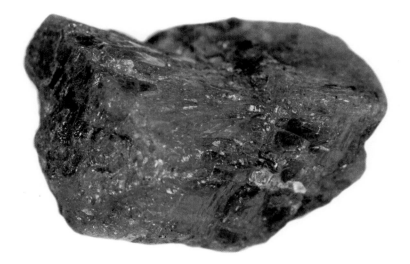

CHAROITE

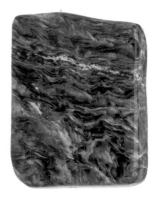

APPEARANCE
—

Charoite exhibits swirls of lilac to purple. It is fibrous in texture, which may create a chatoyant (or cat's-eye) effect. While individual crystals are translucent, charoite is found mixed with other minerals as opaque masses.

RARITY
—

A rare mineral, charoite is found only around the Chara River in eastern Siberia, Russia. The cabochons and beads sold as charoite are actually not pure charoite but a rock with charoite as its dominant mineral.

FORMATION
—

Charoite is a complex silicate mineral containing elements including potassium, sodium, calcium, barium, and strontium. Charoite forms in limestone that meets nepheline- and aegirine-rich syenite rock, a rare occurrence that accounts for the mineral's limited availability.

ATTRIBUTES
—

Charoite enhances intuition and perception. It helps us to integrate those perceptions with our mental and emotional processes. Charoite works against obsessions and controlling behaviors, while helping us to see why these compulsions have become ingrained. Crystal therapists say that charoite helps with problems of the eyes.

HEALING ACTION
—

To help with compulsions and addictive behavior, place on the crown chakra or wear as jewelry. Meditate with charoite to gain a fresh insight on ongoing problems. Hold over any chakra that feels blocked and sluggish to open and reenergize.

COMBINATIONS
—

A combination of charoite and pink lepidolite may help with obsessive compulsions, such as hoarding or handwashing, if you are also receiving help and advice from trained therapists.

CARE
—

Scoring just 5–6 on the Mohs' scale, charoite should be protected from bangs and scratches. Clean with warm, soapy water and a soft cloth. Do not breathe in its dust.

AMETHYST

APPEARANCE
—

Amethyst is a variety of the mineral quartz that ranges from pale lavender to deep purple. It grows as six-sided prisms ending in six-sided pyramids. It is also often found as geodes, which are clusters of small crystals that grow within hollow spherical rocks.

RARITY
—

Prior to the 1700s, amethyst was considered a precious stone. Today, after the discovery of numerous deposits in Brazil, South Korea, the United States, and elsewhere, it is priced as a semiprecious stone.

FORMATION
—

Clear quartz is made purely of silicon and oxygen, but amethyst is tinted by natural irradiation and impurities of iron and other transition metals. Geodes form when cavities in volcanic rock are filled with hydrothermal fluid rich in silicon and oxygen.

ATTRIBUTES
—

Like all varieties of quartz, amethyst is an amplifier of energy. However, this variety is also soothing and balancing. It calms overactive, overstressed, and overworked minds. It eases the heart at times of grief and loss. Some crystal therapists claim that amethyst can help rejuvenate the body during convalescence.

HEALING ACTION
—

To ease a stressed or busy mind, place at the crown chakra. To relieve stress or to recover from loss, wear as a pendant, earrings, or ring. Sleep with an amethyst geode by the bed to help with insomnia, night waking, and troubled dreams.

COMBINATIONS
—

To relieve insomnia, meditate with amethyst and howlite before bed. For fortitude and calm at times of stress, combine with black onyx.

CARE
—

Amethyst scores 7 on the Mohs' scale, which makes it suitable for regular wear as jewelry. However, its color can fade if it is overexposed to light. Do not inhale amethyst dust, which can cause silicosis. Clean in warm, soapy water with a soft cloth.

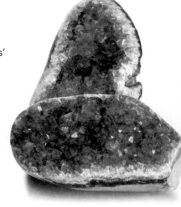

KÄMMERERITE

APPEARANCE
—
Ranging from purple to burgundy and cranberry, kämmererite is translucent to transparent. It is found as hexagonal crystals and crusts.

RARITY
—
Due to this mineral's extreme softness and tendency to separate into thin sheets, faceted kämmererite gemstones are very rare. A specimen is more easily bought as an encrusted rock. Turkey, India, Russia, and the United States are the main sources.

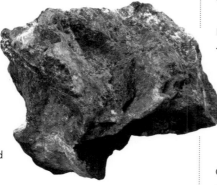

FORMATION
—
This variety of the mineral clinochlore is rich in chromium. It is found in metamorphic rocks and in hydrothermal replacement deposits.

ATTRIBUTES
—
Kämmererite helps us to enter deep meditative states. It allows the mind to travel beyond the bounds of the body, encouraging spiritual growth and heightened awareness. Crystal therapists say that kämmererite's intense vibration helps to release toxin build-up.

HEALING ACTION
—
Place kämmererite at the third eye and crown to activate the higher chakras. Hold kämmererite while attempting contact with angelic beings. Use this crystal during deep relaxation meditation.

COMBINATIONS
—
A powerful combination during deep meditation is kämmererite and blue lace agate.

CARE
—
With a score of just 2–2.5 on the Mohs' scale, kämmererite is too soft to wear in a ring or bracelet. It can be scratched by household dust, so do not wipe with a dry cloth. Avoid excessive handling. If cleaning is necessary, dip in warm, soapy water.

PURPLE SAPPHIRE

APPEARANCE
—
A gem-quality purple sapphire is transparent and may be periwinkle, delicate lilac, or vivid purple. Sapphire is the name for any gem-quality corundum crystal that is not red, with those crystals named "rubies." While sapphires are typically blue, those of other colors, known as "fancy" sapphires, do occur.

RARITY
—
Purple sapphires are rarer than blue sapphires, but usually take a lower price tag as they are not so sought after. Always buy any gem-quality stones from a reputable jeweler. A common source of purple sapphires is Sri Lanka.

FORMATION
—
Corundum forms deep underground under intense heat and pressure. Pure corundum is aluminum oxide, but traces of chromium, iron, and titanium tint it purple.

ATTRIBUTES
—
Sapphires are known as crystals of wisdom. Purple sapphires have particular resonance with spiritual wisdom. This is the wisdom that helps us to know what is truly important in life. Purple sapphires help to free us from materialism, obsessions, and emotional shortsightedness. These sapphires are said to improve the circulation, although there is no scientific proof of this claim.

HEALING ACTION
—
If personal evolution is your goal, meditate with purple sapphire regularly. Wear purple sapphire jewelry to surround yourself with wisdom, allowing yourself to hear wise voices and read wise books. Place purple sapphire in the knowledge corner of the home, which is to the immediate left if you enter by the front door.

COMBINATIONS
—
Crystals that can support the energies of purple sapphire in a quest for spiritual enlightenment are: clear quartz, clear fluorite, tektite, and tiger's eye.

CARE
—
Sapphires are exceptionally hard, scoring 9 on the Mohs' scale. Clean with warm, soapy water and a soft cloth. However, cavity-filled, fracture-filled, or dyed gems should be cleaned only with a damp cloth. Do not use them in gem elixirs.

SUGILITE

APPEARANCE
—

Purple to pink, sugilite is usually found as opaque masses. When well-formed crystals do occur, they are hexagonal and translucent.

RARITY
—

Sugilite is relatively rare, but can be found in Japan, India, Canada, South Africa, Italy, and Australia. Mineral-collectors may call this mineral lavulite, luvulite, or royal azel. Translucent sugilite is extremely rare.

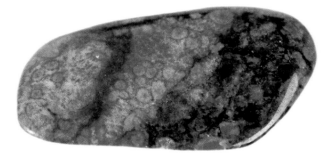

FORMATION
—

This complex mineral is composed of potassium, sodium, iron, aluminum, lithium, silicon, oxygen, and manganese. It forms in manganese deposits, granite, and syenite. It is manganese that bestows the rich purple shade.

ATTRIBUTES
—

Sugilite's warming energy opens the mind to love, allowing us to accept the reality that we are loved and deserve to be loved. It opens the chakras, allowing the flow of positive energy throughout the body. Crystal healers say that sugilite can ease headaches as well as muscle aches and pains.

HEALING ACTION
—

If you are looking for romantic love, place sugilite in the love corner of the home, which is at the back right if you enter by the front door. Wear sugilite jewelry as a constant reminder that you are loveable. Meditate with sugilite to feel suffused by warmth and positivity.

COMBINATIONS
—

If you are feeling unloved and unlovable, build a pink-to-purple grid with sugilite, pink lepidolite, and confidence-building thulite.

CARE
—

Sugilite scores 6–6.5 on the Mohs' scale, so is suitable for jewelry other than rings. Clean in warm, soapy water with a soft cloth.

STICHTITE

APPEARANCE
—

Ranging from pink through lilac to deep purple, stichtite is usually found as masses, but fibrous crystals do occur.

RARITY
—

Stichtite is found in around a dozen localities worldwide, including in Australia, South Africa, and Zimbabwe. It is not facetable, but can be bought as masses, cabochons, and jewelry inlays.

FORMATION
—

A chromium magnesium carbonate, stichtite forms when the minerals serpentine and chromite react with hot fluid.

ATTRIBUTES
—

Stichtite is the crystal of forgiveness. It helps us to overcome the anger and distrust of others. It helps us to forgive ourselves for mistakes and failings, then to gather the strength to be better. Some say that stichtite eases muscular and joint pains, but there is no scientific proof of this claim.

HEALING ACTION
—

If you cannot let go of anger toward those you feel have wronged you, meditate daily with stichtite. Wear stichtite jewelry to feel that, whatever mistakes you have made in the past, every day is a fresh opportunity to be your best self.

COMBINATIONS
—

If you are struggling with feelings of blame and censure toward your life partner, place stichtite and rose quartz in the marriage corner of the home, which is at the back right if you enter by the front door.

CARE
—

Scoring just 1.5–2 on the Mohs' scale, stichtite must be handled very carefully. It dissolves in acids, so should not be used in gem elixirs as it may react dangerously with stomach acid. Clean in warm, soapy water with a soft cloth.

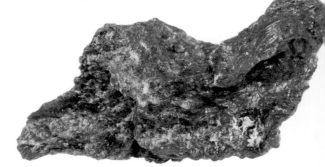

LILAC LEPIDOLITE

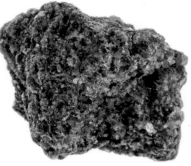

APPEARANCE
—

Gray-lilac lepidolite is an opaque to translucent crystal. It is often found as grains, plates, masses, scaly aggregates, and pseudohexagonal crystals.

RARITY
—

Lepidolite is often sourced from Madagascar, Canada, Brazil, Russia, Zimbabwe, or the United States.

FORMATION
—

Lepidolite grows in granite that is rich in lithium. It is the most abundant lithium-bearing mineral, making it a valuable ore. Traces of manganese cause its lilac-to-pink shades.

ATTRIBUTES
—

Lilac lepidolite clears and focuses the mind, allowing us to focus on what truly matters. When faced with a dilemma, this lepidolite helps us to see the way forward. It also helps to mitigate obsessive or irrational behavior. Lepidolite is said to ameliorate the symptoms of allergies, although there is no scientific proof of this claim.

HEALING ACTION
—

Place at the crown chakra to ease an obsessive desire to collect or hoard objects. Meditate with lepidolite when struggling with confusion or uncertainty. For a good night's sleep, without troubling dreams or stress-induced wake-ups, place lilac lepidolite in the bedroom.

COMBINATIONS
—

If you are plagued by an obsessive need to clean or tidy, combine lilac lepidolite with calming pink petalite and freeing lizardite.

CARE
—

Lepidolite is very soft, scoring just 2.5–3 on the Mohs' scale, so be careful with knocks and scratches. Avoid contact with chemicals, particularly acids, which will dissolve lepidolite. Do not immerse in water or use in gem elixirs. It may react dangerously with stomach acid. If necessary, wipe clean with a soft cloth.

IOLITE

APPEARANCE
—

Iolite is the transparent, gem-quality variety of the mineral cordierite. The name iolite comes from the ancient Greek for "violet." It ranges from lilac to blue to gray and appears to change shade when viewed from different angles.

RARITY
—

Although much softer than sapphire, iolite is often used as a less-expensive substitute for the precious gem. Iolite is found in Australia, Brazil, Canada, India, Madagascar, Myanmar, Namibia, Sri Lanka, Tanzania, and the United States.

FORMATION
—

A magnesium iron aluminum silicate, iolite forms as fine-grained sedimentary rocks are metamorphosed by great heat and pressure.

ATTRIBUTES
—

This crystal defuses conflict. Its effect can be felt in interpersonal conflicts as well as internal battles, between head and heart, reason and intuition, optimism and pessimism. Some crystal therapists say that iolite ease problems of the sinuses and respiratory system.

HEALING ACTION
—

For frequent familial conflict, place iolite in the dining room or family room, where its calming vibrations can soothe anger. When you are torn by two conflicting courses of action, meditate with iolite.

COMBINATIONS
—

For a grid that wards off anger and argument, team iolite with variscite, rhodonite, and aquamarine.

CARE
—

Iolite may react dangerously with stomach acid, so it should not be used in gem elixirs. Scoring 7–7.5 on the Mohs' scale, it is suitable for jewelry. Iolite can be cleaned in warm, soapy water with a soft cloth.

COLORLESS, WHITE, AND CREAM

When used mindfully, these powerful crystals can awaken the higher chakras, the soul star, stellar gateway, and universal mind. White and colorless crystals help us on our way in the journey toward enlightenment. On a more practical level, they engage the mind and eyes, both physically and metaphorically. These bright crystals act as beacons in the darkness, both protecting and comforting our spirits.

White is the color of purity and truth. It is also the color of surrender. Yet this is not a surrender of weakness but of strength—white crystals encourage us to open ourselves bravely to others and to the Universe. White and "colorless" crystals (and objects) reflect all colors equally, making them some of the most powerful crystals there are. They are often well teamed with black crystals, which absorb all colors and reflect none to the eyes. White and colorless crystals can be used as amplifiers of the energy of other crystals.

ATTRIBUTES
—

Diamond is a high-energy crystal that boosts positive feelings and sweeps away the negative. It boosts love and commitment, while driving out fear and doubt. It helps to heal pain and sadness. Crystal therapists say that diamond helps to balance the metabolism.

HEALING ACTION
—

Wear diamond jewelry to enhance feelings of love and bonding. Place at the higher chakras to drive away spiritual doubt and darkness. Place diamond beside the bed to awake feeling energized and optimistic.

COMBINATIONS
—

Place diamond at the heart of a loving grid, surrounded by pyrope, red beryl, thulite, and kunzite.

CARE
—

The hardest natural mineral, diamond scores 10 on the Mohs' scale. Clean with warm soapy water and a soft cloth.

DIAMOND

APPEARANCE
—

Pure diamond is colorless and transparent to translucent. Diamonds may also be yellow, brown, or gray, or, more rarely, any color of the rainbow, or black. Well-formed crystals are octahedral.

RARITY
—

Diamonds are the most common (and least expensive) of the precious stones. Diamonds are priced on their color, clarity, carat, and cut. High-priced diamonds should be bought only from a reputable jeweler.

FORMATION
—

Diamond is pure carbon. Most diamonds are between 1 and 3.5 billion years old. They formed deep in the earth's mantle under extreme heat and pressure, then were carried closer to the surface by volcanic eruptions.

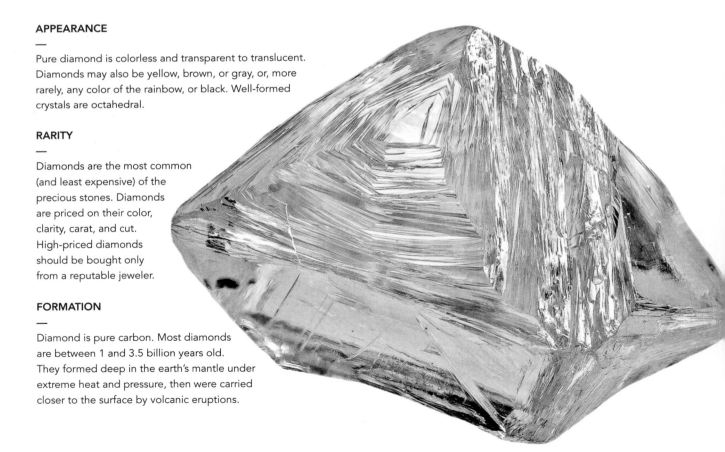

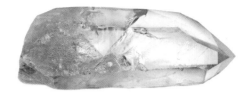

CLEAR QUARTZ

APPEARANCE
—

Pure quartz is colorless and transparent. Quartz crystals often grow as six-sided prisms ending in pointed pyramids. They may be found as single crystals, twinned crystals, or clusters. If a crystal is white and translucent to opaque, it is known as milky quartz. Azeztulite is the tradename for a milky quartz found in North Carolina.

RARITY
—

Quartz is common worldwide. More regularly shaped, transparent crystals take a higher price.

FORMATION
—

Pure quartz is made of silicon and oxygen atoms. Quartz is a common rock-forming mineral, found in felsic rocks such as granite. Milky quartz is caused by tiny bubbles of gas or liquid that were trapped during crystal formation.

ATTRIBUTES
—

Clear quartz is a powerful amplifier of energy. It heightens our awareness of this world and others, while attuning us to notice changes in our own physical and mental state. Quartz purifies, heals, and balances. Some crystal therapists say that it stimulates the immune system. Milky quartz is valuable for situations where a gentler energy is needed.

HEALING ACTION
—

Place at the higher chakras to open the mind to endless possibilities and to reach for true enlightenment. When working with quartz wands, turn their points toward yourself to draw energy inward. Turn wands outward to direct the way to new possibilities. Clear quartz is an ideal crystal for scrying.

COMBINATIONS
—

Combine clear quartz with any other crystals in grids or during meditation to amplify their power.

CARE
—

Quartz is named for the Germanic word for "hard." It scores 7 on the Mohs' scale. Do not inhale quartz dust as it contains silicon, which can cause silicosis. Clean in warm, soapy water with a soft cloth.

HEULANDITE

APPEARANCE
—

Usually colorless or white, heulandite may also be tinted green, yellow, or pink. Crystals are rhombic prisms, barrel-shaped, or plate-like. Heulandite is transparent to translucent.

RARITY
—

Good-quality heulandite is sourced from Iceland, Denmark, India, and the United States. Heulandite is one of the more common members of the zeolite group of minerals. It can be bought from specialist mineral suppliers.

FORMATION
—

Heulandite is a complex hydrous calcium aluminum silicate. Heulandite most commonly forms in cavities within the igneous rock basalt.

ATTRIBUTES
—

A high-vibration crystal, heulandite encourages spiritual and emotional growth. It helps us to be better people and to offer more love, compassion, and empathy to others. It is said to reduce bloating and dispel toxins, although there is no scientific proof of this claim.

HEALING ACTION
—

Place at any chakra that is blocked or sluggish. Meditate with heulandite to open your mind and spirit to others and to other possibilities. Place heulandite in the knowledge and self-cultivation corner of the home, which is to the left if you enter by the front door.

COMBINATIONS
—

Heulandite and angelite make a powerful combination for embarking on spiritual journeys.

CARE
—

Scoring just 3–4 on the Mohs' scale, heulandite should be protected from knocks and scratches. Do not use in gem elixirs and do not breathe in its dust. Clean very gently in warm soapy water.

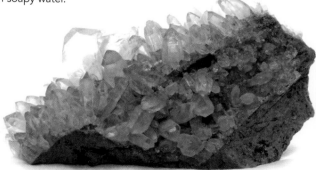

CLEAR FLUORITE

APPEARANCE
—

A transparent to translucent mineral, fluorite grows in well-defined cubes and octahedrons, as well as more haphazard chunks, columns, and fibers. Some crystals fluoresce (a phenomenon named after the mineral) in ultraviolet light.

RARITY
—

A common mineral, fluorite specimens can be sourced worldwide. Clear fluorite is less commonly used for decorative purposes than brightly colored varieties. High-quality transparent and colorless fluorite is used in lenses for microscopes and telescopes.

FORMATION
—

Pure, colorless fluorite contains only the elements calcium and fluorine. It often forms in hydrothermal veins in felsic igneous rocks, which are rich in lighter elements.

ATTRIBUTES
—

Like other varieties of fluorite, this crystal helps us to bring about positive change in our lives. This pure, powerful crystal is for those searching for enlightenment and the higher truths. Yet it also helps us to see what changes we can make in our daily lives to find simple happiness and honesty. Crystal therapists may use clear fluorite externally as a pain-reliever.

HEALING ACTION
—

If you are searching for transformative truths, place fluorite at the universal mind chakra. If you feel that you have lost sight of your goals or that your values are under threat, meditate with clear fluorite on a daily basis. Place in the knowledge corner of the home, which is immediately to the left if you enter by the front door.

COMBINATIONS
—

To enter transformative meditative states, combine with angelite and tanzanite.

CARE
—

Fluorite scores just 4 on the Mohs' scale, so protect it from knocks and scratches. Fluorite is not water safe, so clean with a dry cloth if necessary. It is toxic and may react dangerously with stomach acid, so do not use in gem elixirs and do not ingest.

GOSHENITE

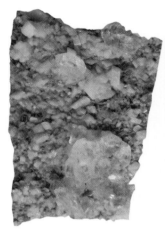

APPEARANCE
—

Goshenite is colorless beryl, ranging from translucent to transparent. It grows in hexagonal crystals, but may also be found as plates, grains, and chunks. Some specimens are bought (as pictured) on the matrix in which they formed.

RARITY
—

Goshenite is one of the most common forms of beryl, found all around the globe. The best-quality specimens often come from Brazil. Unless it is artificially colored, goshenite is not popular for gemstones, making clear stones affordable.

FORMATION
—

Goshenite is named after Goshen, Massachusetts, where it was first found. It is the purest form of beryl, composed of beryllium, aluminum, silicon, and oxygen. Goshenite forms in pegmatites, which are igneous rocks with enlarged crystals.

ATTRIBUTES
—

Beryl helps us to meet our potential. This clear form of the mineral gives its user the clear-sightedness to see how to reach goals and to identify stumbling blocks along the way. It also helps us to combine intuition with intellect as we strive for success. Some say that goshenite relieves eye strain and clears headaches, although there is no scientific basis for this claim.

HEALING ACTION
—

Place goshenite at the crown chakra to stimulate both insight and intellect. Meditate with this beryl when you face a problem that seems insurmountable. Place goshenite in the wisdom corner of the house, which is to the left if you enter by the front door.

COMBINATIONS
—

For enhanced problem-solving ability, combine obsidian with goshenite.

CARE
—

Goshenite is strong and durable, scoring 7.5–8 on the Mohs' scale. Goshenite contains beryllium, a known carcinogen, so do not inhale its dust and do not use in gem elixirs.

CLEAR SELENITE

APPEARANCE

Pure selenite crystals are colorless or white. Transparent specimens are known as selenite. Those that are pearly, silky, and display chatoyance (a cat's-eye effect caused by light reflecting in a fibrous internal structure) are called satin spar. Common crystal forms are plates, prisms, and columns, which are often twinned. Crystals that form curved rosettes may be called gypsum flowers.

RARITY

Selenite is a very common mineral. Delicate and transparent crystals may take a slightly higher price.

FORMATION

Selenite and satin spar are varieties of gypsum. They are calcium sulfate dihydrate, which means they contain molecules of water. Selenite is an evaporite mineral, forming as water evaporates from salt flats, seas, caves, and mud or clay beds.

ATTRIBUTES

Selenite helps us to learn the lessons that life gives us. If we are unhappy, it helps us to pinpoint what is troubling us so that we can make changes. When we are working toward a goal, selenite helps us to see clearly the steps that we must take to get there. This mineral also heightens clairvoyance and telepathy. Some crystal therapists say that selenite is useful for treating joint and muscle pain.

HEALING ACTION

To avoid complacency and to keep nourishing a long-term relationship, meditate with a twinned selenite crystal. For extraordinary insights, use satin spar during scrying. Position selenite at the third eye to heighten awareness of ourselves, others, and the spiritual realm.

COMBINATIONS

Combine with angelite if you are attempting automatic writing.

CARE

Selenite dissolves in acids and water, so do not use in gem elixirs. It scores just 2 on the Mohs' scale, which makes it soft enough to be scratched by a fingernail. If necessary, clean very gently with a soft cloth.

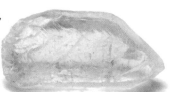

CLEAR PETALITE

APPEARANCE

Also known as castorite, petalite is transparent to translucent. Colorless or white crystals are found as columns or plates.

RARITY

Colorless petalite is often used as a gemstone. Small, cloudy specimens are less highly priced. Petalite is sourced from Australia, Brazil, Namibia, Zimbabwe, and Canada.

FORMATION

Petalite is found in granite pegmatites, which grow oversized crystals as they cool slowly underground. This mineral contains aluminum, lithium, silicon, and oxygen. It is an important ore of lithium.

ATTRIBUTES

This pure, potent stone opens the mind wide for clairvoyance, telepathy, and scrying. It aids focus during meditation. Clear petalite is also purifying, helping us to break free from damaging habits, repetitive thoughts, and worn-out thinking. Petalite is said to aid the endocrine system, although there is no scientific basis for this claim.

HEALING ACTION

In a busy day, a few moments meditating with petalite are both reenergizing and freeing. Position petalite on a table where you are carrying out tarot readings or automatic writing. If you are looking for a fresh start, whether emotional, mental, or practical, wear petalite earrings.

COMBINATIONS

Use with angelite to enhance telepathy and other activities that require mental and spiritual receptivity.

CARE

Since it is fairly easily scratched, petalite should be stored separately from other crystals and jewelry. It scores 6–6.5 on the Mohs' scale. Do not inhale dust. Clean with warm, soapy water and a soft cloth.

APOPHYLLITE

APPEARANCE
—

Usually colorless or white, apophyllite may also be violet, blue, pink, yellow, or green. Crystals are usually plates, pyramids, or cubes. This mineral ranges from transparent to opaque.

RARITY
—

Apophyllite is not a rare mineral, but facetable specimens are scarce. It is found in India, Canada, Mexico, and the United States.

FORMATION
—

This silicate mineral also contains elements including potassium, calcium, and sodium. It is found in basalt and other igneous rocks.

ATTRIBUTES
—

Apophyllite opens the door to the realm of spirits, facilitating out-of-body journeys while also allowing us to see, hear, and feel messages from other worlds. It encourages our minds to become finely attuned to the promptings of the spirit. Some say that apophyllite is beneficial for pain relief after injury and recuperation after illness, although there is no scientific basis for those claims.

HEALING ACTION
—

Clear, transparent apophyllite is an ideal crystal to use for scrying. Meditate with apophyllite regularly to activate the higher chakras. Hold over any chakra that is blocked or sluggish.

COMBINATIONS
—

While scrying with apophyllite, place a wand of protective black tourmaline nearby.

CARE
—

Apophyllite is extremely fragile along certain axes, so handle it with care. It scores 4.5–5 on the Mohs' scale. If exposed to heat, it may flake. It is also soluble in acids, so do not use in gem elixirs as it may react dangerously with stomach acid. Clean in lukewarm, soapy water. Due to its potassium content, apophyllite is mildly radioactive, but at a barely detectable level.

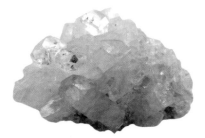

HERKIMER DIAMOND

APPEARANCE
—

These crystals are not actually diamonds, but transparent quartz crystals with unusually regular faceting. A true Herkimer diamond has a termination point at each end, each forming a pyramid of six faces. In the center of the crystal are six more rectangular faces, giving a Herkimer diamond with 18 faces in total.

RARITY
—

Herkimer diamonds are found only in Herkimer County and the Mohawk River Valley, in New York State. Good-quality crystals are expensive.

FORMATION
—

Herkimer diamonds formed during the Carboniferous Period in small cavities called vugs inside dolomite rock. In the heat of the buried dolomite, the crystals of silicon and oxygen atoms formed very slowly, resulting in their exceptional clarity and exact form.

ATTRIBUTES
—

All forms of clear quartz are amplifiers of energy, but Herkimer diamonds are perhaps the most powerful of all. They facilitate dream work, telepathy, and all creative endeavors. Some say that Herkimer diamonds detoxify the body and correct the metabolism.

HEALING ACTION
—

Herkimer diamonds are often used in pairs. If you must be parted from a loved one, give them one crystal while you keep the other, so that your hearts and minds can be bound together by the purest energy. Although Herkimer diamonds are particularly attuned to the crown and third eye chakras, they can be positioned on any chakra to cleanse and balance.

COMBINATIONS
—

To enhance telepathy or automatic writing, combine with angelite, blue obsidian, and shattuckite.

CARE
—

Herkimer diamonds score 7.5 on the Mohs' scale. Clean with warm, soapy water and a soft cloth. Avoid vigorous wear and tear. Do not inhale quartz dust as it can cause silicosis.

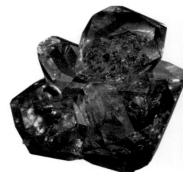

CLEAR ZIRCON

APPEARANCE
—

Specimens range from gem-quality transparent crystals to cloudy. Zircon forms as plates, prisms, or chunks.

RARITY
—

Zircon is common in the earth's crust, but economically important deposits of gem quality are rarer. Most zircons are mined in Australia or South Africa. Transparent, colorless zircons are often used as diamond substitutes in jewelry, but are far less expensive.

FORMATION
—

Zircon, which is zirconium silicate, forms in silicon-rich magma. It is often found in felsic rocks such as granite, which are rich in lighter elements including silicon, oxygen, and aluminum.

ATTRIBUTES
—

Clear zircon has a powerful healing energy. Known traditionally as a promoter of "virtue," zircon helps us to be our best selves. It encourages us to live up to our own moral ideals and to strive to meet our own practical goals. Some say that zircon is helpful for easing vertigo.

HEALING ACTION
—

Hold this crystal over any chakra that is blocked or sluggish. By resonating with each of the lower chakras in turn, clear zircon can also help us access the higher chakras. Meditate with clear zircon when you feel yourself being tested, either morally or spiritually.

COMBINATIONS
—

Combine with high-vibration petalite to open the door to the higher chakras.

CARE
—

Zircon ranks 7.5 on the Mohs' scale, but it can be chipped along faceted edges. Do not use in gem elixirs, as zirconium may be toxic and may react dangerously with stomach acid. Clean only in warm water with a mild soap.

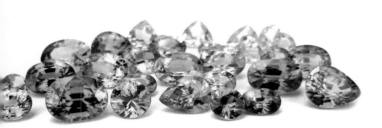

CHALCEDONY

APPEARANCE
—

Transparent to opaque, chalcedony is usually white to gray. It is a microcrystalline mineral, so its individual crystals are not visible. It can often be found in geodes (pictured), lining the cavity with rounded bumps.

RARITY
—

This is a common mineral, found in a wide range of environments worldwide. Colorful varieties of chalcedony, such as agate and jasper, are popular among collectors and craftspeople.

FORMATION
—

Chalcedony is composed of intergrowths of two silica minerals, quartz and moganite, which are chemically identical but distinguished by their different crystal structures. Chalcedony often forms in vugs inside igneous rocks.

ATTRIBUTES
—

This crystal brings the mind and spirit, body and emotions, into harmony. It helps us to hear the promptings of our emotions. It helps us to see when the body is trying to tell us that our spirit is troubled. It wards off psychosomatic symptoms, such as sore necks, headaches, or stomach disorders caused by stress.

HEALING ACTION
—

If suffering from stress-induced irritable bowel syndrome, place on the lower abdomen. Position on the crown chakra to tune into the voice of the body. Place chalcedony in the knowledge and self-cultivation corner of the home, which is to the left as you enter by the front door.

COMBINATIONS
—

When overwhelmed by strong emotion, meditate with chalcedony and calming amazonite.

CARE
—

Chalcedony scores 7 on the Mohs' scale. Do not breathe in chalcedony dust, which can cause silicosis. To clean, dip in lukewarm, soapy water. Do not soak as chalcedony is mildly soluble in water, particularly hot water.

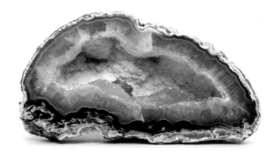

WHITE CALCITE

APPEARANCE
—

Usually white or colorless, transparent to translucent, calcite crystals take countless different forms. Among the most attractive are pyramids and radiating clusters often called "flowers."

RARITY
—

Calcite is ubiquitous, but large, finely shaped crystals take a higher price tag.

FORMATION
—

Calcite is calcium carbonate, which is an essential component of sedimentary rocks such as limestone and chalk. This mineral formed the shells and skeletons of the tiny sea creatures from which these rocks are made. Fine calcite crystals are often found in limestone caves.

ATTRIBUTES
—

Calcite stimulates the intellect, while allowing us to trust our own reasoning and problem-solving. It also enhances our insights and opens the door to telepathy, clairvoyance, and scrying. Some crystal therapists say that white calcite encourages bones, skin, and muscle to heal after injury.

HEALING ACTION
—

Placed at the higher chakras, white calcite aids telepathy. At the crown chakra, it benefits intellectual pursuits, from academic study to chess. Position a calcite wand on the table while carrying out tarot readings.

COMBINATIONS
—

If attempting automatic writing, work with calcite, shattuckite, magnetite, and angelite.

CARE
—

Calcite is brittle and soft, scoring just 3 on the Mohs' scale. It should not be handled excessively. Calcite is not soluble in pure water but is soluble in rainwater, which is slightly acidic. Do not use in gem elixirs. Use pure water and a soft cloth to clean.

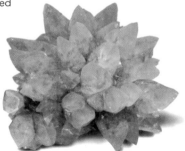

WHITE JADE

APPEARANCE
—

Jade is one of two minerals with similar properties and appearance, jadeite and nephrite. White specimens may be either mineral. They range from translucent to opaque.

RARITY
—

White jade, known in China as "mutton fat" jade, is less common than green varieties. Found in just a dozen locations, jadeite is rarer and more costly than nephrite.

FORMATION
—

Both jadeite and nephrite form during metamorphism, where two tectonic plates are converging. Jade is often found around the rim of the Pacific Ocean, where it may be collected as rind-covered pebbles and boulders in stream valleys.

ATTRIBUTES
—

Jade brings harmony. White jade has particular resonance with the higher chakras, allowing us to balance day-to-day concerns with our desire for connection with the spiritual realm. It encourages us to be the person we were meant to be, before we compromised our ideals because of practical concerns. White jade is said to help balance body fluids and expel toxins.

HEALING ACTION
—

Meditate with white jade if you have lost your spiritual path. Place a white jade carving in the wisdom corner of the house, which is to the left when you enter by the front door. Place on the higher chakras if they are blocked and are causing a feeling of being spaced out.

COMBINATIONS
—

When searching for guidance from the spirit world, combine with celestite.

CARE
—

Nephrite scores 6–6.5 on the Mohs' scale, while jadeite is slightly harder, 6.5–7. Wipe jade clean with a soft, soapy cloth, then rinse with clean water and dry carefully. Jade should not be soaked. Keep jade out of direct sunlight.

HOWLITE

APPEARANCE
—

Well-formed crystals of howlite are rare: this mineral is usually found as white, irregular nodules covered by dark veins resembling spider's webs. Howlite is translucent to opaque.

RARITY
—

Widely available, howlite is usually bought as tumbled and polished stones, but is also dyed and used as inlays and cabochons in jewelry. Sources include Canada and the southwestern United States.

FORMATION
—

This calcium borosilicate hydroxide is found in evaporite deposits in dried-out lakes.

ATTRIBUTES
—

Howlite is famed as the mineral that can give insomniacs a good night's sleep. It eases stress, repetitive thoughts, and compulsions. It also guards against mood swings that result in anger, tetchiness, or prickliness. Some say that howlite can ease back and neck pain caused by tension.

HEALING ACTION
—

Place howlite under the pillow or beside the bed for an unbroken and refreshing night's sleep. Meditate with howlite to cool the temper and ease tension. Wear howlite jewelry to combat stress and intrusive thoughts.

COMBINATIONS
—

If you are suffering from mood swings, meditate with howlite, red jade, and variscite.

CARE
—

Howlite scores 3.5 on the Mohs' scale. It is soluble in acids, so should not be used in gem elixirs as it may react dangerously with stomach acid. Undyed howlite can be cleaned in lukewarm, soapy water. Dyed howlite should not be immersed.

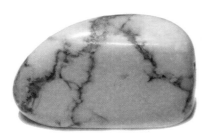

WHITE ARAGONITE

APPEARANCE
—

Although usually white, aragonite may be any color of the rainbow. Aragonite crystals form hexagonal prisms, stalactites, needles, fibers, and branching forms known as *flos ferri*, meaning flowers of iron (pictured). Aragonite is transparent to opaque.

RARITY
—

Aragonite is a very common mineral, but *flos ferri* and other delicately shaped crystals are collector's items.

FORMATION
—

A type of calcium carbonate, aragonite forms through biological and geological processes. It is made naturally in most mollusk shells. Crystals precipitate from saltwater and freshwater, often around hot springs and in caves.

ATTRIBUTES
—

Aragonite gives us patience. It not only helps us to be calm and accepting in our dealings with others, but to be patient with ourselves. Aragonite also helps us to have the composure and fortitude to finish painstaking tasks and to work toward long-term goals. Crystal therapists say that aragonite is helpful with problems of the circulatory and immune systems.

HEALING ACTION
—

To encourage diligence and perseverance, place white aragonite on the desk where you or a loved one work. To engender feelings of calm and forbearance, meditate with aragonite on the floor before you.

COMBINATIONS
—

Build a grid to support a long-term goal using white aragonite, jet, mahogany obsidian, and pink beryl.

CARE
—

Aragonite is fragile, scoring just 3.5–4 on the Mohs' scale. *Flos ferri* should be handled with extreme care. Aragonite is soluble in acids and in water. Do not use in gem elixirs. If cleaning is necessary, dip briefly in lukewarm soapy water.

OKENITE

APPEARANCE
—

Okenite is usually seen as small, round "cotton boll" formations within geodes. The tiny, fibrous crystals that form these balls are translucent and bendy, but fragile. Okenite is usually white but may be tinted pale yellow or blue.

RARITY
—

Okenite is found in India, Greenland, Azerbaijan, New Zealand, Chile, Ireland, and the Faroe Islands. It is popular with mineral collectors.

FORMATION
—

A calcium silicate hydrate, okenite grows inside vugs created by gas bubbles in the common extrusive igneous rock basalt.

ATTRIBUTES
—

Okenite is a highly protective crystal that wards off negative entities and psychic attack. As it protects, it helps us both to heal and to grow, encouraging us to reach out from the shells that we build for ourselves. Some say that okenite calms disorders of the skin, from eczema to acne, although there is no scientific proof of that claim.

HEALING ACTION
—

If you have suffered hurt, meditate regularly with okenite to encourage healing, optimism, and trust. If you have been hurt in love, place okenite in the love corner of the home, which is at the back right if you enter by the front door.

COMBINATIONS
—

For hurts inflicted during past lives, combine with rhodonite.

CARE
—

Okenite scores 4.5–5 on the Mohs' scale. Handle with care as the crystals easily mat together or snap. Avoid cleaning. Do not immerse in water.

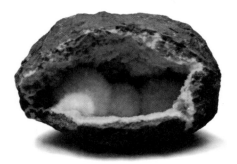

ULEXITE

APPEARANCE
—

Also known as TV rock due to its optical properties, ulexite is colorless to white. Its fibrous crystals act as optical fibers, transmitting light along their length by internal reflection. Although disordered cotton boll formations are common, if ulexite crystals grow parallel to each other and the specimen is cut perpendicular to its fiber growth, it will display an image of the surface on its opposite side.

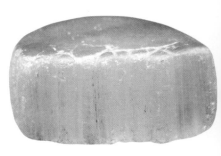

RARITY
—

Ulexite is a fairly common mineral in desert areas, such as in the southwestern United States, but specimens with high-quality parallel crystals are collector's items.

FORMATION
—

This mineral is a sodium calcium borate hydroxide. It forms in desert areas during the evaporation of shallow boron-rich pools.

ATTRIBUTES
—

Ulexite is a crystal of vision. It allows us to look deep inside ourselves to question our motivations and beliefs. It gives us the insight to see others as they truly are. It also opens the third eye to the spiritual world. Some say that ulexite can ease eye strain and conjunctivitis, although there is no scientific basis for this claim.

HEALING ACTION
—

Gently place ulexite at the third eye to see deeply and wisely into the spiritual realm. Meditate with ulexite to increase awareness of yourself, others, and the Universe beyond. Ulexite is an ideal choice for scrying, either for gazing or as an accessory crystal to heighten perception.

COMBINATIONS
—

If engaging in deep emotional introspection using ulexite, keep protective black tourmaline or jet nearby.

CARE
—

Ulexite dissolves in water, so do not soak or use in gem elixirs. To clean, dip in cold, soapy water. Ulexite scores 2.5 on the Mohs' scale, so handle carefully. It contains borate, so do not ingest or breathe in dust.

MAGNESITE

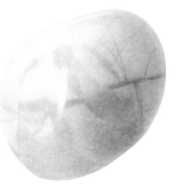

APPEARANCE
—

This colorless, white, lemon, or pastel-tinted mineral commonly forms masses resembling cauliflowers or brains. When well-formed crystals do occur, they are rhombohedrons or hexagonal prisms. Magnesite is transparent to opaque.

RARITY
—

Brain-like masses are widely available, but transparent crystals are far rarer. Faceted stones and cabochons, sometimes dyed, are used in jewelry. Sources include Brazil, India, and South Africa.

FORMATION
—

Magnesite is composed of magnesium, carbon, and oxygen. It forms in veins in magnesium-rich rocks during metamorphosis.

ATTRIBUTES
—

This mineral boosts the brain, improving reasoning, memory, and learning. It also stimulates creative thought processes, from writing to problem-solving. It helps the left and right hemispheres to work together, so that we can combine proficient communication with reasoning, and mathematical ability with artistic flair.

HEALING ACTION
—

Position magnesite on the desk (see also "Care") during work or study to boost performance. Meditate regularly with magnesite to encourage clear, creative, and imaginative thinking.

COMBINATIONS
—

A powerful crystal combination for students is magnesite and black onyx.

CARE
—

Magnesite scores just 3.5–4.5 on the Mohs' scale, so store gems in a soft bag, away from harder minerals. Magnesite is soluble in acids, so do not use in gem elixirs as it may react dangerously with stomach acid. Its dust can irritate the eyes, skin, and respiratory system, so avoid excessive handling. Clean in warm, soapy water with a soft cloth.

PEARL

APPEARANCE
—

A pearl has a body color, as well as overtones of iridescence. Body colors range from white, cream, rose, and pink to black, gray, bronze, blue, green, red, purple, and violet. Pale pearls may have a yellow or pink overtone or none. Dark pearls often have a metallic overtone.

RARITY
—

Today, most pearls are cultivated, although divers still collect wild "natural" pearls in some parts of the world, including the seas off Bahrain and Australia. Natural pearls are rare and cost many times more than a cultivated pearl. Pearls are also graded by their size, shape, color, and luster. Akoya pearls from Japan are among the highest-valued cultured pearls.

FORMATION
—

Pearls form inside the shells of pearl oysters and mussels, in both freshwater and saltwater, when a tiny parasite or grain of sand makes its way inside. The mollusks surround the intruder with layers of nacre. Nacre, often called mother of pearl, is a mix of the mineral aragonite with the horn-like protein conchiolin.

ATTRIBUTES
—

Pearls are associated with weddings and brides. They bless romantic unions, whether formalized by marriage or not, acting as a magnet for love, trust, and honesty. They also encourage loyalty—both loyalty to friends and to our own ideals. Some crystal therapists say that pearls can help to control allergies and skin conditions.

HEALING ACTION
—

Wear pearls in jewelry to engender feelings of love and trust. Place pearl at the heart chakra for the ability to show love without fear. Meditate with pearl when you feel that your love or loyalty is tested.

COMBINATIONS
—

Pearl and gold jewelry make an ideal gift for a newlywed or anyone committing to a life partner.

CARE
—

Pearls may be toxic, so do not ingest or use in gem elixirs. They score 2.5–4.5 on the Mohs' scale, so should be stored in a soft bag away from other gems. Never immerse pearls in water: wipe clean with a wet, soapy cloth.

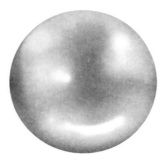

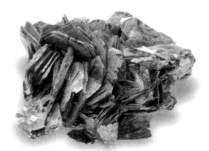

MUSCOVITE

APPEARANCE
—

Although often white, gray, or silvery, muscovite may also be found in green, yellow, violet, or red. Its crystals are flexible and can often be cut into thin pieces with a knife. It is usually found as plates or chunks.

RARITY
—

Muscovite can be bought from most mineral stockists. Much muscovite is sourced from India, Pakistan, Brazil, and the United States.

FORMATION
—

This mineral is composed of potassium, aluminum, silicon, oxygen, and fluorine. It forms in igneous rocks or when clay minerals are transformed by the heat and pressure of regional metamorphism.

ATTRIBUTES
—

Muscovite helps us to compromise and to be emotionally flexible. It also helps us to weather the storms and obstacles that all of us must face as we move through life. It allows us to move forward stronger rather than broken, bitter, or hopeless. Crystal therapists say that muscovite helps to fine-tune the metabolism.

HEALING ACTION
—

If you are feeling battered or broken by conflict, loss, or disappointment, position at the earth chakra to feel strengthened and grounded. Meditate with muscovite to see an emotional problem from all angles, to rethink ingrained thought processes, and to break restrictive self-imposed rules.

COMBINATIONS
—

If you are experiencing conflict with a family member, combine muscovite's flexibility with rhodochrosite's healing love.

CARE
—

Muscovite scores just 2–4 on the Mohs' scale. Do not soak this mineral in water as it may flake apart. Do not use in gem elixirs. If necessary, clean very gently with a dry, soft brush.

METALLIC

Metallic crystals have a dual nature, resonating both with the chakras of the earth and root, as well as with the third eye, crown, and higher chakras. The bright, ethereal glow of these crystals engages with our spirituality and reason. Yet their earthy, elemental nature should never be forgotten. It engages with our basic needs and with our connection to place and time. As a result, these crystals both inspire and comfort.

Culturally and literally, metallic crystals are associated with wealth. Indeed, these crystals are often precious metals or important ores of metals used for construction, machinery, or electronics. Folk wisdom tells us that these crystals bring wealth and prosperity. No crystal can accomplish that "magic bean" feat, yet these crystals do encourage us to make the wise, considered choices and the strong alliances that can lead to financial and emotional security. Note that metals and metallic compounds should not be ingested. If in doubt when working with a mineral with a metallic sheen, do not ingest, do not inhale dust, do not touch it to broken skin, and do not use in a gem elixir.

COPPER

APPEARANCE
—

Copper is a native element mineral—one of the few metallic elements to occur in pure mineral form in nature. It forms cubic and octahedral crystals but is more usually seen as irregular masses. Fresh surfaces are red-orange, but copper weathers over time.

RARITY
—

Native (or pure) copper can be mined from locations including Brazil and the United States. Copper jewelry, spheres, nuggets, and crystals are widely available.

FORMATION
—

Copper is an element, which means it is formed from only one type of atom, in this case atoms with 29 protons in their nucleus. Copper is the 25th most common element in the earth's crust.

ATTRIBUTES
—

Copper combats lethargy, passivity, and low mood, replacing them with energy and optimism. Copper bracelets are said to aid arthritis symptoms, although there is no scientific basis to this belief. However, there is broad scientific proof that copper has antimicrobial properties.

HEALING ACTION
—

When your mood is low, meditate with copper. Wear copper jewelry to encourage initiative-taking and enhance emotional stamina. Place copper on the root chakra to banish feelings of powerlessness.

COMBINATIONS
—

Wear jewelry with lapis lazuli set in copper for a powerful combination against feelings of purposelessness and pessimism.

CARE
—

Copper scores just 3 on the Mohs' scale, but is highly bendable. Copper reacts with oxygen in the air to form a layer of darker copper oxide. If left outdoors for a considerable time, copper will take a green coating known as verdigris. Since excess copper is toxic and may be linked with Alzheimer's disease, do not use in gem elixirs. Clean in warm, soapy water with a soft cloth.

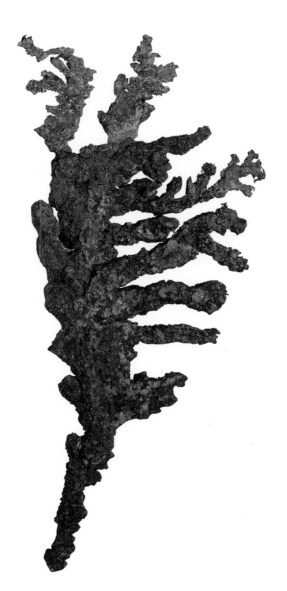

BRONZITE

APPEARANCE
—

Not related to the alloy bronze (which is primarily composed of copper and tin), this green-to-brown mineral has a bronze luster. It is usually found as masses that can be polished to a high shine.

RARITY
—

This mineral is found in locations including England, Greenland, India, South Africa, and the United States. Bronzite is occasionally used as an ornamental stone for cabochons and beads.

FORMATION
—

Bronzite is a form of enstatite (composed of magnesium, silicon, and oxygen) that is rich in iron. On the mineral's surface, the iron separates into oxides and hydroxides. It is light reflecting between these layers that creates the metallic schiller. Bronzite is found in igneous rocks such as peridotite.

ATTRIBUTES
—

Bronzite gives us the courage to trust our emotions and to follow their promptings. It gives us strength to alter our course in life. It is also a highly protective stone, being said to ward off curses and hexes. Some crystal therapists claim that bronzite strengthens the body after illness and at times of particular exhaustion.

HEALING ACTION
—

Meditate with bronzite to tune in to your true emotions. Wear bronzite jewelry for the strength to follow your heart, no matter what critics or doubters say. Place by the bedside while recuperating from illness or overwork.

COMBINATIONS
—

Use bronzite and jet as a protective talismanic combination against negative entities and psychic stress.

CARE
—

Bronzite scores 5–6 on the Mohs' scale. Since it contains silicon, its dust should not be inhaled. Do not soak and do not use in gem elixirs. Clean with a soft cloth and warm soapy water, then dry carefully.

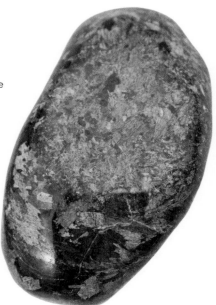

SILVER

APPEARANCE
—
A native element mineral, silver occurs as pure grains, nuggets, and branching, tree-like formations. It is white-gray with a shiny surface.

RARITY
—
Pure silver is rare in nature, with most of our silver obtained by smelting ores. Among the world's biggest silver producers are Mexico, Peru, Canada, and the United States. Silver nuggets and jewelry are widely available.

FORMATION
—
Silver is composed of atoms that have 47 protons in their nucleus. Native silver is found in basalt and hydrothermal veins.

ATTRIBUTES
—
Silver opens the door to the higher chakras, allowing us to direct our minds outward into the spiritual plane. Silver encourages us to be our best self, overcoming our own flaws and fears. Like copper, silver has antimicrobial properties, leading to its use in medical applications. However, see "Care" for safety advice.

HEALING ACTION
—
Use native silver to activate the higher chakras by first opening and engaging the lower chakras, working from the earth upward. To feel self-confident in your own abilities and wisdom, wear silver jewelry.

COMBINATIONS
—
A potent combination at the higher chakras is silver and celestite.

CARE
—
Silver is a soft and bendy metal, scoring 2.5–3 on the Mohs' scale. Do not ingest or inhale silver particles, which can cause argyria. When exposed to air, silver develops a tarnish, which can be removed with a specialist polish.

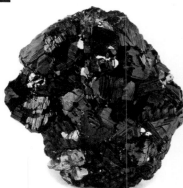

MAGNETITE

APPEARANCE
—
This mineral is black, gray, or gray-brown with a shiny surface. It is found as grains, chunks, and octahedral crystals. It is the most magnetic of all naturally occurring minerals.

RARITY
—
Large deposits of magnetite are found in Chile, Uruguay, Mauritania, Australia, and the United States. A naturally magnetized magnetite specimen is known as a lodestone.

FORMATION
—
Magnetite is an iron oxide, composed of iron and oxygen. It is found in igneous and sedimentary rocks, where it often takes the form of banded iron formations, produced by oxygen combining with dissolved iron in ancient oceans.

ATTRIBUTES
—
Magnetite's natural magnetism can be used to align the chakras. Just as a magnet has north and south poles, this mineral exhibits seemingly opposing properties: it both grounds us deeply in the earth and attracts visitors from other realms.

HEALING ACTION
—
For alignment of the chakras, seek treatment from an experienced crystal therapist. Place at the third eye to enhance telepathy, clairvoyance, and lucid dreaming. Place at the earth chakra to feel centered and rooted in the reality of the present moment.

COMBINATIONS
—
To experience transcendent dreams, place magnetite and blue agate by the bedside. To enhance clairvoyance, combine with azurite.

CARE
—
This mineral scores 5.5–6.5 on the Mohs' scale. Its black surface will fade to brown over time. To avoid rusting, do not soak in water or leave in a damp place. Do not ingest or breathe in magnetite dust, which may be toxic. To clean, dip in water then dry thoroughly.

MOLYBDENITE

APPEARANCE
—

This black to gray mineral has a silvery luster. It is found as grains, plates, chunks, and hexagonal crystals. It is opaque, but translucent in flakes. Molybdenite feels greasy and leaves gray marks on the skin when touched.

RARITY
—

Although chunks of molybdenite can be bought at a low price, it is a relatively rare mineral and the most important ore of the metal molybdenum. It is frequently mined in the United States.

FORMATION
—

This mineral, composed of molybdenum and sulfur, is found in rocks such as granite, rhyolite, and pegmatite.

ATTRIBUTES
—

A brightly shining mineral, it teaches self-reflection. It encourages us to look at ourselves, at our strengths and weaknesses, and our hopes and fears. Molybdenite also encourages us to examine our lives, weighing up factors such our relationships and work–leisure balance.

HEALING ACTION
—

Hold molybdenite at each chakra in turn for a thorough appraisal of emotional and spiritual well-being. Place this mineral in the knowledge corner of the home, to the left of the front door, to facilitate self-reflection.

COMBINATIONS
—

If you are feeling dissatisfied with your life, meditate with molybdenite and black obsidian for a thorough examination of the root causes of your feeling.

CARE
—

Molybdenite scores just 1–1.5 on the Mohs' scale, so avoid excessive handling. Since molybdenum may be toxic, do not use this mineral in gem elixirs or breathe its dust. If cleaning is necessary, dip in lukewarm soapy water.

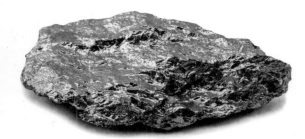

GALENA

APPEARANCE
—

A dark gray mineral, galena has a bright silvery luster, but tarnishes quickly in air. Crystals grow as plates, cubes, and octahedra. Galena is opaque.

RARITY
—

Galena is a fairly common mineral that is mined in Germany, Bulgaria, Australia, and the United States.

FORMATION
—

Composed of lead and sulfur, galena is the world's main ore of lead. Galena forms in hydrothermal veins.

ATTRIBUTES
—

Galena is a challenging crystal that makes us question our assumptions, habits, and preconceived ideas. It helps those wishing to make a break with the past, who are embarking on a journey or a new episode in life.

HEALING ACTION
—

Due to its lead content, galena should be used only under the direction of a qualified crystal therapist.

COMBINATIONS
—

A crystal therapist may use galena in combination with aegirine to overcome deeply ingrained negative behaviors.

CARE
—

Keep galena away from children and pets. Galena contains lead, which is highly toxic if inhaled as dust or ingested. If skin is not broken, the mineral is considered reasonably safe to handle, provided it is not dusty. Wash hands after touching. Do not use in gem elixirs. Galena scores 2.5–2.75 on the Mohs' scale.

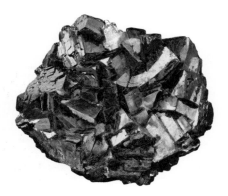

HEMATITE

APPEARANCE
—

Hematite is gray to rust-red with a steely luster. Its crystals take many forms, from plates, columns, and radiating fibers to rosettes. Hematite is opaque.

RARITY
—

This ubiquitous mineral can be bought as tumbled stones or fine crystal rosettes (pictured), often called iron roses. It is occasionally used as a decorative stone. Hematite is frequently sourced from Brazil, England, Italy, or Canada.

FORMATION
—

An iron oxide, hematite is found widely in rock and soils. It usually precipitates from seawater or standing freshwater, but can also crystallize in hot magma.

ATTRIBUTES
—

Hematite is a strongly grounding crystal, tethering the spirit when we are spaced out or emotionally lost. It is highly beneficial for concentration. Hematite helps us to focus on the here and now, breaking free from the past and viewing the future with equanimity. Some say that hematite helps with blood disorders, but there is no scientific proof of this claim.

HEALING ACTION
—

Meditate with hematite when feeling emotionally lost or confused. Place a hematite crystal on the desk to benefit study or work. Position on the earth chakra to ground a wandering or yearning spirit.

COMBINATIONS
—

To help with focus during a lengthy course of study, meditate with hematite and black onyx.

CARE
—

Hematite scores 5.5–6.5 on the Mohs' scale, but is brittle. Clean in warm, soapy water with a soft cloth. Hematite will rust if left damp. Due to its iron content, hematite should not be ingested or used in gem elixirs. It is soluble in acids, so may react dangerously with stomach acid.

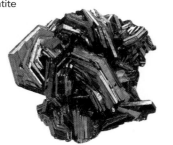

CASSITERITE

APPEARANCE
—

Although usually black or gray with a metallic luster, cassiterite is more rarely brown, red, yellow, or white. It is found as pyramids, crusts, and masses. While masses are opaque, thin crystals are translucent. Translucent crystals can split light into a rainbow of colors, giving a "fire" seen in diamonds.

RARITY
—

A major ore of tin, cassiterite is considered a conflict mineral, due to fighting over cassiterite deposits in the Democratic Republic of the Congo. Other sources include Bolivia, Malaysia, Thailand, and Indonesia. Facetable, gem-quality cassiterite is extremely rare.

FORMATION
—

Cassiterite is a tin oxide that is found in metamorphic and igneous rocks as well as stream and shoreline sediments. Economically important quantities of cassiterite usually form in hydrothermal veins.

ATTRIBUTES
—

This is a crystal that helps us to see the good in others and in ourselves. When times are hard, it encourages us to see the light at the end of the tunnel. It draws in strength and energy, replenishing our stores when we are in need. Cassiterite is said to help with hormonal imbalances.

HEALING ACTION
—

To build up reserves of strength, place at the earth chakra. Place at the third eye to take a fresh, optimistic view of your life and resources. Place at the center of the home as a constant source of resilience and hope.

COMBINATIONS
—

If struggling with empty nest syndrome or the demise of a long relationship, build a grid with cassiterite, black onyx, danburite, and amethyst.

CARE
—

Scoring 6–7 on the Mohs' scale, cassiterite should be protected from knocks and scratches. It can be cleaned in warm, soapy water with a soft cloth.

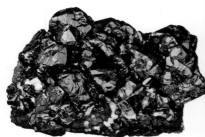

GOLD

APPEARANCE

—

Gold is a bright, shining yellow. A native element mineral, gold is one of the few metals to occur naturally in pure form. It is most commonly found as grains and nuggets. Gold is highly malleable and ductile.

RARITY

—

Pure gold can be bought as jewelry, grains, and nuggets. Gold is a relatively rare element, the 75th most common in the earth's crust. China is the world's largest producer of gold.

FORMATION

—

Gold is an element, formed only from atoms with 79 protons in their nucleus. Pure gold is found as grains in rock, as well as in alluvial deposits after erosion.

ATTRIBUTES

—

Gold is said to be a great healer, expelling toxins and improving blood flow. It enhances emotional stability and positivity while reducing stress and mild depression. It attracts love, friendship, and happiness. Some say that it attracts wealth, although it is more likely that it attracts the positive outlook and alliances that can lead to financial security.

HEALING ACTION

—

Wear gold jewelry to enhance feelings of serenity and happiness. Position at the solar plexus chakra to encourage engagement and good communication with friends and family. Place a gold nugget in the wealth and prosperity corner of the home, which is at the back left if you enter by the front door.

COMBINATIONS

—

To attract love and happiness, wear amethyst in a gold setting.

CARE

—

Gold scores just 2.5 on the Mohs' scale, but bends rather than breaks. In very high doses, gold can be toxic. Clean in warm, soapy water with a soft cloth.

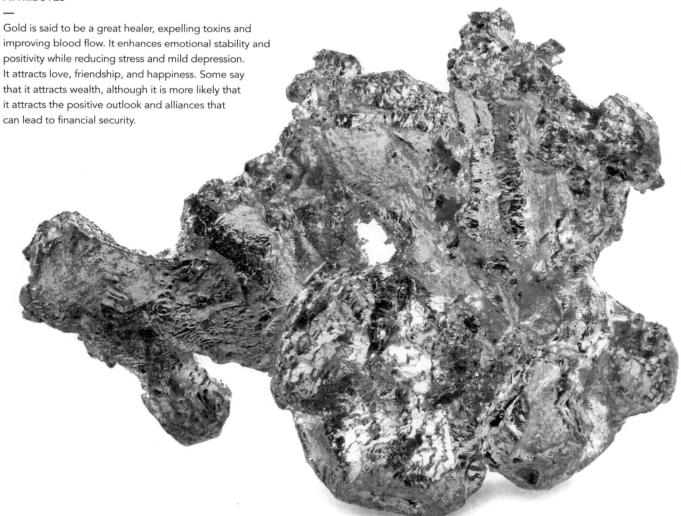

CHALCOPYRITE

APPEARANCE
—

This yellow, opaque, and shiny mineral forms tetrahedrons as well as masses that resemble bunches of grapes. It shares a similar appearance to gold and pyrite, but it is harder than gold and softer than pyrite.

RARITY
—

Found worldwide, chalcopyrite is a major ore of copper. Mineral specimens are often sourced from Canada or Australia. Some specimens are treated with acid to display an iridescence similar to bornite (see page 138).

FORMATION
—

Chalcopyrite is composed of copper, iron, and sulfur atoms. It forms in a variety of ways and environments, including in cooling magma and hydrothermal veins.

ATTRIBUTES
—

Chalcopyrite dispels mental confusion and emotional disorientation. It helps us to focus on what is important and meaningful, helping with decision-making and priority setting. This crystal can also remove blockages from any chakra, as well as harmonizing energy flow between them. It is also said to boost vitality and stamina.

HEALING ACTION
—

Place chalcopyrite at the crown chakra to boost mental resources and perception. If you are torn between two different paths in life, meditate with chalcopyrite for clarity. To boost energy flow, position at each chakra in turn, starting with the earth.

COMBINATIONS
—

During times of extreme emotional turmoil, meditate with both chalcopyrite and pink petalite.

CARE
—

This mineral scores 3.5 on the Mohs' scale. Due to its copper and sulfur content, it should not be used in gem elixirs. Do not inhale chalcopyrite dust. Clean in warm, soapy water with a soft cloth. Do not soak. Over time, chalcopyrite may weather to a dull gray-green.

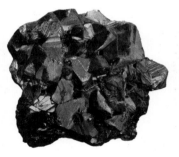

PYRITE

APPEARANCE
—

Also known as fool's gold, thanks to its deceptively similar appearance to gold, pyrite is pale yellow and shiny. Its crystals form cubes, often with striated faces. It may also be found as octahedra, stalactites, globes, and masses.

RARITY
—

Pyrite is the most common sulfide mineral. It is widely available from specialist mineral suppliers, who should give advice on its toxicity and storage.

FORMATION
—

Pyrite is composed of iron and sulfur. It is found in metamorphic, igneous, and sedimentary rocks. It forms by a variety of processes, including contact metamorphism (the intrusion of hot magma) and diagenesis (chemical and physical changes) in sediments rich in organic matter.

ATTRIBUTES
—

This crystal is highly motivating. It encourages us to aim high and dream big. It helps us to work hard to achieve our goals, no matter what obstacles we have to overcome. It encourages mental and emotional resilience. Pyrite is also a grounding crystal, helping us to engage closely and positively with reality. It is said to be rejuvenating and energizing.

HEALING ACTION
—

Due to its toxicity, pyrite should be used only under the direction of a qualified crystal therapist.

COMBINATIONS
—

A crystal therapist may combine pyrite with gold to enhance success in a business venture.

CARE
—

Keep pyrite specimens away from children and pets. Pyrite may contain the poison arsenic. On no account should it be ingested, inhaled, or used in gem elixirs. Keep specimens dry and in a plastic box to avoid decomposition, which will release hydrochloric acid. Do not wash. It scores 6–6.5 on the Mohs' scale.

COLOR-CHANGING, PATTERNED, AND COMBINATION

Many of these extraordinary minerals, mineraloids, rocks, and fossils resonate with the higher chakras: the soul star, stellar gateway, and universal mind. Their pure, high vibrations direct us toward spiritual growth, imaginative freedom, and true enlightenment. Yet plenty of these versatile stones resonate with multiple chakras, including the lowest, helping us to combine creativity with practicality, or to combine clairsentience with the common sense to use it wisely.

Color-changing stones may be magical and transformative, ideal for those who desire to change their life or to become their best self. When choosing a patterned stone, pick the one that draws you in with its colors, shapes, and pictures. Patterned stones speak to those they will most benefit. Finally, combination stones are an ideal addition to any crystal portfolio, as they combine the properties of two or more extraordinary crystals, making them exceptionally powerful.

PRECIOUS OPAL

APPEARANCE
—

Precious opal is a mineraloid, a mineral-like substance without a regular crystal structure. It displays iridescence, or flashes of colored light, caused by the diffraction of white light into its different shades. An opal's background color may be any shade.

RARITY
—

Precious opal is much rarer and more costly than common opal (see page 75). Black precious opals are the rarest of all, with white or gray more easily obtained. Sources of precious opal include Australia, Ethiopia, Mexico, and Nevada.

FORMATION
—

Opal contains up to 20 percent water, with the mineraloid's silicon dioxide containing clusters of water molecules. Opal forms as water trickles through rocks such as sandstone and claystone, collecting particles of silicon dioxide. Over time, the solution forms opal in cracks and holes. Areas within an opal that display iridescence, also called play-of-color, have a more orderly structure than the rest of the opal: they are made up of millions of minuscule silica spheres in a close-packed lattice. This structure diffracts light into the colors of the spectrum.

ATTRIBUTES
—

Precious opal is powerful and transformative. It releases us from the constraints that we impose on ourselves, allowing us to be spontaneous, freethinking, creative, and adventurous. However, precious opal should be used wisely as it may encourage changeability, hasty decision-making, and risk-taking.

HEALING ACTION
—

To allow yourself to shine in a job interview, wear precious opal jewelry. Meditate with precious opal to engage your creativity for problem-solving or artistic pursuits. Precious opal may be an ideal gift for someone embarking on a new and exciting chapter in their life, such as retirement or relocation.

COMBINATIONS
—

To counteract precious opal's tendency to encourage hastiness, combine with grounding crystals such as black tourmaline, shungite, and smoky quartz.

CARE
—

Opal scores 5.5–6 on the Mohs' scale, so care must be taken to avoid chips and breaks. Do not expose to extremes of temperature. Never immerse in water. Opal can be cleaned with a soft cloth dipped in lukewarm, soapy water. Dry thoroughly. Do not use in gem elixirs.

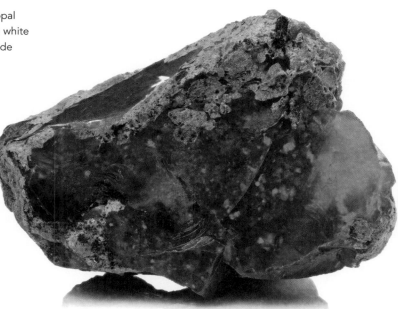

MOONSTONE

APPEARANCE
—
Also known as hecatolite, moonstone displays an effect called adularescence or schiller. This is a milky, usually bluish glow that looks like moonlight on water. Although moonstone is usually white, it can be brown, gray, pink, blue, and green.

RARITY
—
Moonstone can be sourced worldwide, including from Armenia, Australia, Mexico, Madagascar, Myanmar, India, Sri Lanka, and the United States. Jewelry inlaid with moonstone, often in the style of René Lalique, is widely available.

FORMATION
—
Moonstone is a combination of two closely related minerals in the feldspar group, orthoclase and albite. The intergrown minerals stack in alternating layers, which create this gemstone's adularescence as light bounces off these microstructures. Moonstone forms from hydrothermal deposits.

ATTRIBUTES
—
Moonstone is powerfully attuned to the female reproductive system and is said to ease premenstrual syndrome and menopausal mood changes. This is a calming crystal that can also ease stress and insomnia. It encourages emotional healing and serenity.

HEALING ACTION
—
Meditate daily with moonstone if you are experiencing the menopause. Place moonstone under the pillow or by the bedside for a deep and refreshing night's sleep. Wear moonstone jewelry during times of emotional stress.

COMBINATIONS
—
A powerful combination for easing insomnia is moonstone, gray kyanite, and blue topaz.

CARE
—
Moonstone scores 6–6.5 on the Mohs' scale. It is quite easy to fracture, so it is best suited to pendants or earrings than rings. Clean by dipping in warm, soapy water.

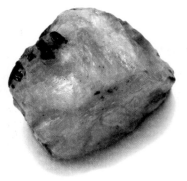

BORNITE

APPEARANCE
—
Also known as peacock ore, bornite initially has a copper to bronze luster but soon tarnishes in air to an iridescent display of purple, turquoise, and blue. It is usually found as opaque masses.

RARITY
—
Bornite is a fairly common mineral and an important ore of copper. Attractively tarnished specimens are valued as collector's items, but this mineral is too soft for most jewelry uses. It is sourced from Italy, Germany, South Africa, Madagascar, Chile, Peru, Canada, and the United States.

FORMATION
—
Bornite is composed of copper, iron, and sulfur. It grows in copper ore deposits formed by hydrothermal fluids, often in igneous rocks rich in iron.

ATTRIBUTES
—
Bornite brings happiness and healing. If we are unhappy, it helps us to identify what is troubling us and find the strength to make changes. It encourages flexibility of thought and behavior so that we are able to make the best of whatever life throws at us. Some crystal therapists suggest bornite as a pain reliever.

HEALING ACTION
—
Meditate with bornite to feel warmed and comforted even in the face of intense stress or loss. To enable positive self-reflection, place bornite on the third eye chakra. Position bornite in the self-cultivation area of the home, which is to the left of the front door.

COMBINATIONS
—
Bornite and sunstone make a powerful happiness-enhancing combination. To encourage flexibility of thought in yourself or a loved one, combine with tangerine quartz.

CARE
—
Bornite scores just 3 on the Mohs' scale, so handle with care. Clean in warm, soapy water with a soft cloth. It will rust if left damp. Due to its copper content, it should not be ingested or used in gem elixirs. It is soluble in acids, so may also react dangerously with stomach acid.

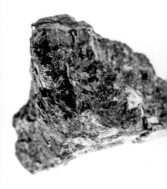

LABRADORITE

APPEARANCE
—

The mineral labradorite has a background color of gray, brown, green, blue, or yellow, but is known for its particular iridescence, known as labradorescence, usually in shades of blue, purple, turquoise, and gold. Labradorite is found as plates and masses.

RARITY
—

Labradorite is named after Labrador, in Canada, where it was first identified. It is also sourced from Australia, China, Madagascar, Slovakia, and the United States. The mineral is often cut as a cabochon to show off its labradorescence.

FORMATION
—

Formed in igneous rocks such as basalt and gabbro, labradorite is a member of the feldspar group of minerals. It contains atoms of calcium, sodium, aluminum, silicon, and oxygen. Its labradorescence results from the reflection of light between layers of crystals that all face in one direction. These crystals are too small to be seen under an ordinary microscope.

ATTRIBUTES
—

Labradorite is a powerful crystal that heightens perception, intuition, and clairvoyance. It opens our consciousness, leading us one step closer to true understanding. It brings messages from the spirit world and our unconscious, allowing them to surface in dreams. Some say that labradorite also helps disorders of the eyes and brain.

HEALING ACTION
—

Hold labradorite at the third eye to awaken clairvoyance. Use it to open the higher chakras (first working on the lower chakras in turn) to widen consciousness. Place labradorite by the bedside for wonderfully lucid dreams.

COMBINATIONS
—

Labradorite and super seven quartz make a high-vibration combination for increasing energy flow through the soul star, stellar gateway, and universal mind chakras.

CARE
—

Labradorite scores 6–6.5 on the Mohs' scale. Do not soak labradorite in water as it will dissolve. Do not use it in gem elixirs. It can be cleaned by wiping with a damp, soft cloth, then drying thoroughly.

PAUA SHELL

APPEARANCE
—

Paua shell is neither rock nor mineral but organic: it is the shell of New Zealand abalone in the *Haliotidae* family. The inside of the shell shines in greens, blues, purples, and gold.

RARITY
—

Paua shell is sourced from New Zealand, where it has long been used in traditional Maori artworks. It is essential that paua shell is bought from a reputable source. There are strict catch limits on wild harvesting of paua. Beware: some paua shells may have been illegally poached and sold on the black market. Since the 1980s, sustainable and responsible paua aquaculture—for shells, meat, and pearls—has been a growing industry.

FORMATION
—

New Zealand haliotis sea snails are up to 7 in (18 cm) across. The inner surface of their shells is nacre, composed of hexagonal platelets of the mineral aragonite, a form of calcium carbonate. Nacre is iridescent because its platelets interfere with different wavelengths of light, creating different colors when seen from different angles.

ATTRIBUTES
—

Paua shell expands our consciousness. It frees us from habits of thought, allowing us to learn new skills and embrace new ideas. It also allows our spirit to break free from its earthly body, allowing us to experience lucid dreams or even astral travel. It is said that paua shell is useful for treating stress-induced headaches.

HEALING ACTION
—

Meditate with paua shell to enter a deeper and more enlightened meditative state. Wear paua shell to help with learning new skills during a course of study or in the workplace.

COMBINATIONS
—

A strong combination for students following a demanding course is paua shell and black onyx.

CARE
—

Paua shell scores around 3–3.5 on the Mohs' scale, so jewelry should be protected from knocks and scratches. Do not breathe in shell dust. Paua shell can be cleaned in warm, soapy water with a soft cloth.

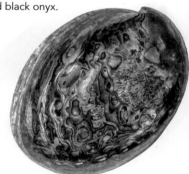

AMMOLITE

APPEARANCE

This organic gemstone may be black or gray, but displays iridescence in shades of red, orange, yellow, and green. It may also be known as *aapoak*, calcentine, and Korite (a mining company tradename).

RARITY

Ammolite is found on the eastern slopes of the Rocky Mountains in Canada and the United States. The value of an ammonite specimen is determined by its thickness, brightness, and iridescence. Most ammolite is impregnated with resin before cutting to avoid flaking.

FORMATION

Ammolite is formed of the fossilized shells of Cretaceous Period ammonites called *Placenticeras*. When they died, these cephalopods sank to the bottom of the Western Interior Seaway, which bordered the Rocky Mountains. After being covered by sediment, the shells fossilized.

ATTRIBUTES

Ammolite aids emotional health and healing. It is helpful for those who have suffered trauma or loss, particularly during childhood. Ammolite helps us to express our hurt, to feel comforted, and to begin to grow. Some say that it can improve energy levels after illness or intense exertion.

HEALING ACTION

During times of intense emotional stress, meditate with ammonite to find relief and comfort. Place at the throat chakra for the ability to express repressed feelings. Display ammolite in the self-cultivation corner of the home, which is to the left of the front door.

COMBINATIONS

To overcome trauma inflicted in past lives, combine with jet.

CARE

Scoring 3.5–4.5 on the Mohs' scale, ammolite can be used in earrings, pendants, and brooches, rather than in rings. Do not use in gem elixirs, as it may be toxic. Clean in warm, soapy water with a soft cloth.

TIGER'S EYE

APPEARANCE

Tiger's eye is red-brown to gold and displays chatoyancy, often called a cat's-eye effect. It has a silky luster.

RARITY

Tiger's eye is usually cut into cabochons to show off its chatoyancy. Jewelers who cut and grind tiger's eye must take precautions as its amphibole fibers include asbestos. Tiger's eye is sourced around the world, including from Australia, Myanmar, Namibia, South Africa, and the United States.

FORMATION

Tiger's eye is formed of chalcedony (a combination of the silica minerals quartz and moganite), with embedded fibers of amphibole minerals that have mostly turned to limonite, an iron ore. It is these fibers that create the cat's-eye effect as they reflect the light.

ATTRIBUTES

In many parts of the world, tiger's eye is believed to ward off the evil eye. It is a strongly protective crystal, keeping dark entities and curses at bay. It also gives us the strength to withstand temptation, as well as the self-confidence to weather confrontation and criticism. Tiger's eye is said to speed the mending of broken bones.

HEALING ACTION

This stone should be used under the direction of a qualified crystal therapist.

COMBINATIONS

Under the care of a qualified crystal therapist, tiger's eye may be combined with smoky quartz to give us strength and bolster our defenses.

CARE

Keep tiger's eye away from children and pets. Tiger's eye contains silicon and asbestos. Asbestos fibers cause lung cancer and asbestosis. Cut and finished cabochons of tiger's eye are considered low risk to display. However, do not ingest, do not use in gem elixirs, and do not breathe in tiger's eye dust if it shatters. Handle infrequently and wash hands afterward. Tiger's eye scores 6.5–7 on the Mohs' scale. Clean in warm, soapy water with a soft cloth.

ALEXANDRITE

APPEARANCE
—

This variety of chrysoberyl is strongly pleochroic, appearing different colors when viewed at different angles or in different lights. In daylight, a top-quality crystal appears emerald-green, but it appears red to purple when viewed in incandescent light.

RARITY
—

Crystals that show intense color change are rare and sought after, taking a high price. Some specimens are grown in laboratories. Natural alexandrite is sourced from Russia, India, Sri Lanka, Madagascar, Tanzania, and Brazil.

FORMATION
—

Chrysoberyl is composed of beryllium, aluminum, and oxygen atoms. It forms in igneous rocks called pegmatites, which formed by slow crystallization at high temperatures. Alexandrite's color change results from some replacement of aluminum by chromium, which causes intense absorption of yellow light. Since our vision is most sensitive to green light, alexandrite appears green in daylight, which contains the full spectrum of visible light, and red in incandescent light, which emits less green light.

ATTRIBUTES
—

Alexandrite enhances creativity, intuition, and empathy. It helps us to be flexible and sensitive, responding to different people and situations with delicacy and diplomacy. Some crystal therapists say that it purifies the blood and strengthens blood vessels, but there is no scientific proof of this claim.

HEALING ACTION
—

Place chrysoberyl on the crown chakra to encourage creativity. When placed at the higher heart chakra, it enhances empathy and compassion. Wear alexandrite jewelry to show charm and kindness in social situations.

COMBINATIONS
—

If engaged in a creative project, meditate with alexandrite and anyolite.

CARE
—

Alexandrite is extremely hard, scoring 8.5 on the Mohs' scale. Clean in warm, soapy water with a soft cloth.

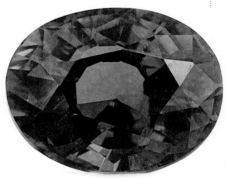

RAINBOW FLUORITE

APPEARANCE
—

Transparent to translucent, rainbow fluorite features bands or zones of green, turquoise, blue, and purple. It is found in cubes, octahedrons, columns, and masses. Many crystals fluoresce (a phenomenon named after the mineral) in ultraviolet light.

RARITY
—

Fluorite is an extremely common mineral, but gem-grade specimens of rainbow fluorite may be priced as semiprecious stones. It is popular among mineral collectors.

FORMATION
—

Fluorite commonly forms in felsic igneous rocks, which are rich in lighter elements. It is composed of calcium and fluorine. Pure fluorite is colorless, but impurities—usually caused by variations in hydrothermal fluid—can tint it any shade.

ATTRIBUTES
—

All varieties of fluorite help us to make positive changes in our lives. Rainbow fluorite helps us to find much-needed balance in our hectic lives. It allows us to balance work and home, love and friendship, intellect and senses.

HEALING ACTION
—

If you are feeling burned out by work or caring for loved ones, meditate with rainbow fluorite. Place on the desk as a constant reminder that there is more to life than the next deadline. Place in the center of the home to bring together all its different people and pursuits.

COMBINATIONS
—

If you are concerned by your work–life balance, build a grid with rainbow fluorite, clear-sighted obsidian, and transformative charoite.

CARE
—

Fluorite scores just 4 on the Mohs' scale, so take care when wearing fluorite jewelry. Fluorite is not water safe, so clean with a dry cloth if necessary. It is toxic, too, so do not use in gem elixirs and do not ingest. Do not expose to acids.

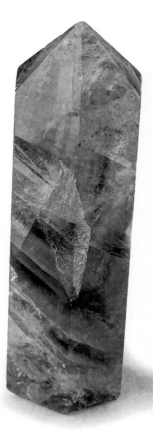

AMETRINE

APPEARANCE
—

Ametrine, also known as trystine or bolivianite, is a combination of amethyst and citrine, which are both tinted varieties of quartz. While citrine ranges from yellow to orange to brown, amethyst is lavender to deep purple. Citrine grows as six-sided prisms and also inside geodes, which are hollow, spherical rocks.

RARITY
—

Natural ametrine is rare, found only in Bolivia. Lower-priced ametrine specimens may be artificial, formed either from partially irradiated citrine or from differentially heat-treated amethyst.

FORMATION
—

Pure quartz is made purely of silicon and oxygen atoms. Both citrine and amethyst contain traces of iron, with citrine containing oxidized iron and amethyst containing non-oxidized iron. The different oxidation states occur when there are variations in temperature across the crystal as it grows.

ATTRIBUTES
—

This combination crystal combines the best of both amethyst and citrine. While amethyst calms and balances, citrine clears the mind. Ametrine is ideal for those suffering from burnout, anxiety, and stress. It also encourages us to seek harmony and agreement with others.

HEALING ACTION
—

Meditate with ametrine at times when familial relationships or friendships are stormy. Wear ametrine as a pendant to calm and soothe in the workplace or when faced with challenging people and intolerance. Sleep with an ametrine geode by the bed to aid an unbroken night's sleep.

COMBINATIONS
—

To restore trust in a relationship that has tested your loyalty, meditate with ametrine and rose quartz.

CARE
—

Ametrine scores 7 on the Mohs' scale. Wash in soapy water with a soft cloth. Do not inhale ametrine dust, which can cause silicosis.

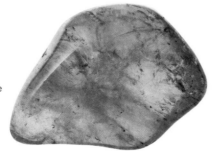

WATERMELON TOURMALINE

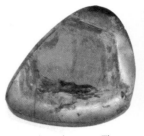

APPEARANCE
—

This variety of tourmaline has zones of both pink and green. The most prized specimens have an outer layer of green, with pink nestled inside, as in the fruit. Translucent to opaque, tourmaline grows in columnar, radiating, or needle-shaped forms, often triangular in cross section.

RARITY
—

Watermelon tourmaline is highly prized for gems and mineral collections. The more closely the colors match the shade of real watermelon, the higher the price. Watermelon tourmaline is often sourced from Brazil, Madagascar, Nigeria, Afghanistan, and the United States. Cut gemstones with distinctly different color zones are known as parti-color gems. Zoned gems may have less clarity in the color-change area.

FORMATION
—

Tourmaline grows in metamorphic rocks such as schist and marble. Tourmaline is a complicated silicate mineral, containing a high number of elements, including aluminum, boron, iron, lithium, magnesium, potassium, and sodium. Even small changes in the mineral structure result in a dazzling array of colors. Changing conditions during tourmaline crystal growth result in bicolored crystals.

ATTRIBUTES
—

Like all tourmalines, this variety offers spiritual protection. It also combines the attributes of pink and green tourmaline. While pink tourmaline encourages love, trust, and generosity, green tourmaline encourages cooperation and awareness. These qualities make watermelon tourmaline an extraordinarily nurturing and positive stone.

HEALING ACTION
—

Watermelon tourmaline is an ideal gift for someone who works with others—in a caring profession, such as teaching or nursing, or in a creative role, such as acting. Meditate with this crystal to strengthen your bonds with others.

COMBINATIONS
—

Combine with sunstone to strengthen a parent–child relationship by engaging love, trust, and good communication.

CARE
—

Tourmaline rates 7–7.5 on the Mohs' scale. Clean in warm, soapy water with a soft cloth.

MARBLE

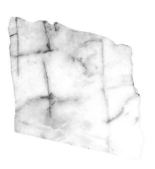

APPEARANCE
—

This rock is often white with dark, swirling patterns, but is also commonly green, pink, bluish-gray, or black. It is fine-grained and translucent when cut into thin slices, and can be polished to a high shine.

RARITY
—

Marble is sought after for flooring, carvings, and artworks. Notable sources include Turkey, Italy, and Greece.

FORMATION
—

Marble is a metamorphic rock that is usually created when limestone or dolomite rock is subjected to extreme heat and pressure. Pure limestone forms white marble, but impurities in the limestone, such as clay or sand, create dark swirls. More widespread impurities, including iron oxides or magnesium, result in a range of colors.

ATTRIBUTES
—

This rock brings strength and self-control. It gives us the fortitude to withstand emotional knocks and challenges. It also aids physical training by helping with mental and physical stamina. It helps with our ability to enter a deep meditative state. Some crystal therapists say that marble is useful for balancing body systems.

HEALING ACTION
—

Meditate with marble to block out external stimuli and enhance the depth of meditation. Place marble nearby during workouts and training to improve focus and the will to succeed. Place on the root chakra to boost self-control and emotional strength.

COMBINATIONS
—

To build the willpower to break free from problem habits, from emotional eating to social media addiction, meditate with marble and aegirine.

CARE
—

Marble scores 3–5 on the Mohs' scale, so can be fairly easily chipped. Do not ingest, as marble reacts with acids, including possibly stomach acid. Do not use acidic cleaning products. Marble left outdoors may slowly by damaged by acid rain. Clean with a specialist stone cleaner or wipe with a wet, soapy cloth.

JASPILLITE

APPEARANCE
—

Also known as jasper taconite, this rock displays swirling bands of red with gray to black rings.

RARITY
—

Used as an ornamental stone, jaspillite is most often sourced from Brazil, Canada, Ukraine, and the United States.

FORMATION
—

A sedimentary rock, jaspillite is usually composed of bands of chert (a sedimentary rock composed of tiny crystals of quartz) and iron ore, either hematite or magnetite. It formed on the ancient seabed, as a result of cyclic oxygenation of seawater by cyanobacteria. The oxygen combined with dissolved iron in the water to form iron oxides, which formed thin layers on the seabed.

ATTRIBUTES
—

Jaspillite helps to separate dreams from reality. It is a deeply grounding rock that keeps our feet on the ground and helps us to focus on the here and now. It also stabilizes our energy fields. Some say that it ameliorates anemia, although there is no scientific proof of this claim.

HEALING ACTION
—

Place on the root chakra to feel grounded, secure, and peaceful. Pass over each chakra in turn, working upward from the earth, to balance energy fields. To generate positive, comforting energy, position jaspillite at the very center of the home.

COMBINATIONS
—

When feeling spaced out or emotionally lost, a grounding grid can be built with jaspillite, black tourmaline, shungite, and smoky quartz.

CARE
—

Jaspillite scores 5–6 on the Mohs' scale. Do not ingest, use in gem elixirs, or inhale dust. Do not soak. Wipe clean with a wet, soapy cloth, rinse, then dry thoroughly.

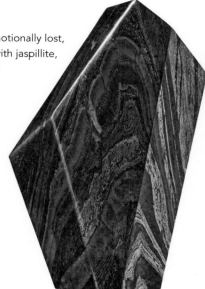

SARDONYX

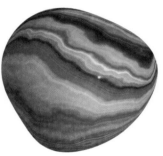

APPEARANCE
—

Sardonyx is a variety of onyx with parallel bands of translucent red and orange.

RARITY
—

This semiprecious stone is widely available worldwide, with sources including India, Brazil, and the United States. It is often bought as tumbled stones or cabochons. Ensure that any sardonyx you buy has not been artificially colored.

FORMATION
—

Sardonyx is a form of chalcedony, a cryptocrystalline (with microscopically small crystals) blend of the silicate minerals quartz and moganite. The colored bands are created as fluid with differing amounts of dissolved iron, which crystallizes over time.

ATTRIBUTES
—

This stone helps us to find willpower in matters of the heart. When loyalty to a partner or friendship is wavering, sardonyx can help us find the strength to stay true. It brings stability to marriages, families, and working relationships. Some say that sardonyx helps strengthen the cardiovascular system.

HEALING ACTION
—

Wear sardonyx in a ring as a constant reminder of the importance of loved ones. Place a sardonyx wind chime outside your door to welcome all friendly visitors. If traveling far from home, take a moment every day to meditate with this comforting, revitalizing stone.

COMBINATIONS
—

Use with shungite to help with making the virtuous choice when it seems most difficult. Meditate with red jade and sardonyx to release anger and reinforce love toward a loved one who has hurt us.

CARE
—

With a hardness of 6.5–7 on the Mohs' scale, sardonyx is durable provided it is not scratched by harder minerals or dropped. Do not inhale onyx dust, which can cause silicosis. Clean with warm, soapy water and a soft cloth.

PETRIFIED WOOD

APPEARANCE
—

Petrified wood is ancient wood that has been turned to stone ("*petro*" in Latin). It has a glassy shine and may display a range of colors, including red, yellow, and blue-gray.

RARITY
—

Petrified wood is found in numerous locations worldwide, with particularly famous "petrified forests" in Arizona, California, Argentina, and Greece. Petrified wood must not be taken from state or national parks, but must be bought from a reputable supplier. Not all "petrified wood" sold online is genuine.

FORMATION
—

Thousands or millions of years ago, wood such as tree trunks was buried under sediment, then soaked with mineral-rich water. Silica minerals and mineraloids—including quartz, chalcedony, and opal—replaced all the living material in the wood.

ATTRIBUTES
—

This fossil works against anxiety and fear. It soothes nightmares and night terrors. It eases anxieties that stop us from living our lives to the full. It can also ameliorate phobias, helping us to understand their root cause and numb their terror. Some say that petrified wood aids problems with the back, including sciatica.

HEALING ACTION
—

Meditate with petrified wood when you need to confront "irrational" fears, from public speaking to spiders. Petrified wood may aid the work of a professional therapist in treating phobias.

COMBINATIONS
—

Petrified wood and moonstone are an ideal combination for calming troubled sleep.

CARE
—

Petrified wood scores 7 on the Mohs' scale. Do not breathe in its silica-rich dust, which could cause silicosis. Do not ingest and do not use in gem elixirs. Wash hands after touching. Clean in warm, soapy water with a soft cloth.

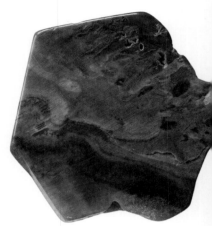

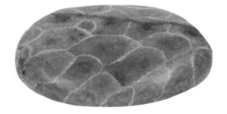

FOSSILIZED CORAL

APPEARANCE
—
Fossilized coral is often found as a pebble-shaped rock that shows the mottled pattern of ancient coral. When the coral creates a hexagonal pattern, revealing that the original coral was rugose Hexagonaria, the fossil is known as a Petoskey stone (pictured).

RARITY
—
Although these fossils are relatively rare, they are well known in particular localities of the United States, including Michigan, where Petoskey stone is the state stone. Always buy fossils from a reputable supplier.

FORMATION
—
Corals are invertebrate animals. The oldest-known fossils date back around 500 million years. Ancient coral may be preserved in the sedimentary rock, limestone. Pebbles were usually plucked from the bedrock by glaciers, then tumbled smooth, before being left on beaches and in sand dunes.

ATTRIBUTES
—
Fossilized coral can help us to collaborate, both in the workplace and during leisure time. It helps us to make and keep friends. It is also a powerful stone for helping to rebuild bridges with estranged family members or old friends. It is also said to treat disorders of the joints, such as arthritis.

HEALING ACTION
—
Meditate with this fossil if you want to reconnect with an estranged sibling or parent: its promptings will bring the humility, empathy, and strength to do what is needed. Position fossilized coral in the family area of the home, midway through the left side of the house, to encourage good communication and cooperation.

COMBINATIONS
—
Fossilized coral and loving pink tourmaline make a strong combination for taking the first step to overcoming estrangement from a parent or child.

CARE
—
These fossils score 3–4 on the Mohs' scale, so they should be handled carefully. They can be cleaned in warm, soapy water.

ORBICULAR JASPER

APPEARANCE
—
This opaque stone holds circular or spherical inclusions. When the inclusions have jagged edges, it is known as brecciated jasper.

RARITY
—
Beautiful, patterned specimens of orbicular jasper are priced as ornamental stones or semiprecious stones. Depending on provenance, orbicular jasper may be known as poppy jasper (usually from California) or ocean jasper (from Madagascar).

FORMATION
—
Jasper is a mixture of quartz and chalcedony, which is itself composed of fine intergrowths of quartz and moganite. Both these minerals are composed of silicon and oxygen atoms but have different molecular structures. Jasper often forms where fine, soft sediments are cemented by silicon dioxide. When inclusions diffuse from a central point, the orbicular pattern is created. Brecciated jasper is formed when fragmented rock is cemented.

ATTRIBUTES
—
While jasper is supportive and protective, orbicular and brecciated jaspers are particularly nurturing of family bonds. It also supports kinships other than through blood, from friendship groups to workplaces and clubs. Some crystal therapists use orbicular jasper for disorders of the digestive system.

HEALING ACTION
—
Place orbicular jasper in the workplace or classroom to draw people together as a team working toward a common goal. At home, position this stone in the family corner of the house, which is on the center left if you enter by the front door. Meditate with orbicular jasper when family relationships are fraying.

COMBINATIONS
—
Combine with blue obsidian to encourage honest and open discussion between family or friends.

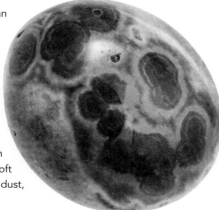

CARE
—
Jasper scores 6.5–7 on the Mohs' scale. Clean with warm, soapy water and a soft cloth. Do not inhale jasper dust, which can cause silicosis.

PICTURE JASPER

APPEARANCE

—

This variety of jasper contains patterns, such as bands, that create pictures, from landscapes to cloudy skies.

RARITY

—

Picture jaspers are found worldwide, often with different names from different localities, such as Idaho's Bruneau jasper or Indonesia's Purbalingga. Note that other striped or banded stones may sometimes be offered as picture jasper.

FORMATION

—

Bands form in jasper's silicon dioxide where sediment has been laid down in layers or by the flow of hydrothermal fluid. Other patterns are created by diffusion.

ATTRIBUTES

—

It is key when buying a picture jasper to choose a stone with a picture that speaks to you. Picture jasper nurtures our dreams and life goals. A picture that suggests rolling hills and cloudy skies will draw you nearer to a dream of living a more self-sufficient and healthy life. A picture that suggests bright activity and bursts of energy will draw you to a life of incident and excitement. Some crystal therapists say that picture jasper can help revitalize the body after a long illness.

HEALING ACTION

—

To see a path toward the life you wish to lead, meditate with your chosen picture jasper at the third eye chakra. Place your jasper on your desk or on a safe shelf in the kitchen to remind yourself of your goals.

COMBINATIONS

—

When your dream seems farthest from your grasp, meditate with picture jasper and practical sphalerite.

CARE

—

Jasper is fairly hard, scoring 6.5–7 on the Mohs' scale. Do not inhale its dust, which can cause silicosis. Clean with warm, soapy water and a soft cloth.

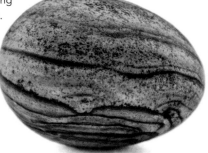

MOOKAITE

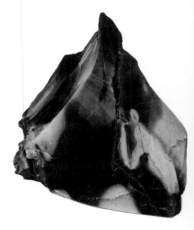

APPEARANCE

—

Mookaite exhibits flame-like patterns and colors, from cream and yellow through orange to brown and purple. It is opaque and often found in sharp-edged chunks.

RARITY

—

Often called mookaite jasper because of its silicon dioxide content, this rock is sourced only from the Windalia Radiolarite Formation, in Western Australia. It can be bought as chunks, cabochons, or carvings. Mookaite is named after the Mooka Station on which it was first found.

FORMATION

—

Mookaite is a type of sedimentary rock known as radiolarian chert. It was formed from the remains of tiny protozoa called radiolarians, cemented together by silica-rich ooze. Changing sediment influx—with waves of clay and carbonates—creates the rock's flame-like patterns.

ATTRIBUTES

—

Sharp-edged and flame-like, mookaite is a passionate and incisive rock. It gives a burst of sensuous vitality to romantic relationships. It helps us to cut through unimportant details to get to the crux of any matter, whether it is a work problem or a family dispute. Some say that mookaite can speed the healing of wounds and strengthen the immune system.

HEALING ACTION

—

To reawaken passion in a romantic relationship, place mookaite in the bedroom or in the love and marriage corner of the home, which is at the back right if you enter by the front door. Place on the root chakra, the source of our sexual energy.

COMBINATIONS

—

Combine mookaite and black obsidian for insight into a problem that seems unbearably convoluted or insolvable.

CARE

—

Mookaite scores 6–7 on the Mohs' scale. Do not inhale its dust, which can cause silicosis. Clean with warm, soapy water and a soft cloth.

FIRE AGATE

APPEARANCE
—

This variety of agate contains bands or zones of orange to red. The translucent stone displays flashes of internal "fire," or iridescent rainbows of colors.

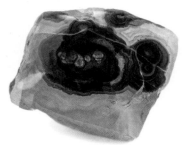

RARITY
—

Fire agate is found only in Mexico and the southwestern United States. All known fire agates formed 36–24 million years ago when this region saw high volcanic activity.

FORMATION
—

Agate is a translucent form of quartz and chalcedony, which is made of tiny intergrowths of quartz and moganite. These minerals are composed of silicon and oxygen, but have different molecular structures. Fire agates were formed when a hot solution of silica and iron oxide filled small voids in the surrounding volcanic rock, then slowly crystallized in layers. Alternating silica and red iron oxide layers diffract the light, creating an effect similar to opalescence.

ATTRIBUTES
—

All forms of agate heighten vision, concentration, and memory. Fire agate is also a deeply energizing stone, giving us the strength, power, and courage to act on our insights. It encourages us to turn dreams into reality; memories of past failures into the determination to succeed. Some say that fire agate heals the stomach, when applied externally.

HEALING ACTION
—

Position at the root chakra to stimulate conviction and self-belief. When you meet with disappointment or lost opportunity, meditate with fire agate for the insight and strength to create new opportunities.

COMBINATIONS
—

To turn pessimism into optimism, build a glowing, golden grid with fire agate, amber, golden topaz, and sunstone.

CARE
—

Fire agate scores 5–7 on the Mohs' scale. Clean with warm, soapy water and a soft cloth. Dry thoroughly. Do not inhale dust from agate, which can cause silicosis.

TURRITELLA AGATE

APPEARANCE
—

This rock contains the fossilized shells of ancient snails. While the shells are creamy, the translucent to opaque matrix is brown to black.

RARITY
—

The popular collector's item and gem known as Turritella agate is actually a chalcedony-rich sedimentary rock containing *Elimia tenera* freshwater snail shells (originally mistaken for *Turritella* sea snails). It is found in Wyoming. Agate containing true *Turritella* fossils has been found in Texas and California.

FORMATION
—

About 50 million years ago, snail shells were deposited in shallow lakes, then overlaid with sediment. Dissolved silica in the groundwater crystallized in the cavities of the snail shells and the spaces between them.

ATTRIBUTES
—

Turritella agate is a powerful stimulator of memory, both the practical memory that allows us to pass exams or master musical instruments and the emotional memory that makes us who we are. This agate allows us to access memories of past lives. It is said that this variety of agate is beneficial to bones and joints.

HEALING ACTION
—

When revising for exams or learning lines for performances, wear Turritella as a pendant or place on your desk. Place this agate on the third eye chakra when trying to awaken memories of this life, but place on the higher chakras when working with past lives.

COMBINATIONS
—

If searching for the memories of past lives, combine this agate with jet.

CARE
—

Turritella agate is durable, scoring 6.5–7 on the Mohs' scale, but should be cleaned with a damp cloth after handling or wearing. Do not inhale dust from agate. Do not use in gem elixirs.

CONDOR AGATE

APPEARANCE
—

Condor agate displays bands of bright primary colors. The agate's priming layer can often be seen surrounding the translucent stone. This was the first layer deposited on the cavity walls as the agate started to form.

RARITY
—

This variety of agate is found only in the mountains near the city of San Rafael, in western Argentina. In 1993, a plentiful supply of condor agate was discovered for surface collection. Today, the agate must be mined, resulting in higher prices.

FORMATION
—

This agate formed as nodules within extrusive igneous rock. Cavities in the lava were filled with silica-rich fluid, which formed solid layers as it crystalized on the walls then worked its way inward. Variations in the solution and conditions created the bands of vibrant shades.

ATTRIBUTES
—

Condor agate offers immense creativity and intellectual versatility. It encourages us to take leaps of thought, to think of new forms of expression, and to dream of new methods and possibilities. Some crystal therapists use condor agate for cleansing the lymphatic system.

HEALING ACTION
—

This stone is an ideal gift for an artist, author, or anyone who works in a creative field, either professionally or in their spare time. Place condor agate in the creativity corner of the home, which is on the right and midway through the house if you enter by the front door.

COMBINATIONS
—

If you or a loved one are pursuing a demanding course of study, combine condor agate with aquamarine to stimulate the intellect and faculties for creative thinking.

CARE
—

Like other forms of agate, condor agate scores 6.5–7 on the Mohs' scale. Wash in warm, soapy water with a soft cloth. Do not inhale dust from agate.

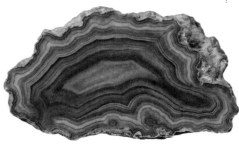

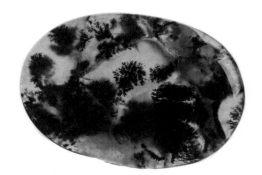

TREE AGATE

APPEARANCE
—

Also known as dendritic agate, this agate displays dark, branching patterns in a white or colorless translucent matrix.

RARITY
—

Tree agate is often sourced in Brazil, Iceland, India, Morocco, and the United States.

FORMATION
—

The branching patterns in this variety of agate were formed by inclusions of manganese or iron oxide in the silica matrix. As with other forms of agate, this matrix is composed of quartz and moganite, types of silicon dioxide with different molecular frameworks.

ATTRIBUTES
—

This form of agate has particular resonance with activities such as gardening, farming, forestry, and conservation. As with other forms of agate, tree agate stimulates the vision and intellect—but in this case, the agate works on our ability to understand the natural cycles of plants and how our own actions, both positive and negative, can affect them. This variety of agate is said to help with neuralgia, although there is no scientific proof of this claim.

HEALING ACTION
—

Meditate with tree agate to open your heart and mind to the natural world. Place this powerfully grounding stone at the earth chakra. Tree agate is an ideal purchase for any gardener, farmer, or eco-activist.

COMBINATIONS
—

If you are longing for a greener, healthier lifestyle, meditate with tektite and tree agate to find the way forward.

CARE
—

This agate scores 6.5–7 on the Mohs' scale. Do not inhale dust from agate. Wash in warm, soapy water with a soft cloth.

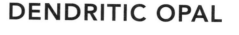

POLYHEDROID AGATE

APPEARANCE
—

This agate is shaped in polyhedrons, or three-dimensional shapes with straight edges and sharp corners. When sliced, the agate's internal banding is in the form of concentric polygons.

RARITY
—

An extremely rare form, polyhedroid agate is sourced only from one location, in Paraiba, Brazil. Since there is a limited supply, specimens take a high price.

FORMATION
—

Many mineralogists believe that this agate grew in the polyhedral spaces between other straight-edged crystals, such as calcite, that later dissolved.

ATTRIBUTES
—

Polyhedroid agate, like other forms of agate, enhances our intellects, memories, and insights. This form has particular resonance with finance, business, and academic studies. It is particularly powerful when invoked during decision-making, as it helps us to consider the causes and effects of our decisions. It is said to help with skin disorders.

HEALING ACTION
—

Place on your desk to offer support with calculations and planning. Position in the wealth and prosperity corner of the home, which is in the back right if you enter by the front door. Meditate with polyhedroid agate when you need to think a decision through to every possible conclusion.

COMBINATIONS
—

To encourage success in a business venture, build a grid with practical and clear-thinking carnelian and red jasper.

CARE
—

Like other forms of agate, this crystal scores 6.5–7 on the Mohs' scale. Do not inhale dust from agate. Wash in warm, soapy water with a soft cloth.

DENDRITIC OPAL

APPEARANCE
—

Often called merlinite, this form of common opal (see page 75) does not usually display iridescence but contains dark, fern-like or tree-like patterns, usually against a pale white or cream background. Dendritic opals are often found as rounded masses.

RARITY
—

These opals are found in many locations, including Australia, Brazil, Guatemala, Honduras, Indonesia, Japan, Mexico, and the United States. They take a lower price than precious opals (see page 137). However, dendritic opals are difficult to work with for artisans, due to the opal's soft, watery nature and the hardness of its metallic inclusions.

FORMATION
—

The dark patterns in a dendritic opal are made of metallic oxides of manganese or iron, which grow in the mineraloid's watery silicon dioxide. Dendritic opal forms as water trickles through rocks such as sandstone and claystone, collecting particles of silicon dioxide and metallic oxides.

ATTRIBUTES
—

Dendritic opal gained the name of merlinite because it is a bringer of magic. It helps us to develop our psychic knowledge and to make contact with spirits. It is essential for shamanic journeying. It acts as a talisman, warding off negative energies and dark spirits. Some claim that dendritic opal can relieve headaches caused by stress, eye strain, or poor posture.

HEALING ACTION
—

Place on the third eye to enhance clairvoyance and clairsentience. Hold during shamanic journeying. Place at the entrance to the home to welcome all those who come to help and soothe the hearts of those who come to hinder.

COMBINATIONS
—

To facilitate contact with the angelic realm, combine with angelite. Combine with protective jet during out-of-body journeys.

CARE
—

Scoring just 5.5–6 on the Mohs' scale, dendritic opals should be handled with care. Do not expose to extremes of temperature. Never immerse in water. Opals can be cleaned with a soft cloth dipped in lukewarm, soapy water. Dry thoroughly. Do not use in gem elixirs.

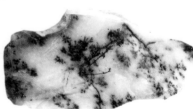

K2 STONE

APPEARANCE

—

This rock contains orbs of bright blue, up to 1 in (2.5 cm) in diameter, in a matrix of pale stone dotted with dark crystals.

RARITY

—

Named after the world's second-highest peak, this rock is sourced only from the base of K2, in the Skardu region of Pakistan's Karakoram Range. Despite its limited source, K2 stone is not highly expensive. It can be bought as tumbled stones, palm stones, cabochons, and wands.

FORMATION

—

K2 stone is a pale granite marked by spheres of the blue mineral azurite. Granite is a common igneous rock composed of quartz, plagioclase, muscovite, and biotite. Azurite stained the rock, working like a dye, after the granite had solidified from magma.

ATTRIBUTES

—

This rock combines the spiritual properties of azurite with the grounding of granite. It facilitates scrying, channeling, telepathy, and clairvoyance. It helps us to integrate spiritual perception into our everyday lives, putting wisdom to practical effect. K2 stone may also help with stress-induced headaches and stomach upsets.

HEALING ACTION

—

K2 is particularly beneficial during meditation, when holding the stone can deepen feelings of peace and acceptance. Place nearby during scrying and channeling. Hold at the third eye to enhance psychic abilities.

COMBINATIONS

—

When attempting to make contact with the realm of spirits, use with celestite.

CARE

—

This rock scores 6–7 on the Mohs' scale. Since the azurite in K2 stone contains copper, this rock should not be ingested or used in gem elixirs. Keep away from sunlight to preserve its bright blue shade. Dip in cold water to clean.

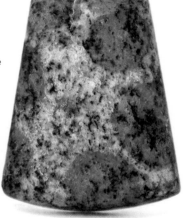

CHRYSANTHEMUM STONE

APPEARANCE

—

Chrysanthemum stone displays chrysanthemum-like flowers in milky white, against a dark gray or black background. The stone is opaque and matte.

RARITY

—

This ornamental stone is often sourced from Liuyang City, in China's Hunan Province, as well as Guangxi and Jiangxi. Japanese chrysanthemum stone comes from Gifu Prefecture. Specimens are often selectively painted or carved to enhance the flower pattern. Since source of the stone are limited, large and well-formed specimens are expensive

FORMATION

—

The pale flower of chrysanthemum stone is usually either celestite or calcite and chalcedony. The rest of the rock is carbon-rich limestone. Chrysanthemum stone formed as thick layers of organic-rich mud were heated and pressed on the seabed. Celestite (strontium sulfate) or calcite (calcium carbonate) found their way into the mix. A small crystal started to grow at the center of each flower, then further crystals grew outward—forming petals.

ATTRIBUTES

—

Chrysanthemum stone encourages us to be more empathic and less judgmental of others. It helps us to live in harmony with others, taking strength from positive relationships. Likewise, it encourages us to protect the natural world and to draw strength from nature's beauty and harmony. Chrysanthemum stone is said to treat connective tissues, including bones, muscles, ligaments, and skin.

HEALING ACTION

—

Meditate with chrysanthemum stone to open the spirit to the beauty and peace of the natural world. Display chrysanthemum stone in the family room, where its harmonious energy can be a constant source of serenity.

COMBINATIONS

—

For deep and peaceful meditation, combine with marble.

CARE

—

Chrysanthemum stone scores just 3–4 on the Mohs' scale. Do not ingest and do not use in gem elixirs. Do not soak, as some of its minerals may dissolve. It may be wiped with a damp, soft, clean cloth, then dried thoroughly.

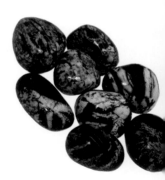

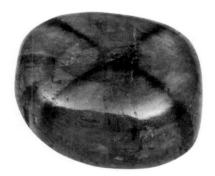

CHIASTOLITE

APPEARANCE
—
Named for the ancient Greek for "arranged crossways," this rock displays a dark cross pattern against a background that is reddish-brown, olive-green, cream, or pinkish. It is translucent to opaque.

RARITY
—
Chiastolite is found in Spain, Chile, and Russia. Tumbled stones or palm stones are inexpensive.

FORMATION
—
Chiastolite forms in metamorphic rock. It is a variety of the mineral andalusite that contains dark particles of graphite. The graphite was pushed aside by andalusite crystals as they grew, with the graphite collecting at crystal interfaces.

ATTRIBUTES
—
Chiastolite was carried by medieval pilgrims, as a protective amulet and sign of their faith. This is a highly protective stone. It also deeply resonates with both death and birth. It soothes the hearts of those moving between life and death. At the other end of life's journey, it is said to ease labor pains.

HEALING ACTION
—
Wear chiastolite jewelry as a protective talisman. Place by the bedside of a loved one who is nearing the end of their life. Hold, or place nearby, during labor. Meditate with chiastolite for comfort and reassurance at times of transition.

COMBINATIONS
—
Meditate with chiastolite and super seven quartz to be reassured by nature's eternal patterns of birth and death.

CARE
—
Scoring 5–5.5 on the Mohs' scale, chiastolite can be cleaned in warm, soapy water with a soft cloth. Do not breathe in andalusite dust.

UNAKITE

APPEARANCE
—
Unakite contains patches of mottle-pink, green, and colorless crystals.

RARITY
—
This rock is named for the Unaka Mountains of North Carolina. Outside the United States, it is also sourced from Australia, Brazil, China, and South Africa. Good-quality unakite is used for beads, cabochons, and artworks.

FORMATION
—
Unakite contains crystals of pink orthoclase feldspar, green epidote, and colorless quartz. It forms when the igneous rock granite is altered by hydrothermal fluid. The dominant mineral in the granite, plagioclase, is changed to epidote.

ATTRIBUTES
—
This stone helps us identify the root causes of our problems, then points the way to making changes. However, this is not a cruel or uncompromising stone: It facilitates slow, incremental, positive change. It helps us to grow like a plant reaching for the light. It is also said to be very beneficial for hair growth, healing wounds, and recovering from illness.

HEALING ACTION
—
Meditate with unakite when you are troubled and unsure how to proceed. Place in the knowledge and self-cultivation corner of the house, which is to the left of the front door. To examine close relationships with empathy and insight, place on the higher heart chakra.

COMBINATIONS
—
When you are troubled by conflict in the workplace, combine with gray kyanite.

CARE
—
Do not use in gem elixirs, as unakite may react dangerously with stomach acid. Do not inhale unakite dust. Clean in warm, soapy water with a soft cloth. Unakite scores 6–7 on the Mohs' scale.

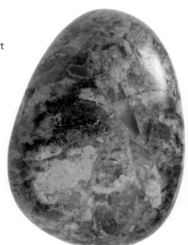

BIRD'S EYE RHYOLITE

APPEARANCE
—

This pale rock is patterned by eye-like circles of pink, orange, brown, and burgundy. Dark lines pattern the rock, giving it the appearance of an abstract work of art.

RARITY
—

This form of rhyolite is frequently sourced from Mexico. It may be mistakenly described as bird's eye jasper. It is cut into jewelry inlays, cabochons, beads, and palm stones.

FORMATION
—

Rhyolite is an extrusive igneous rock, formed of cooled lava rich in silica and low in iron and magnesium. The eye-like circles are the result of mineral inclusions that crystallized in radial aggregates. Natural fissures formed as the rock cooled, then were filled with iron ores.

ATTRIBUTES
—

This is a powerful stone for vision, both spiritual and creative. It aids clairvoyance, lucid dreaming, and scrying. It also helps artists, designers, decorators, gardeners, and anyone else who tries to create visual beauty. It is said to aid eye complaints, from conjunctivitis to eye strain.

HEALING ACTION
—

Rub gently during scrying to enhance visions. Place in the workroom, or wherever you are conceiving an artistic project, to awaken creativity and free the mind to conceive new forms.

COMBINATIONS
—

Gardeners will find that bird's eye rhyolite and black tourmaline make a creative and nurturing combination.

CARE
—

Rhyolite scores 6–6.5 on the Mohs' scale. Do not breathe in its silica-rich dust, which could cause silicosis. Wash in warm, soapy water with a soft cloth, then dry thoroughly.

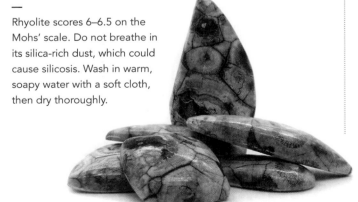

SNOWFLAKE OBSIDIAN

APPEARANCE
—

This variety of the volcanic glass is marked with white snowflake-like patterns. Snowflake obsidian is often found as small, tumbled stones.

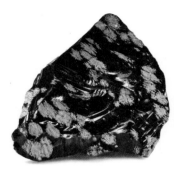

RARITY
—

Snowflake obsidian is widely available. It is sourced in areas of heavy volcanic activity, either past or present, including the western United States.

FORMATION
—

Obsidian forms when felsic lava—rich in aluminum and silicon—cools too quickly to form crystals, resulting in its glass-like texture. The snowflakes are spherulites, small, rounded bodies composed of radiating fiber-like crystals of cristobalite, a silicon dioxide.

ATTRIBUTES
—

Jet-black obsidian is an incisive, powerful stone. When speckled with snowflakes, its sometimes-caustic strength is softened. Snowflake obsidian offers clarity, along with the ability to forgive flaws, mistakes, and imperfections. It is said to treat the veins and improve circulation, although there is no scientific proof of that claim.

HEALING ACTION
—

Place at the root chakra to encourage self-acceptance without blindness to one's own mistakes and poor habits. Wear as a pendant if you are constantly troubled by self-doubt and self-criticism, as its quiet, soothing strength will allow you to accept your own failings and move forward.

COMBINATIONS
—

Place with amethyst to encourage love and forgiveness for the mistakes of loved ones. Try meditating with snowflake obsidian and smoky quartz if you are suffering from writer's block caused by self-doubt.

CARE
—

With a hardness of 5–6 on the Mohs' scale, obsidian is prone to conchoidal fractures. Do not use in gem elixirs or breathe in dust, which may cause silicosis. It can be cleaned in warm, soapy water with a soft cloth.

CALLIGRAPHY STONE

APPEARANCE
—

Also known as miriam stone, elephant skin jasper, and Arabic stone, this brown rock contains yellow swirls and snakes that resemble Arabic calligraphy. It is opaque and can be polished to a pleasing shine.

RARITY
—

Calligraphy stone is often sold as spheres, eggs, palm stones, carvings, and tumbled pebbles. It is usually sourced from the Himalayas.

FORMATION
—

This rock formed as the Himalayas were pressed upward by the movement of tectonic plates. The heat and pressure concreted a mixture of fossilized bivalve shells and iron-rich mud.

ATTRIBUTES
—

Calligraphy stone is a useful rock for writers, as well as anyone who needs creative inspiration for work or leisure pursuits. This rock also enhances automatic writing sessions. Some crystal therapists say that calligraphy stone is useful for reducing stress and high blood pressure, although there is no scientific proof for this claim.

HEALING ACTION
—

Gently rub a palm stone to escape writer's block and for inspiration while engaged in any creative project. Place on the table during automatic writing. Meditate with calligraphy stone to awaken creativity and to open the mind to new ideas and possibilities.

COMBINATIONS
—

Calligraphy stone and condor agate make a powerful combination for enhancing creativity.

CARE
—

Calligraphy stone scores around 3.5 on the Mohs' scale, so protect from knocks. Do not use in gem elixirs. If necessary, wipe clean with a damp, soapy cloth.

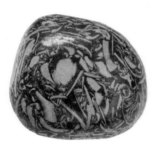

STAR SAPPHIRE

APPEARANCE
—

This type of sapphire exhibits a star-like reflection of light, known as an asterism, particularly when viewed under a single, overhead light source. Star sapphires are translucent and may be any shade apart from red, when they are known as "star rubies." The stars are usually six-rayed, although twelve rays are not unknown.

RARITY
—

Star sapphires are rare and valuable, with the color and clarity of the stone having more impact on price than the strength of the asterism. Always buy from a reputable jeweler. Be aware that the more perfect the star pattern, the less likely the gem is to be genuine. Sources include Sri Lanka, Myanmar, Cambodia, and India. Star sapphires are cut as cabochons.

FORMATION
—

Sapphires are a variety of the mineral corundum, an aluminum oxide. Corundum forms deep underground under intense heat and pressure. A whitish star pattern is usually created by intersecting needles of the mineral rutile embedded in the crystal. Needles of hematite cause a golden star.

ATTRIBUTES
—

Like other sapphires, star sapphires bring wisdom. These gems also act as a beacon, helping us to set goals—of knowledge, acceptance, or achievement—and then guiding us as we reach them. Star sapphires attract the help we need to reach those goals, whether that is knowledgeable teachers or supportive friends. Some crystal therapists say they aid the cardiovascular system.

HEALING ACTION
—

Place on the third eye chakra to enhance learning, whether academic or spiritual. Wear as jewelry to act as a constant guide and support as you strive to build a better, truer, and more spiritually fulfilling life.

COMBINATIONS
—

To support academic studies, whether your own or a family member's, build a grid with memory-enhancing Turritella agate and problem-solving white calcite.

CARE
—

Sapphire scores 9 on the Mohs' scale, so is very durable. Clean with warm, soapy water and a soft cloth.

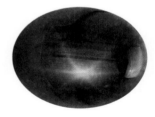

DUMORTIERITE QUARTZ

APPEARANCE
—

Dumortierite quartz is quartz that contains large quantities of dumortierite inclusions, usually making the resulting rock opaque. The rock is speckled, banded, or otherwise marked in blues and grays. The dumortierite often forms parallel, fibrous aggregates of needles, causing an almost fur-like appearance.

RARITY
—

These stones are usually sourced from Austria, France, Russia, Madagascar, or the United States. They are often shaped into round or oval cabochons.

FORMATION
—

Quartz contains silicon and oxygen, while dumortierite also contains boron and aluminum. Dumortierite is colored blue by traces of iron, zinc, and manganese. Dumortierite commonly forms as inclusions in quartz, in high-temperature metamorphic rocks and boron-rich granite.

ATTRIBUTES
—

Combining the attributes of dumortierite and high-energy quartz, this rock offers the gift of powerful speech, the ability to convince and fascinate others with our words. It enhances vocal performance, from singing to acting and public speaking. Some say that it aids ailments of the throat, such as laryngitis.

HEALING ACTION
—

Place at the throat chakra to empower speech and performance. A dumortierite quartz paperweight on a desk or in an office will encourage creative discussion or writing. Meditate with this stone if you are searching for the words to voice your needs or fears.

COMBINATIONS
—

For those with speech impediments, wearing blue agate or blue obsidian with dumortierite quartz will enhance self-confidence at times of stress.

CARE
—

This rock scores 7 on the Mohs' scale. Avoid constant direct sunlight and remove jewelry when gardening or in the sauna. Do not inhale dust. Wash in warm, soapy water with a soft cloth.

SUPER SEVEN QUARTZ

APPEARANCE
—

Also known as melody stone, super seven is composed of clear quartz, smoky quartz, and amethyst (purple quartz), which encase inclusions of four other minerals: cacoxenite, goethite, lepidocrocite, and rutile. The translucent to transparent matrix has streaks and fibrous needles of purple, red, and black.

RARITY
—

Genuine super seven is mined only from one mine in Espirito Santo, Brazil, resulting in high prices. Ensure that you buy from a reputable source.

FORMATION
—

As the quartz crystal grew, it encased the other crystals, in most cases keeping their needle-like form intact. The smoky quartz and amethyst portions of the crystal are caused by natural irradiation of traces of aluminum or iron in the crystal structure.

ATTRIBUTES
—

This high-energy, complex crystal helps us to open our minds to the contemplation of life's most difficult metaphysical questions. It offers understanding and acceptance of our place in the Universe. On a personal level, super seven encourages connection and empathy with others. It is said to powerfully reenergize the body after illness.

HEALING ACTION
—

Position at the higher chakras during meditation to further your search for enlightenment. Place at the crown chakra if you are searching for the strength to make a large change in your life, such as moving abroad or changing career. A super seven cabochon is an ideal gift for a loved one embarking on a new course of study.

COMBINATIONS
—

If spiritual growth is your quest, combine with tektite and blue obsidian.

CARE
—

The quartz matrix of super seven scores 7 on the Mohs' scale. Do not inhale quartz dust. Wash in warm, soapy water with a soft cloth.

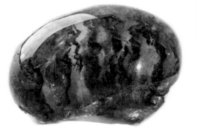

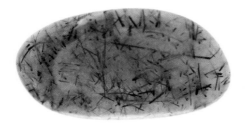

TOURMALINE QUARTZ

APPEARANCE
—

This stone is composed of clear or milky quartz encasing needles of black tourmaline.

RARITY
—

Tourmaline quartz is found worldwide. It is often purchased as tumbled, polished stones or cabochons.

FORMATION
—

Quartz is a ubiquitous silicate mineral, while closely associated tourmaline is a boron silicate. The tourmaline crystals were engulfed by the quartz as it grew.

ATTRIBUTES
—

This stone combines the grounding qualities of black tourmaline with the high energy of quartz, making it ideal for those who want to engage fully and practically with the world, particularly anyone working as a parent, teacher, doctor, or other carer. Tourmaline quartz frees us from inaction and doubt, turning negative energy to positive. It is said to be useful for detoxifying the body.

HEALING ACTION
—

Tourmaline quartz is particularly powerful for clearing blockages and dispersing negative energy. Position at any chakra to cleanse and balance. Meditate with tourmaline quartz for the strength and energy to pursue work, whether inside or outside the home, with dedication.

COMBINATIONS
—

Those who care for babies or young children will find that meditating with loving sugilite and tourmaline quartz will help to renew energy, patience, and devotion.

CARE
—

Wash in warm, soapy water as necessary. Do not inhale quartz dust. Like other varieties of quartz, this rock scores 7 on the Mohs' scale.

RUTILE QUARTZ

APPEARANCE
—

This variety of quartz contains needle-like inclusions of the mineral rutile. The needles may appear randomly scattered, aligned, or starlike. The rutile may be red, gold, silver, or black. The quartz crystals themselves usually grow as six-sided prisms ending in pyramids, as single wands, twins, or clusters.

RARITY
—

While rutile quartz is fairly common, a good-quality crystal with attractively arranged needles is priced as a semiprecious gemstone.

FORMATION
—

Rutile is titanium dioxide. It forms easily in high-temperature and high-pressure metamorphic and igneous rocks. Quartz is a common silicate mineral that often encloses other minerals without significantly altering their structure.

ATTRIBUTES
—

This gem allows us to overcome difficulties and challenges, ranging from physical feats such as mountain climbs and marathons to emotional endeavors, such as surmounting our own fears and failings. Some crystal therapists say that rutile quartz is helpful for impotence, although there is no scientific proof of this claim.

HEALING ACTION
—

Meditate with rutile quartz to enhance motivation during times of low energy and lethargy. Wear a rutile quartz pendant or earrings when courage is needed, whether that is when challenging phobias or facing up to mistakes.

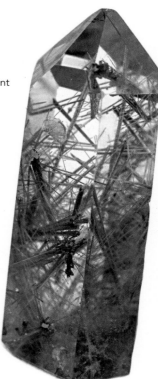

COMBINATIONS
—

In the dark of long winter nights, when energy is at a low ebb, build a grid containing rutile quartz, carnelian, amber, and sunstone.

CARE
—

This is a tough and durable stone, scoring 7 on the Mohs' scale. Do not inhale quartz dust. Wash in warm, soapy water with a soft cloth.

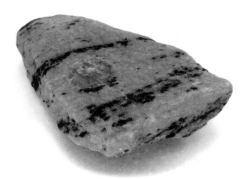

ANYOLITE

APPEARANCE
—
Anyolite is a combination stone, composed of green zoisite studded with ruby, as well as small amounts of black or dark green pargasite.

RARITY
—
This rock is mined only from limited regions in Kenya and Tanzania. It is usually sold as chunks of rough rock, polished cabochons, or small carvings.

FORMATION
—
Anyolite forms in metamorphic rocks that are rich in aluminum. While the zoisite contains atoms of silicon, aluminum, calcium, oxygen, and hydrogen, the ruby is formed from aluminum, oxygen, and chromium.

ATTRIBUTES
—
This combination stone offers the properties of zoisite combined with ruby. Zoisite is a stone of positive energy, turning negative feelings of sadness, anger, and fear to happiness and calm. Ruby motivates love, passion, and creativity. In combination, these minerals are said to heal the immune system and enhance potency.

HEALING ACTION
—
Anyolite carvings are an ideal gift for someone suffering from mild depression, creative block, or listlessness. Position anyolite at the heart chakra to encourage feelings of love. At the root chakra, anyolite engenders self-confidence and self-motivation.

COMBINATIONS
—
For those suffering from lost love, combine with lapis lazuli to encourage hope and self-belief. If you are lacking motivation, meditate with aquamarine and anyolite.

CARE
—
Anyolite scores 6–7 on the Mohs' scale. Note that the rubies in anyolite are not of gem quality and can shatter. Do not inhale dust. Wash in warm, soapy water with a soft cloth.

BLOODSTONE

APPEARANCE
—
Also called heliotrope, bloodstone is a mineral aggregate consisting of a green matrix studded with red speckles that resemble drops of blood. It is usually opaque and found as tumbled stones.

RARITY
—
Bloodstone is found in numerous locations across the globe, from Scotland's Isle of Rum to Western Australia.

FORMATION
—
Bloodstone is a green variety of chalcedony, with inclusions of red hematite, which is iron oxide. Chalcedony is composed of fine intergrowths of the silicon dioxide minerals quartz and moganite, which are differentiated by their crystal structures at the microscopic level.

ATTRIBUTES
—
Bloodstone combines the qualities of green chalcedony, also known as chrysoprase, with hematite. While the chalcedony encourages lateral thinking and creativity, the hematite is grounding and realistic. It is also a particularly useful stone when trying to analyze dreams for their personal truths and meanings. Some say that bloodstone cleanses and strengthens the blood.

HEALING ACTION
—
Bloodstone is an ideal gift for someone trying to turn a creative hobby, such as pottery or writing, into a money-making business. To wake with an understanding of one's dreams, sleep with a tumbled bloodstone under the pillow.

COMBINATIONS
—
If faced with a seemingly unsolvable problem, meditate with bloodstone and a wand of black tourmaline.

CARE
—
Wash in warm, soapy water with a soft cloth. Hematite can rust if left damp. Do not inhale bloodstone dust, which can cause silicosis. Do not use in gem elixirs, as this stone may react with stomach acid. Bloodstone scores 7 on the Mohs' scale.

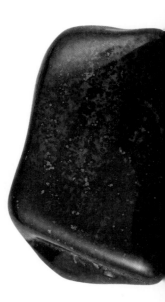

SEPTARIAN NODULE

APPEARANCE
—

The word septarian comes from the ancient Greek word *septa*, meaning "division." These nodules, which may be chunks or carved into balls, are concretions of rock with dark lines, or septa, running through them like spiders' webs.

RARITY
—

Well-known sources of septarian nodules are Madagascar; the coast near Moeraki, South Island, New Zealand; the south coast of England; and Utah. Nodules from Madagascar are sometimes known as dragon stone.

FORMATION
—

These concretions usually form in a calcium-rich clay that hardened into limestone. As the rock dried out, it shrank, creating cracks that filled with calcium-carbonate-rich water in which calcite solidified.

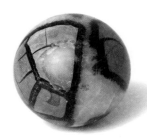

ATTRIBUTES
—

Septarian nodules help us to achieve balance. They support us in balancing conflicting demands—of family, work, hobbies, and friends. These nodules also assist with balance in the mind, emotions, and spirit. They prevent us from either being overwhelmed by our emotions or unable to acknowledge them. Some say that septarian nodules can help to balance the metabolism.

HEALING ACTION
—

If you are suffering from mood swings, place a septarian nodule at the solar plexus chakra while practicing a breathing exercise. Meditate with a nodule at times when you need to balance head and heart.

COMBINATIONS
—

When work–life balance is a problem, place a septarian nodule and a piece of uvarovite in the career area of the home, which is immediately inside the front door.

CARE
—

Depending on its exact composition, a septarian nodule scores around 3 on the Mohs' scale, so should be protected from knocks. A nodule is not soluble in pure water but is soluble in rainwater, which is slightly acidic. Do not use in gem elixirs. If cleaning is necessary, wipe with a clean, soft cloth.

ECLOGITE

APPEARANCE
—

This dense rock displays pink to red speckles against a green matrix. Sometimes blue, white, or other speckles can also be seen.

RARITY
—

This relatively rare rock occurs in locations including western North America, Italy, Norway, and Australia. Eclogite can be bought from specialist rock and mineral suppliers as chunks and tumbled stones.

FORMATION
—

Eclogite is a metamorphic rock formed when igneous rock rich in magnesium and iron is subjected to intense pressure. The green matrix is composed largely of the mineral omphacite, while the pink speckles are garnet. Other possible inclusions are blue kyanite and white quartz.

ATTRIBUTES
—

Eclogite is a grounding stone. It encourages us to reconnect with our roots, with old friends, and the place where we were born. It helps us to draw strength from ancestral spirits. It encourages us to gain satisfaction and serenity from working with our hands. Some say that it benefits the bones.

HEALING ACTION
—

If searching for the guidance and love of ancestral spirits, meditate with eclogite. Position at the root and earth chakras to combat feelings of insecurity and listlessness.

Eclogite makes an ideal gift for anyone who enjoys working with their hands, from gardeners to mechanics, carpenters, and potters.

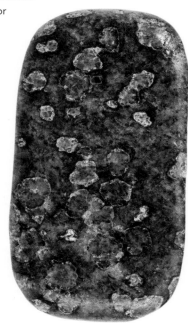

COMBINATIONS
—

To sense the promptings of ancestral spirits, work with eclogite and seraphinite.

CARE
—

Eclogite scores 7–7.5 on the Mohs' scale. It can be cleaned in warm, soapy water.

CHAROITE WITH TINAKSITE

APPEARANCE
—
Displaying psychedelic colors and swirls, this combination stone has patches of orange, purple, and white. It is translucent to opaque.

RARITY
—
Charoite–tinaksite can be bought from specialist mineral suppliers as chunks, pebbles, eggs, and palm stones. These are sourced from northern Russia. Larger specimens or artisanal work demand a higher price.

FORMATION
—
This aggregate is a combination of silicate minerals, including pale-to-orange tinaksite and purple charoite. Tinaksite is almost always found growing inside charoite. They form where limestone has been altered by the intrusion of magma.

ATTRIBUTES
—
Charoite–tinaksite is a stone of partnerships. Just as tinaksite cannot thrive alone, it helps us to focus on—and grow with—the essential partnerships in our lives, whether romantic, platonic, or business. Its positive energy helps us to work well with others, communicating honestly and kindly, while listening wisely and receptively. Some say that this aggregate benefits the kidneys.

HEALING ACTION
—
If you would like to draw positive energy into your marriage or other life partnership, place charoite–tinaksite in the love corner of the home, which is at the back right if you enter by the front door. If you would like to focus on friendships, place at the front right of the home. Place at the throat chakra to improve communication and openness.

COMBINATIONS
—
A beneficial friendship grid can be centered on tinaksite, surrounded by rhodonite, thulite, amber, and sunstone.

CARE
—
This combination scores 5–6 on the Mohs' scale. Do not inhale its dust and do not use in gem elixirs. Clean in warm, soapy water with a soft cloth.

DALMATIAN STONE

APPEARANCE
—
Sometimes called dalmatian jasper, although it is not a jasper, this is a pale, usually creamish, rock with dark black or brown markings, like the well-known dogs.

RARITY
—
Dalmatian stone is often sourced from Mexico. It can be bought as spheres, palm stones, beads, and carvings.

FORMATION
—
This igneous rock is composed primarily of pale perthite, an intergrowth of feldspar minerals. The dark speckles are the rare mineral arfvedsonite (not tourmaline, as was once widely believed).

ATTRIBUTES
—
Dalmatian stone brings out the child in us. It encourages playfulness, laughter, and joy in the moment. It helps us to be trusting, loving, and enthusiastic. Its light, quickly moving energy is useful for improving energy flow through sluggish or underused chakras. Some crystal therapists use dalmatian stone for purifying the blood.

HEALING ACTION
—
Hold over each chakra in turn to quicken energy flow and release blockages. If suffering from low mood, wear dalmatian stone jewelry to feel lighter and more joyful. Meditate with this kind and playful stone when feeling overworked, bad-tempered, or listless.

COMBINATIONS
—
If you feel that you have laughed too little recently, place a sunstone and a dalmatian stone in each pocket and take a break from work and chores—to chat with a friend, walk in the park, or watch a movie.

CARE
—
Keep dalmatian stone away from children and animals. Do not use in gem elixirs, do not inhale dust, and do not ingest. Wash hands after touching. It scores 6–6.5 on the Mohs' scale. Clean in warm, soapy water.

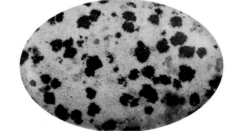

LLANITE

APPEARANCE
—

An igneous rock, llanite contains large blue and gray-to-orange crystals against a black or dark-brown, fine-grained background.

RARITY
—

Llanite is named after Llano County, in Texas, the only known occurrence of this rock. It can be bought as reasonably priced spheres and tumbled stones.

FORMATION
—

This is a porphyritic rock, which means it is made up of crystals with widely different sizes. It is a variety of the rock rhyolite that contains quartz, colored blue by ilmenite, and perthitic feldspar. The llanite formed when a rising column of super-hot magma cooled in two stages: first quickly, resulting in the very small crystals of the matrix, then more slowly, allowing time for the enlarged crystals of quartz and feldspar to grow.

ATTRIBUTES
—

This rock helps us to be emotionally stronger. It is particularly beneficial for those who have a problem saying "no" to other people's requests. It overcomes shyness and lack of self-confidence. It helps us heal after emotional shocks. Llanite is said to help crystal healers detect where there is a problem in the body.

HEALING ACTION
—

Position at the sacral chakra to build self-confidence and self-belief. Hold at the throat chakra to overcome shyness and speak up for your own needs. Meditate with llanite after an emotional blow or a loss.

COMBINATIONS
—

A strong combination for overcoming shyness is llanite and amber.

CARE
—

Llanite scores 6–6.5 on the Mohs' scale. Do not breathe in its silica-rich dust, which could cause silicosis. Wash in warm soapy water.

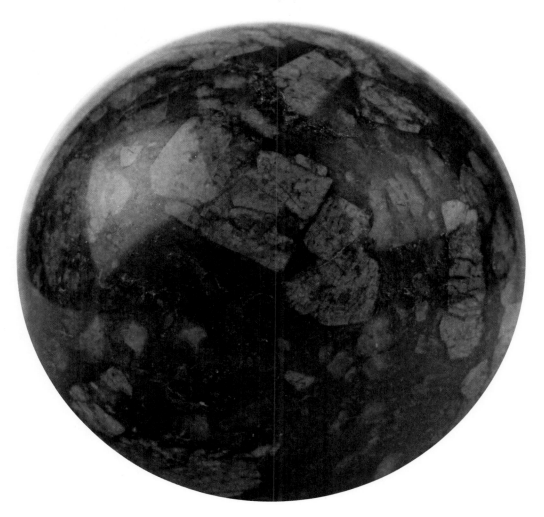

CRYSTAL
REMEDIES

PART THREE

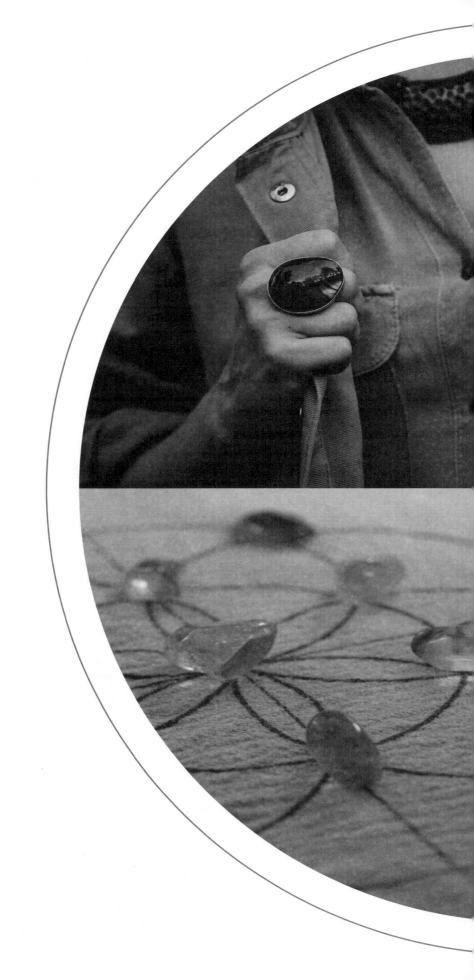

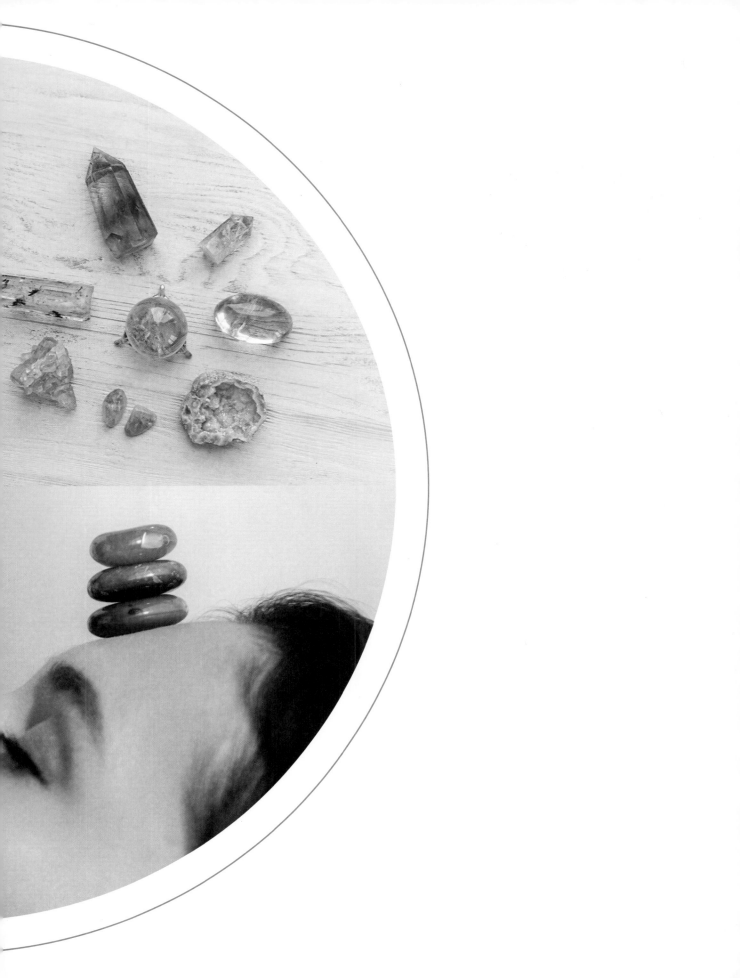

A GUIDE TO USING CRYSTAL REMEDIES

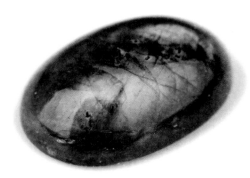

Labradorite is a powerful crystal that is understood to help with disorders of the eyes and brain, heightening perception and the unconscious.

Crystals can be used as a form of holistic healing. They're not an alternative to conventional medication—especially treatments, therapies, or medications prescribed by a doctor—but they can be used alongside it to add an extra dimension of support and healing.

Crystal remedies work in a different way to conventional medicine, focusing on subtle energies and vibrations, and working on the emotional, mental, and spiritual levels. They can be used to help balance and strengthen the chakras and the aura, which can reflect back on your physical health.

There are various ways in which you can use crystals, including:

• Placing crystals directly onto your body, at points of pain or discomfort.
• Placing crystals around your body.
• Wearing crystal jewelry.
• Creating crystal grids or layouts and using the dowsing method over them.
• Placing crystals onto or near your chakras to unblock and re-balance them.
• Making an indirect crystal gem elixir and bathing in it, spraying it around you and your aura, or putting it directly onto your skin.
• Using a crystal wand, point, or crystal egg to gently massage points on your body, such as reflexology or acupuncture points.
• Balancing crystals on your own body can be tricky, so they can be temporarily held in place using medical tape.

If you're going to try placing crystals directly onto or around your body, aim to keep them in place for a maximum of 10 to 20 minutes. The energies of crystals are all different, but some can have powerful effects, so it's important not to over-use them without professional advice and guidance. If at any time you feel uncomfortable whilst using crystals, stop immediately and remove them.

Depending on the crystals you've used, you might feel slightly spaced out or tired after using crystal remedies. If possible, take it easy and drink plenty of water to hydrate yourself. If you have any concerns about using crystals, always consult a qualified crystal therapist.

HOW TO CHOOSE THE RIGHT REMEDY FOR YOU

—

In the following pages you'll find a guide to some of the key crystals that could help with a range of common ailments. They're split into categories, such as skin and hair, bones and muscles, and mental and emotional issues, so that you can easily identify the type of condition for which you're looking for extra support. Each condition included has some of the key crystals listed, along with ways in which they could be used or chakras on which

they could be placed. Plus you'll find details of other crystals that could be used as part of grids or layouts.

Choosing the right remedy isn't always straightforward, though. Sometimes there are multiple underlying causes of symptoms—some that you're able to identify, and others you're unaware of. A headache, for example, can be caused by eyestrain, alcohol, or stress, so focusing on the underlying cause may be helpful.

When you're choosing which remedy to try, be honest with yourself and think about how it could have been caused. If your headache is down to stress, try some of the crystals that can be used to ease stress (see page 250). If you have a crystal pendulum, you could use the dowsing method to try to find the right crystal for you.

If you don't find the perfect remedy for your ailment straightaway, be patient and try again. Not every crystal works in the same way for everyone and it can be a matter of trial and error to find the right one for you. Plus, crystals work through subtle vibrations and energies and it's possible you might not immediately notice benefits, but they do become apparent at a later stage.

Crystals work in mysterious ways, so enjoy using them and letting them work their magic on you.

Learn to remain positive and open-minded when working with crystals; the results may surprise you.

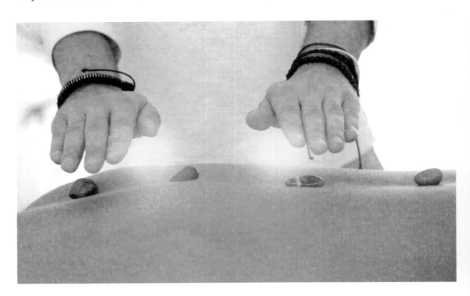

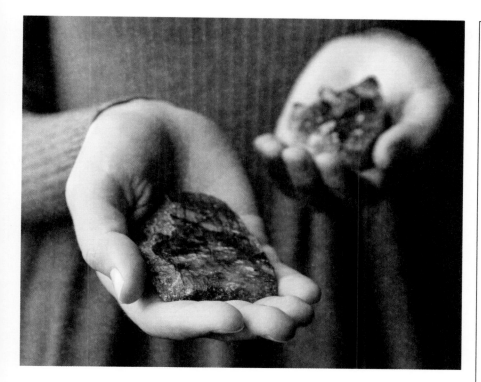

Crystals can add an extra dimension of support and healing.

WHEN TO SEEK HELP
—

Crystals are great to use in conjunction with other treatments, medications, and therapies in a holistic manner, as they can add an extra dimension to mental, spiritual, and emotional healing. But you do need to keep in mind at all times that crystals are not an alternative to conventional medicine and should never be regarded as one.

WHEN TO SEEK HELP FROM A QUALIFIED MEDICAL PRACTITIONER
—

You should always consult a qualified medical practitioner as a first port of call for any health or medical conditions. This is especially so if you:

• Experience sudden, unexpected symptoms for the first time.
• Experience new symptoms for an existing condition.
• Have an existing condition that suddenly worsens.
• Need first aid treatment.
• Are experiencing a medical emergency.
• Have sudden pain or discomfort in your chest that doesn't go away.
• Experience breathing difficulties.

• Have sudden severe pain anywhere in your body that doesn't go away.
• Suddenly lose the feeling in your arms or legs for no apparent reason.
• Suddenly develop a rash, particularly if it's red-hot, rapidly spreading, and doesn't fade if you press the side of a clear glass against the skin.

Always follow any medical advice you've been given by a medical practitioner, take medicines as prescribed and take a full course of antibiotics, even if the condition seems to improve before the end of the course of medication.

WHEN TO SEEK HELP FROM A PROFESSIONAL CRYSTAL THERAPIST
—

There are times when making contact with a professional crystal therapist or crystal healer could be beneficial. As a result of their training, they'll have more in-depth knowledge about certain crystals and could have ideas as to treatments, layouts, or grid combinations that could work effectively for you.

Some crystals are best used and handled by a professional, as they can potentially be toxic and could cause you more harm than good if you're unaware of their true properties.

DOS AND DON'TS OF USING CRYSTALS

To summarize, here are some useful dos and don'ts to keep in mind as you explore and work with healing crystals.

DO:

• Enjoy experimenting with crystals and learning about the many different types.

• Put crystals in your home, car, and workplace, as it's good to have the energies around you.

• Learn to be guided by intuition and tune into crystal vibrations when choosing and working with crystals.

• Remain positive and open-minded when working with crystals, the results may surprise you.

• Make indirect crystal gem elixirs, as they offer a safe way of harnessing the power of crystals.

• Remember to cleanse and purify your crystals after use. This keeps them in tip-top condition and ensures all negative energies are removed.

• Take care to look after delicate crystals, as some can be more fragile than others.

• Reach out for additional help and advice from a crystal therapist or medical practitioner when you need it.

DON'T:

• Use crystal remedies for serious conditions before seeing a medical practitioner.

• Use crystals as an alternative to proper first aid treatment.

• Rely on the crystals to heal all physical, mental, or emotional ailments.

• Give up—if one crystal doesn't work for you, try another one.

• Worry about the size of crystals or not being able to afford large specimens—even small stones can be powerful!

• Abandon prescribed medications or therapies in favor of only using crystals instead—they work better in harmony with other treatments, rather than as an alternative.

• Leave small crystals in accessible places if you have children or animals in your home—they should not be put in mouths or swallowed.

• Leave crystals in direct sunlight unattended—they run the risk of being a fire hazard if the direct rays of the sun shine onto them.

Do make sure that you ask a crystal therapist in advance what training and qualifications they have, plus how long they've been practicing. Some might use crystals alongside other holistic health treatments. Most professional crystal therapists will charge an hourly fee for a consultation.

HOW TO USE THIS SECTION

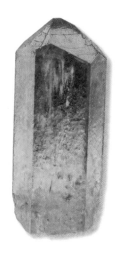

This section on getting the most from crystal remedies sets out a comprehensive reference of ailments of the mind, body, and spirit, suggesting the best crystals and methods for effective treatment.

Within each entry, there is a list of key crystals that are most effective, especially when used directly on the body. This is shown on the body layout outline on the bottom right of the page, simply and clearly instructing where the crystal is best placed. Examples of this include placing lapis lazuli directly on the forehead to treat headaches caused by stress or tiredness, amethyst placed directly on facial skin to soothe irritation from acne, green aventurine directly on the solar plexus to ease stress, and more.

Next, there is a suggested list of further crystals for use on crystal grids or for additional use. The crystal grid found on the bottom left of each entry shows where best to place the suggested crystals. Crystal grids are part of a special technique used to amplify crystals' healing powers. The grid is an arrangement of crystals in a set geometric pattern with a specific intention in mind. The grid serves to bring together crystals' individual energetic properties, which are enhanced by working together, creating an even more powerful effect. These grids are often based on sacred patterns of geometry, but you can use any patterns you feel an attachment to, and there are crystal grid templates on page 290. For further details of the best methods for setting up and activating a crystal grid, turn to page 31. Many crystal grids benefit from a clear quartz crystal for use as an amplifier. Please note that it is not necessary to include all of the suggested crystals on the grid. It's best to keep it as focused as possible, depending in part on the symptoms being treated. For beginners, the fewer crystals used on a grid, the easier it is to get the hang of the method. Additionally, some crystals are more expensive or more difficult to source. With this in mind, it's often not practical for multiple crystals to be used concurrently on a grid. Neither do you have to lay out your crystals in the exact same positions. Use your intuition and be guided to the grid pattern layout that feels right for you. The grids shown in this section are examples of how you could use some of the crystals, as an inspirational starting point.

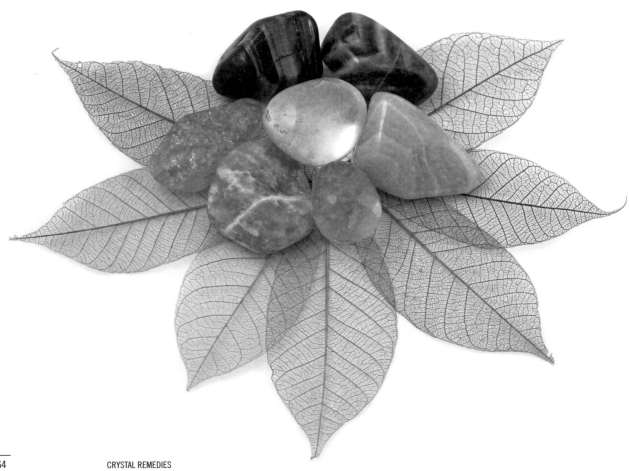

HEADACHES

Headaches are often caused by eyestrain, tiredness, stress, sinusitis, low blood sugar, alcohol, drugs, caffeine, food allergy, or poor posture—the last of which causes muscular tension in the head, neck, or shoulders. Sometimes headaches are the result of a head injury or a symptom of a more serious disorder.

There are many types of headaches, each with a different intensity, type, and duration of pain. Migraines are throbbing headaches, usually on one side of the head, caused by the narrowing of blood vessels on that side of the brain. Migraines may be a hereditary condition or can be caused by stress, hormonal changes, particular foods and medications, or changes in temperature, lighting, or noise. Cluster headaches, most often suffered by men, are short, severe attacks of pain, usually over one eye, which occur many times a day, perhaps over some months. They may be caused by a disorder in histamine metabolism.

KEY CRYSTALS

—

Lapis lazuli—Place on the forehead to draw away pain, particularly in the case of headaches caused by stress, emotional repression, or tiredness. Wear these stones as earrings if headaches are recurrent, as long as a physical cause has been ruled out by your practitioner.

Blue aventurine—For headaches caused by constriction, either as the result of sinusitis (after a bad cold) or poor posture, position blue aventurine at the site of the pain. If suffering from a lengthy migraine, sleep with blue aventurine under your pillow to reduce the duration of the episode.

OTHER GRID AND LAYOUT CRYSTALS

—

• Turquoise (for hangover headaches)
• Emerald (for eyestrain)
• Charoite (for stress)
• Amethyst (for tiredness)

ADDITIONAL THERAPIES

—

If a headache is severe, long-lasting, or recurrent, seek the advice of a qualified medical practitioner. If eyestrain is suspected as a cause, an eye test—and more frequent screen breaks—is required. Regular exercise and meditation may be of great benefit to those suffering with stress headaches. The Alexander Technique and yoga are both recommended for headaches caused by poor posture.

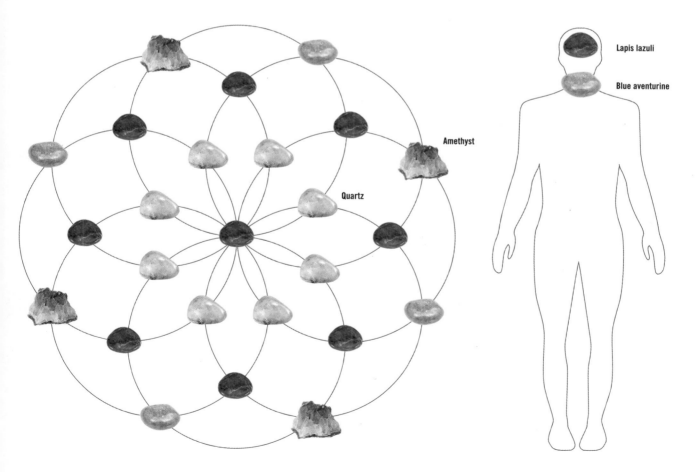

Amethyst

Quartz

Lapis lazuli

Blue aventurine

NEURALGIA

Neuralgia is the term for any pain originating in a nerve. The most common forms are trigeminal neuralgia, caused by damage to the trigeminal facial nerve and resulting in chronic one-sided facial pain; sciatica, caused by spinal nerves being trapped between vertebrae, causing pain in the back that may extend down to the foot; and post-herpetic neuralgia, caused by a previous attack of shingles that results in a burning pain at the site of the rash. In general, neuralgia is caused by damage, constriction, or infection along the route of a nerve. The pain may be intermittent or continuous.

KEY CRYSTALS
—

Quartz—Place or wear this powerful healing stone on the site of the pain. Cathedral quartz, with one tall, spire-like point surrounded by smaller, parallel points, will be particularly effective at drawing away the pain. Quartz may be of use in easing the "burning" pains associated with post-herpetic neuralgia.

Fluorite—Position at the site of the pain to draw it away and also help to rebalance and soothe the body. All varieties of fluorite will be of benefit, but clear fluorite will also amplify the healing properties of other stones and calm the mind during episodes of severe pain.

OTHER GRID AND LAYOUT CRYSTALS
—

• Amber (for pain relief)
• Chiastolite (for protecting the nerves)
• Malachite (for alignment)
• Blue calcite (for fear of pain)

ADDITIONAL THERAPIES
—

If neuralgia is suspected, seek the advice of a qualified medical practitioner to ascertain the cause and to rule out any more serious conditions. In the case of trigeminal neuralgia, an MRI scan may be necessary. If the problem is severe, medication and surgery may be recommended. Trigeminal neuralgia can also be treated by percutaneous procedures, including glycerol injection or balloon compression. Sciatica may improve with gentle stretching exercises under the care of a physical therapist, chiropractor, or osteopath.

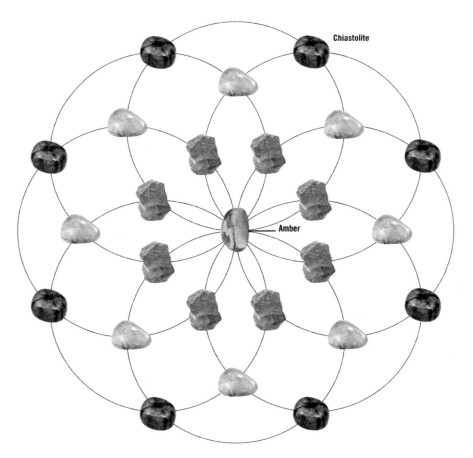

Chiastolite

Amber

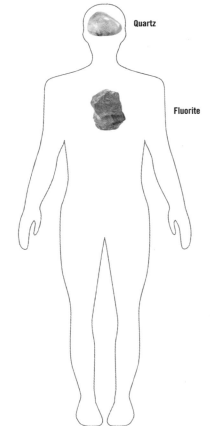

Quartz

Fluorite

LIVING WITH MULTIPLE SCLEROSIS

Multiple sclerosis (MS) is a serious lifelong condition that affects the spinal cord and the brain. It can develop at any age, but women are more likely to be affected than men. For some people it can be mild and the symptoms can be largely controlled, but for others it can cause severe disability. Symptoms of MS can vary considerably, too, but may include fatigue, muscle stiffness, spasms, problems with balance and coordination, numbness, tingling, walking problems, bladder and bowel issues, and problems with thinking. MS can be relapsing or gradually progressing.

KEY CRYSTALS
—

Rhodonite—Place rhodonite on your heart chakra to help rebalance chakras

that are out of sorts. The gentle energies of rhodonite can help release negative emotions and anger directed at long-term chronic pain and suffering and promote feelings of self-love instead. As well as placing it on the heart chakra, try positioning it at any point on your body where you're experiencing pain or discomfort. It's a good all-rounder to use regularly and may help ease inflammation.

Watermelon tourmaline—Place or wear this calming stone on the heart chakra to aid with healing and encouraging the relief of nerve pain. It can boost feelings of inner security, ease stress, and lift the mood.

Scolecite—Make a gem elixir using the indirect method and spray around the aura. The crystal may help to rebalance neurological issues and nerve damage.

OTHER GRID AND LAYOUT CRYSTALS
—

• Carnelian (for energy and motivation)
• Lapis lazuli (for balance and cleansing the body)
• Rose quartz (for emotional healing)
• Red jasper (for cleansing, balancing, and strengthening; good to use on the base chakra)

ADDITIONAL THERAPIES
—

Looking after yourself and developing self-care routines is important and can help quality of life. Eating a healthy balanced diet can help with some symptoms, such as bowel problems and fatigue, and regular activity and exercise can aid strength and mobility. If you smoke, quitting may help to reduce the progression of MS.

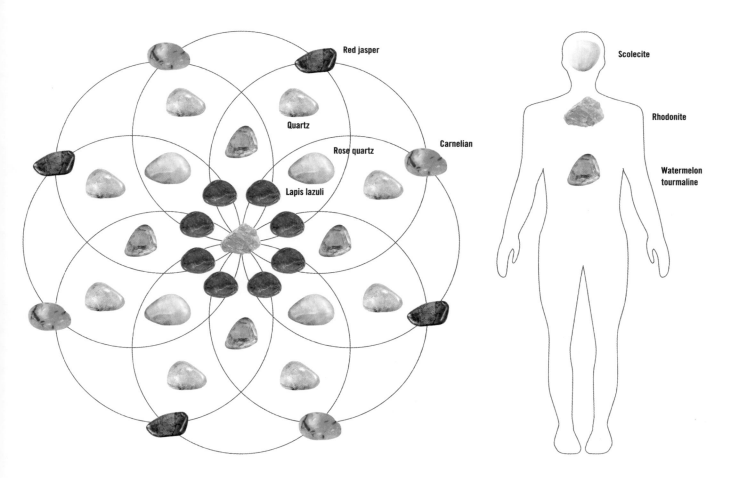

Red jasper

Quartz

Rose quartz

Carnelian

Lapis lazuli

Scolecite

Rhodonite

Watermelon tourmaline

RECUPERATION AFTER STROKE

A stroke is a major medical condition from which it can take time to recover, even when the initial treatment has been completed. Depending on the individual symptoms and severity of the stroke, the recuperation process may start in the hospital and continue at home, and may involve helping you regain your independence. Strokes cause injuries to the brain that can result in a multitude of aspects to deal with, including physical movements, cognitive thought processes, communication, swallowing, and visual issues. It can affect a person psychologically, too, causing feelings of depression, anxiety, fear, frustration, and anger at what has happened. Medical support and help from professionals is essential.

KEY CRYSTALS
—

Black moonstone—Hold or place on the body (if one side is more affected, place it there) to improve stamina, boost motor difficulties, and aid coordination.

Melanite—Place on the heart or throat chakra to help release blockages and aid with communication, which can sometimes be affected by a stroke.

Cleavelandite—This rare crystal from Pakistan may help deal with damage caused by a stroke. Place it near your bed or, if you are able to, hold it in your hand.

OTHER GRID AND LAYOUT CRYSTALS
—

• Red jasper (for strength and balance)
• Amber (for bladder issues and stress)
• Red calcite (for fear)
• Cerussite (to strengthen muscles and for energy)
• Charoite (for frustration)

ADDITIONAL THERAPIES
—

In addition to any medical therapies, physiotherapy can help with muscle strength where a stroke has caused weakness to one side of the body. Counseling and cognitive behavioral therapy (CBT) may help with the psychological aspects, such as depression and anxiety. Lifestyle changes, such as diet improvements, exercise, stopping smoking, and cutting down on alcohol consumption may also help lower the risk of a further stroke and support health in general.

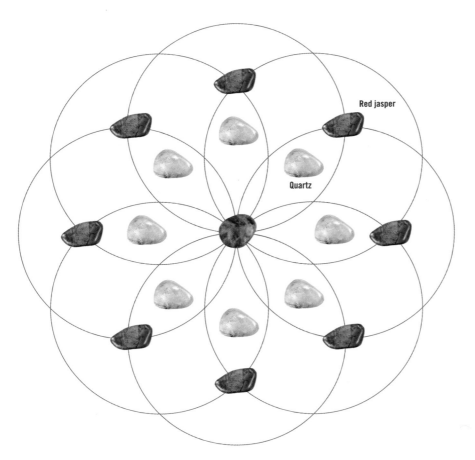

Red jasper

Quartz

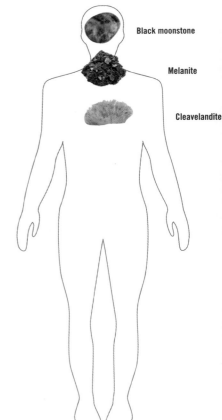

Black moonstone

Melanite

Cleavelandite

ECZEMA AND DERMATITIS

Dermatitis is a common form of skin condition that causes irritated, itchy, dry skin or swollen red rashes. Examples of dermatitis include atopic eczema and contact dermatitis.

Atopic eczema causes skin to become dry, cracked, sore, and itchy. It can affect any part of the body, but most frequently the hands, face, scalp, inside the elbows, or behind the knees and the neck. It often develops in childhood and can be a chronic, long-term condition, sometimes improving and at other times flaring up.

Contact dermatitis occurs when your skin has been in contact with substances that irritate the skin, such as perfumes, chemicals, cleaning products, or jewelry. It causes a red, stinging, and itching rash that may develop into blisters.

KEY CRYSTALS

—

Amethyst—Hold or wear an amethyst crystal, as this purple stone could help ease skin inflammation and swelling.

Calcite—Hold or wear a piece of calcite to stimulate healing. Its cleansing properties can be calming to irritated skin.

Chrysoprase—The calming energy of chrysoprase can soothe irritated skin, so hold or wear this crystal, or try making an indirect gem elixir and bathe in it.

OTHER GRID AND LAYOUT CRYSTALS

- Agate (aids skin healing)
- Green aventurine (for all-round healing)
- Selenite (for skin protection)

ADDITIONAL THERAPIES

—

Both eczema and contact dermatitis can be reduced by developing a regular skin-moisturization habit, ideally with an unscented product. Avoid known skin irritants where possible and investigate whether allergies, such as certain foods, could be linked to eczema symptoms.

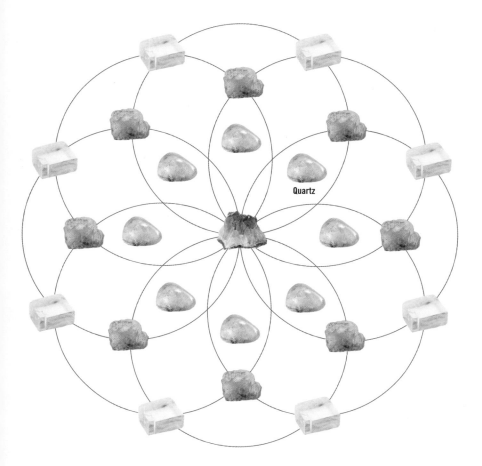

Quartz

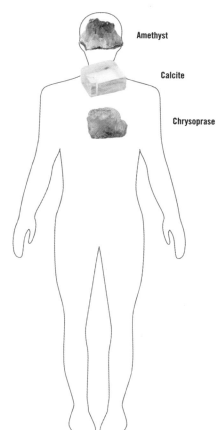

Amethyst

Calcite

Chrysoprase

ACNE

The skin condition acne causes spots to form on the skin. The skin can become oily and, in some cases, painful or hot to touch. Acne most commonly affects the face, back, and chest and, although it's common in teenagers during puberty, it can affect anyone of any age. Changes in hormones, such as during pregnancy, menstruation, or menopause, can cause acne, plus a predisposition to it may run in families. Although it may be tempting to pick or squeeze the spots, this could lead to scarring.

KEY CRYSTALS

—

Aventurine—Place an aventurine crystal on or near an affected area of skin. This soothing stone can have anti-inflammatory properties and help aid the healing of skin eruptions.

Idocrase—If you're feeling self-conscious or low about having acne on your face, hold an idocrase crystal to help banish negative emotions.

Amethyst—If your skin is hot or painful to touch, the soothing energies of amethyst could help ease inflammation. Hold an amethyst crystal or, if able to, place it on or near the affected area.

OTHER GRID AND LAYOUT CRYSTALS

—

• Okenite (to help ease skin eruptions)
• Galena (for skin eruptions)
• Moss agate (to soothe irritated skin)

ADDITIONAL THERAPIES

—

Conventional over-the-counter remedies are available to assist in treating mild acne, but severe acne may need prescription medication to help clear it up. Look after your skin by using self-help methods, such as completely removing makeup at night and washing affected areas with lukewarm water and a mild soap. Choose water-based makeup products that are less likely to block skin pores. Shower after exercising to remove sweat, as sweat can irritate acne, and look for skincare products that are soothing for irritated skin.

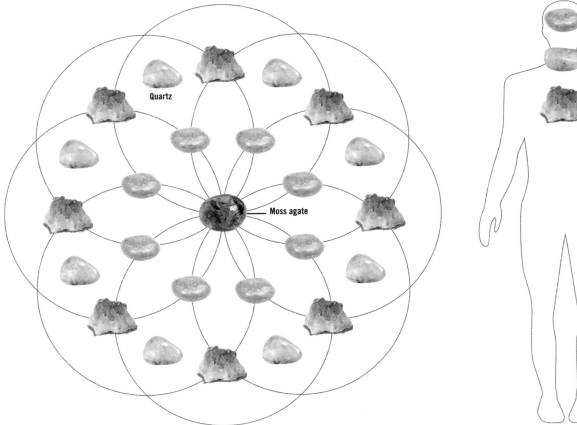

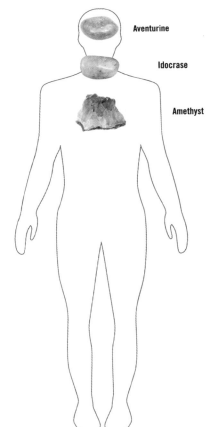

CELLULITE

Cellulite is a common and harmless skin condition that causes a dimpled and bumpy area of skin. It's often described as looking a bit like orange peel. It's commonly experienced by women and is most prevalent on the hips, thighs, and bottom, but can also be found on other areas of the body. Cellulite occurs when fat cells underneath the skin begin to push up, creating a dimpling effect on the surface of the skin. Hormone changes are linked to cellulite, as are genetics. Weight and muscle tone play a part, too (although body type is not a factor, as fit and thin people can also have cellulite).

KEY CRYSTALS

—

Citrine—Placing a citrine crystal on the solar plexus or sacral chakras, or wearing a crystal close to your skin, can help circulation and may help encourage the elimination of cellulite. Plus, the sunny and positive disposition of this crystal can be beneficial in helping you feel better about the appearance of your skin and encourage the realization that there's more to you and your body than a patch of cellulite.

Yellow apatite—Place yellow apatite on the affected area of skin to encourage the elimination of toxins from your body.

OTHER GRID AND LAYOUT CRYSTALS

—

• Carnelian (to balance hormones and revitalize the skin)
• Clear topaz (to support lymphatic health)
• Poppy jasper (for gentle skin stimulation)

ADDITIONAL THERAPIES

—

Eat a healthy, nutritious diet and exercise regularly, aiming to build up muscle tone. Muscle won't make your cellulite disappear, but it may help make the skin look more even. Losing weight may also help the appearance of cellulite. If you smoke, quit the habit, as smoking affects the blood supply to your skin and makes skin thinner and cellulite more visible. Massage your skin in the shower, or with a dry brush, to improve blood flow to your skin.

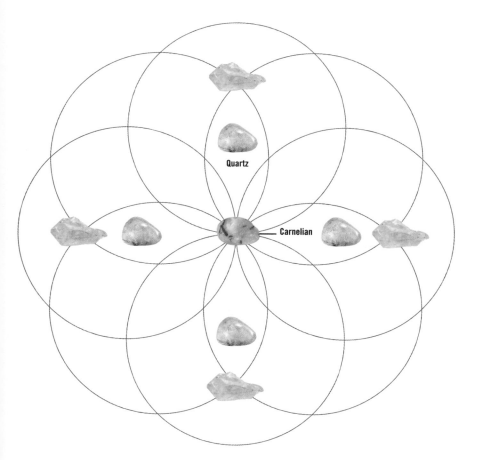

Quartz

Carnelian

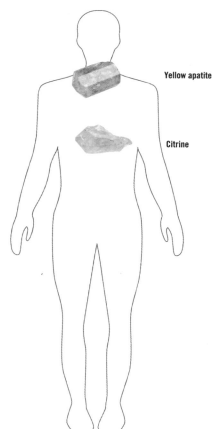

Yellow apatite

Citrine

HAIR LOSS

A small amount of hair loss is normal; in fact, you can lose up to 100 hairs a day without really noticing. But if your hair suddenly starts falling out in clumps or you develop bald patches, something could be amiss. Hair loss can be caused by a range of factors, such as iron deficiency, weight loss, stress, illness, or as the result of cancer treatment. In some cases it may be temporary, but in other situations it may be a long-term change. Baldness, for example, can run in families and be related to age, and although it's more common in men, it can also affect women.

Crystal remedies focus on subtle energies and vibrations, working on the emotional, mental, and spiritual levels. They can be used to help balance and strengthen the chakras and the aura, which can reflect back on your physical health.

KEY CRYSTALS
—

Magnetite—The anti-inflammatory properties of magnetite can soothe and reawaken sluggish hair follicles. Place on the back of the neck or around the head.

Moonstone—Place on or around the crown chakra to stimulate hair growth. Try gently massaging the aura around your head with moonstone to eliminate toxins. Make a crystal gem elixir using the indirect method and use the water while washing your hair.

Unakite—Place unakite on the crown chakra to encourage the growth of hair. Make an indirect gem elixir and use it to wash your hair.

OTHER GRID AND LAYOUT CRYSTALS
—

• Galena (to stimulate hair growth)
• Muscovite (useful if hair loss is linked to a health condition)
• Zincite (for hair loss linked to menopause)

ADDITIONAL THERAPIES
—

In addition to prescribed medication that may help to encourage hair growth, you might find it beneficial to take an iron supplement. For severe hair loss that affects your confidence and self-esteem, real hair and synthetic wigs are worth considering. If the loss of hair has been particularly upsetting, a talking therapy such as counseling may help. There are also online groups for people with alopecia where you can connect with others in a similar position.

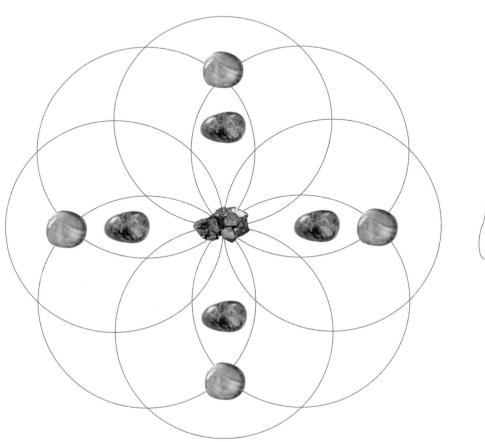

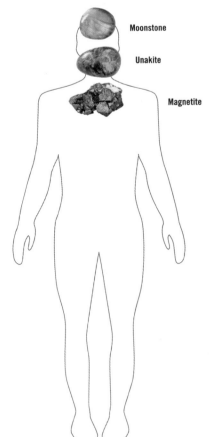

Moonstone

Unakite

Magnetite

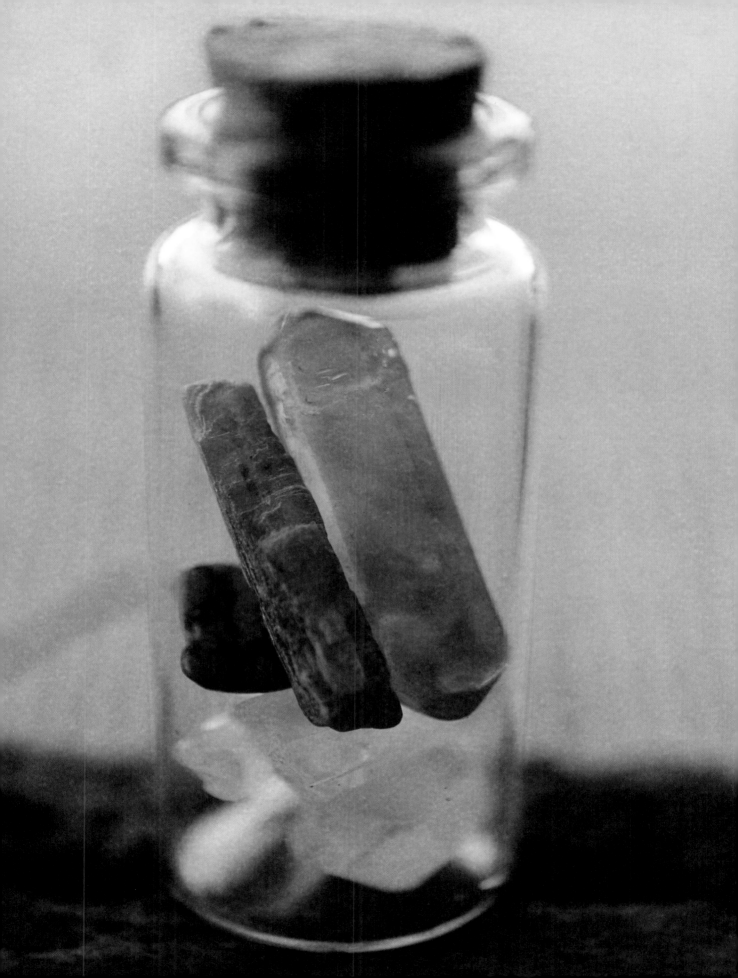

EYESTRAIN

Eyestrain occurs when you've been doing activities that involve using your eyes intensely for a long period of time without a break, such as using a computer, reading, sewing, or driving. It can also occur if you've been straining your eyes in dim light or have been in very bright light. Eyestrain can make your eyes feel tired, sore, watery, dry, or itchy. You may experience blurred or double vision, have a headache, and be sensitive to light. Sometimes your back, neck, or shoulders might feel sore and achy, too. It can sometimes be caused by underlying eye issues, such as changes in your eyesight or conditions such as a dry eye syndrome. Most eyestrain is temporary and not serious, but if you experience prolonged or severe symptoms, always see a qualified medical practitioner.

KEY CRYSTALS

—

Blue lace agate—Use the gentle, calming energy of a blue lace agate stone to ease eyestrain, by placing it on the third eye chakra on your forehead.

Emerald—Place an emerald on the third eye chakra, or around the outside of your head, to soothe eyestrain and tired eyes. You may also like to make an indirect crystal elixir and gently dab the mixture above your eyes (don't put it directly on the eyes).

OTHER GRID AND LAYOUT CRYSTALS

- Amber (for pain relief)
- Amethyst (for tiredness and fatigue)
- Charoite (for stress)

ADDITIONAL THERAPIES

—

If eyestrain has been caused by extended periods of driving, reading, sewing, or using a computer or tablet screen, try to cut back and have regular breaks when doing so. Make sure you have your eyes tested regularly to see if you need glasses or new prescription lenses. Improve lighting, rather than straining to see in dim light, and make sure you get plenty of sleep, to avoid eyestrain due to being tired or stressed. Gentle yoga or the Alexander Technique may be beneficial if you also have related back, neck, or shoulder problems.

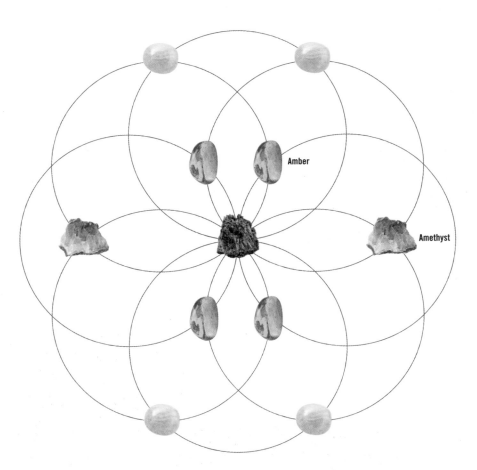

Amber

Amethyst

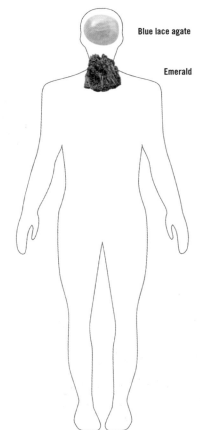

Blue lace agate

Emerald

EARACHE

Earache can have various causes, such as a buildup of wax in the ear, referred pain from toothache, a perforated eardrum, or a sore throat or cold. If you also have a fever with earache, it could be caused by an ear infection or flu. Always avoid putting cotton buds in your ear to try to clean them, as it can compress and push earwax further into your ear, rather than removing it. If you think you could have something stuck in your ear, have ear swelling, have a lot of fluid coming out of your ear, experience a change in hearing, or a very high temperature and shivering, always seek the advice of a medical practitioner.

KEY CRYSTALS
—

Celestite—Place celestite on or near the ear, as its cleansing energies may help to ease the discomfort of earache and encourage the dissipation of any toxins or infections.

Blue chalcedony—Place a blue chalcedony stone on or near the source of the pain, or hold it in the palm of your hand. The cleansing and balancing may help to ease discomfort.

Rhodonite—Wear rhodonite crystal earrings to gently ease earache caused by blocked ears. Rhodonite is also said to help fine-tune hearing.

OTHER GRID AND LAYOUT CRYSTALS
—

• Sardonyx (for generalized earache)
• Apatite (for toothache-related earache)
• Moss agate (for earache due to a cold or flu)
• Clear quartz (to amplify the benefits of the other crystals; also useful to hold while other crystals are placed on or near the ear)

ADDITIONAL THERAPIES
—

Alongside any treatments prescribed by a medical practitioner, placing a warm flannel on the ear could help to relieve some discomfort. If you have a fever with your earache, you may benefit from a cooling flannel instead. A few drops of olive oil can be used to soften hard earwax. Some people suggest specially designed Hopi ear candles can help, too, but it's best to go to a trained holistic therapist for an ear candling session.

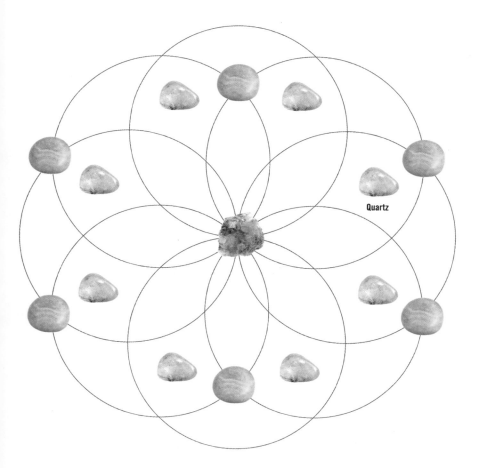

Quartz

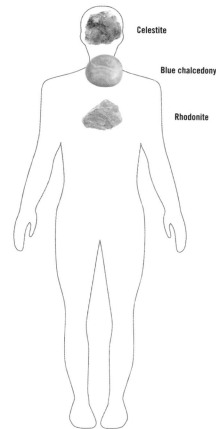

Celestite

Blue chalcedony

Rhodonite

SINUSITIS

Sinusitis is a nasal problem that causes swelling, pain, and tenderness in the sinuses. The sinuses are air-filled cavities located in the cheekbones, the sides of the nose, the forehead, and between the eyes. It's normally caused by an infection and is commonly experienced after colds and flu. Other symptoms caused by sinusitis include a continuous blocked nose, a headache, toothache, mucus in the nose, a reduced sense of smell, and a high temperature. For sinusitis that doesn't clear or gets worse after two to three weeks, medication such as steroid nasal sprays or drops may be necessary, so seek help from a medical practitioner.

KEY CRYSTALS

—

Fluorite—Make a crystal elixir using the indirect method, then add it to warm water to make a steam inhalation bath. Or put the water and elixir in a bowl of water, cover your head with a towel, lean over the bowl, and inhale. Fluorite may well reduce mucus and nasal swelling.

Azurite—Place azurite on the third eye chakra to cleanse it, as it can become blocked with sinusitis. This healing crystal can also help recovery from sinusitis caused by an infection.

Aventurine—Place aventurine on or near the source of discomfort, as its gentle, anti-inflammatory properties could help recovery.

OTHER GRID AND LAYOUT CRYSTALS

- Emerald (to ease nasal discomfort)
- Iolite (for headaches associated with sinusitis)
- Jet (to ease general discomfort)
- Sodalite (for throat issues caused by sinusitis or postnasal drip)

ADDITIONAL THERAPIES

—

Cleaning your nose with a saline saltwater solution may help ease nasal congestion (but it shouldn't be used regularly). Add a few drops of eucalyptus essential oil to a steam inhalation to help clear nasal passages. If an allergy is causing your symptoms, try to reduce contact with potential allergens. Smoke can also irritate sinusitis, so it's best to avoid smoking or exposure to smoke.

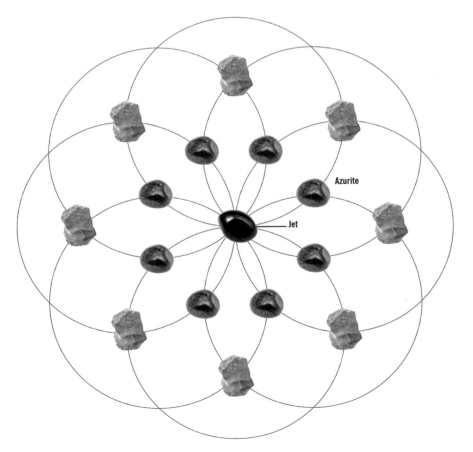

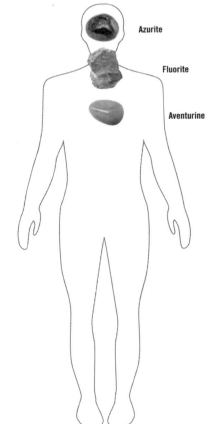

CATARRH

A buildup of mucus in your nose, back of the throat, or in your sinuses is called catarrh. It's commonly experienced with a cold, flu, or infection, but can also be caused by allergies such as hay fever or animal fur, or conditions such as nasal polyps. Catarrh causes symptoms such as a blocked, stuffy nose, a runny nose, a feeling that your throat is blocked, a cough, mucus running down the back of your throat, headache, and a reduced sense of smell or taste. In most cases, catarrh is temporary and will clear up without issues. But if you have chronic catarrh that occurs on a long-term basis and doesn't clear, see a medical practitioner for advice.

KEY CRYSTALS

—

Amber—Place on the third eye chakra or the throat chakra to cleanse and rebalance blockages and ease mucus buildups.

Blue lace agate—Place on the throat chakra, or wear as a crystal necklace, to aid the release of congestion in the nose and throat. For a very blocked nose, consider making an indirect crystal gem elixir and adding it to a steam inhalation bath.

OTHER GRID AND LAYOUT CRYSTALS

- Blue sapphire (to help remove impurities)
- Topaz (for a loss of taste)
- Rose quartz (for a cough caused by a constant need to try to clear the throat)
- Emerald (for a blocked nose)

ADDITIONAL THERAPIES

—

Do things that make you feel good and fill you with joy, gratitude, faith, hope, and happiness. Cleanse your environment with sage. Use meditations and visualizations to surround yourself with a pure white light that protects you at all times. Use chakra and aura healing methods to clear blockages and strengthen your personal energy systems.

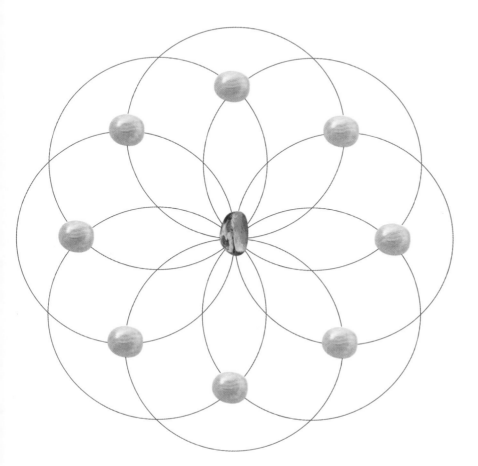

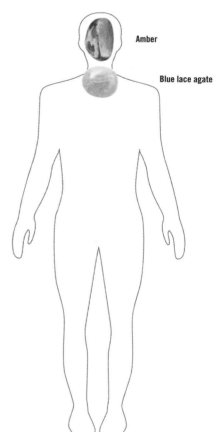

Amber

Blue lace agate

TOOTHACHE

Toothache can be caused by a broken or lost filling, a cracked or damaged tooth, tooth decay, a problem with braces, an infection, or an abscess. Sometimes you can have referred pain that goes up into your head causing a headache, or down into your neck or shoulders. If you have persistent or severe toothache that doesn't abate, especially if it doesn't ease with painkillers, causes swelling in your cheek or jaw, or you have a high temperature, visit a dentist. If you have a dental or gum infection, it should not be left untreated and you may need prescription medication to clear it.

KEY CRYSTALS
—

Amber—Place amber on the throat chakra to release blockages and rebalance the chakra. A blocked throat chakra can sometimes lead to toothache. Wear dangly amber earrings to keep the stone close to your face for continued benefits.

Aquamarine—Make a crystal gem elixir using the indirect method and use the water as a mouthwash. This will help flush out any toxins from your teeth and gums, particularly if there's an infection present.

Citrine—Place citrine on the throat chakra to encourage the release of toxins. You could also make a crystal elixir using the indirect method, or use a special crystal-infused water bottle, and slowly sip the water during the day.

Fluorite—Place fluorite crystals on or around your face and head to direct healing energies to your teeth and gums.

OTHER GRID AND LAYOUT CRYSTALS
—

• Lapis lazuli (to ease toothache, especially if it's also causing a headache)
• Malachite (to stimulate the release of toxins from dental infections)
• Amazonite (for gentle healing and to help amplify the benefits of the other crystals in a grid)

ADDITIONAL THERAPIES
—

While you have toothache, it may help to eat soft foods and brush and floss your teeth regularly (at least twice a day) to help keep them clean and healthy and reduce the risk of infection. Have regular dental checkups and cut down on foods and drinks containing high levels of sugar.

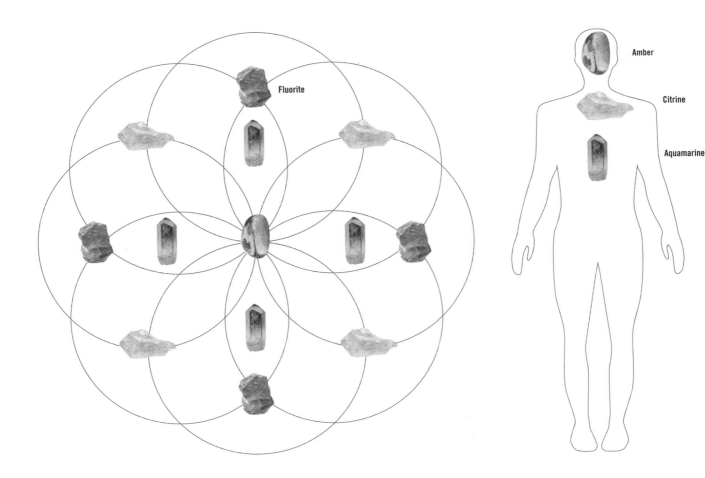

SORE THROAT

Sore throats are common and are usually caused by a virus, so are often experienced in conjunction with a cold or flu. Sometimes smoking can cause sore throats and occasionally a bacterial infection may be to blame. A sore throat can be uncomfortable and disruptive, causing symptoms such as a dry, scratchy throat, pain when swallowing, a cough, redness in the back of the mouth, and swollen glands in the neck. Although unpleasant, a sore throat generally gets better relatively quickly, or within around a week. If you have symptoms that persist, seek advice from a medical practitioner.

KEY CRYSTALS
—

Amber—Hold or wear amber near the throat to help ease the discomfort of a sore throat.

Aquamarine—Place an aquamarine crystal on the throat chakra to help release blockages in the chakra and ease swollen glands.

Blue tourmaline—Place on or around the throat area to help ease a scratchy, dry throat with the soothing energies of blue tourmaline.

Blue lace agate—Make a crystal elixir using the indirect method and gargle with it.

OTHER GRID AND LAYOUT CRYSTALS
—

• Blue jasper (to balance the aura and chakras)
• Lapis lazuli (to aid communication when a sore throat is causing difficulties talking)
• Green opal (to strengthen the immune system)
• Sardonyx (to boost immunity)

ADDITIONAL THERAPIES
—

Soothe the discomfort of a sore throat by sucking on ice cubes or ice lollies or try gargling with warm saltwater. Smoke can irritate throats, so avoid being in smoky environments or stop smoking. Keep hydrated by drinking plenty of water, rest to let your body recover, and aim to eat soft foods that are easy to swallow. Eat foods rich in vitamin C to boost your immune system.

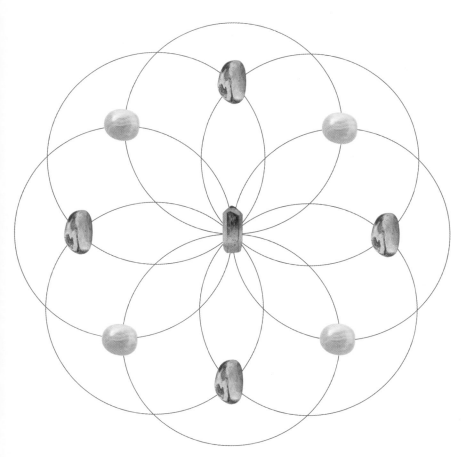

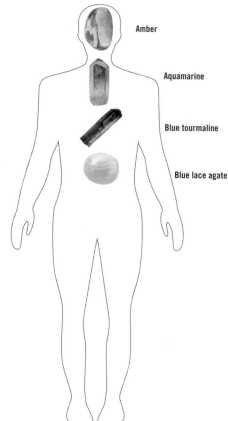

Amber

Aquamarine

Blue tourmaline

Blue lace agate

ASTHMA

Asthma is a common long-term lung condition that occurs when the tubes that carry air in and out of the lungs become inflamed and sensitive. Symptoms include breathlessness, coughing, a tight feeling in the chest, and wheezing when you breathe. It can be caused by allergies, such as pollen or animal fur, exposure to smoke or pollution, cold air, or infections such as flu or colds. Asthma needs to be formally diagnosed by a medical practitioner and you may need prescribed reliever and preventer inhalers. If asthma is well-controlled, the symptoms are manageable. Asthma that isn't controlled can have severe effects on your daily life. If you have symptoms that could be asthma, always see a medical professional for advice. If existing asthma symptoms worsen, or you have a sudden bad asthma attack, seek medical help.

KEY CRYSTALS
—

Amber—Place on the throat chakra to balance and align the chakras. Wear amber jewelry, such as earrings or necklaces, or use the indirect method to make a crystal elixir.

Chrysocolla—Place on or around the body to calm and reenergize the throat and chest. It may help relax the chest muscles and lungs, improving the ability to breathe.

Moss agate—Place moss agate stones around your body, as they may help relax the bronchia and lungs, plus aid inflammation in the airways.

OTHER GRID AND LAYOUT CRYSTALS
—
• Ametrine (to cleanse the aura and reenergize the body)

• Apophyllite (for the respiratory system and asthma caused by allergies)
• Chrysocolla (to calm and reenergize the throat and chest)
• Morganite (to help clear the lungs)
• Rutilated quartz (for lung support for chronic asthma)

ADDITIONAL THERAPIES
—

Make sure you have regular asthma reviews to monitor your progress and treatments. Avoid known allergens where possible. Breathing exercises, such as the Buteyko Breathing Technique or pursed lip breathing technique, may be useful to learn to help you breathe more efficiently with asthma. Improve your physical activity by exercising regularly—as research shows that raising your heart rate can reduce breathlessness—and eat a healthy diet to maintain a healthy weight.

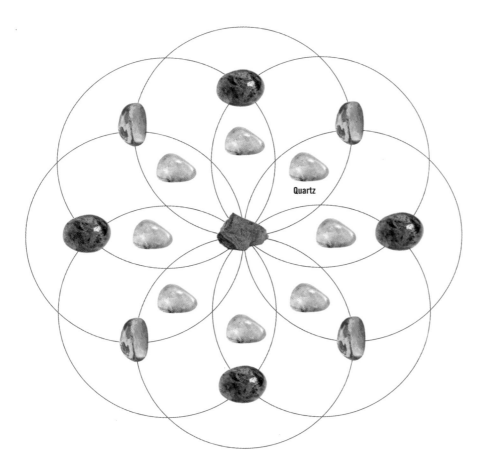

Quartz

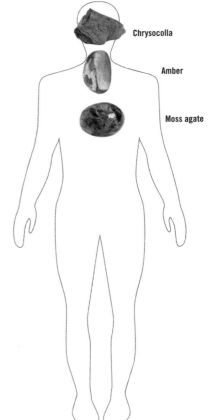

Chrysocolla

Amber

Moss agate

COUGHS

Coughs can be annoying, but the majority tend to be caused by colds or flu and are relatively harmless, usually clearing up within weeks. Other common causes of coughs include acid reflux heartburn or smoking, allergies such as hay fever, or infections such as bronchitis. Coughs can be dry, tickly, chesty, or productive (where you cough up mucus). If you have a sudden, continuous cough, find it hard to breathe, have chest pain, feel very unwell, the glands in your neck become swollen, or your cough rapidly gets worse, seek advice from a medical practitioner.

KEY CRYSTALS
—

Amber—Unleash the immune-boosting benefits of amber by placing it on the solar plexus chakra. It can cleanse and detox your body and bring relief from coughing.

Ametrine—Make an indirect gem elixir and add it to a warm bath. Soak in the bath to ease your body, especially when you're feeling tired from coughing.

Aquamarine—Hold an aquamarine crystal in your hand or place it on the throat chakra to ease tickly, annoying coughs with mucus production.

Blue lace agate—Place on or around your body to rebalance, stabilize, and cleanse your aura.

OTHER GRID AND LAYOUT CRYSTALS
—

• Carnelian (for easing congestion)
• Topaz (for strength in fighting illness)
• Clear quartz (for cleansing toxins)

ADDITIONAL THERAPIES
—

A hot drink made from lemon and honey can ease a tickly cough and there's some evidence that the herbal remedy pelargonium may be helpful. If your cough is making you feel under the weather, get as much rest as you can and drink plenty of fluids to keep you hydrated. Add more vitamin C to your diet, for example by eating oranges, to boost your immune system.

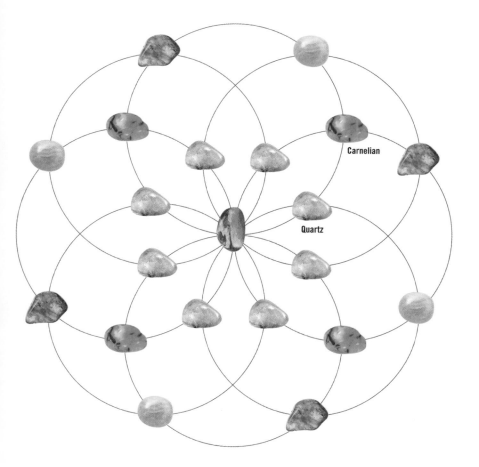

Carnelian

Quartz

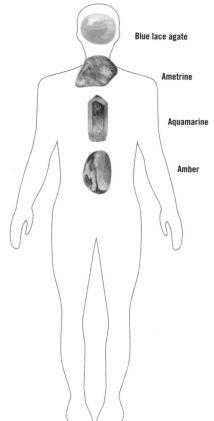

Blue lace agate

Ametrine

Aquamarine

Amber

LIVING WITH EMPHYSEMA

Emphysema is a chronic lung condition caused when the air sacs in the lungs become damaged. It causes severe breathing difficulties and shortness of breath and many people with emphysema also have chronic bronchitis (long-term inflammation of the airways). Exposure to airborne irritants, such as air pollution, smoke, or chemical fumes, is one of the leading causes of emphysema; rarely, it can be an inherited disease. While emphysema can't be cured, there are effective medications and treatments that can be prescribed to help manage the symptoms and improve quality of life.

KEY CRYSTALS
—

Chrysocolla—Hold or place chrysocolla on your throat chakra to help calm and reenergize the throat and chest. It might help the lungs to relax and make breathing easier.

Amber—Place on or around your body to aid healing and discomfort in the lungs. Placed in a room, it will also absorb negative energies and turn them into positive ones.

Rhodonite—Place on or around your body to help balance physical and mental energy, giving you strength to cope with your long-term lung issues.

OTHER GRID AND LAYOUT CRYSTALS
—

• Morganite (to help damaged cells and ease the lungs)
• Moss agate (for inflammation)
• Rhodochrosite (for the respiratory system)
• Kunzite (for the respiratory system)
• Rose quartz (to help if you're feeling low or down)

ADDITIONAL THERAPIES
—

In addition to prescribed medications and treatments, breathing techniques may help you to manage your breathing more effectively and improve your ability to do some exercise. Eating healthily and losing weight, especially in the early stages, may offer benefits.

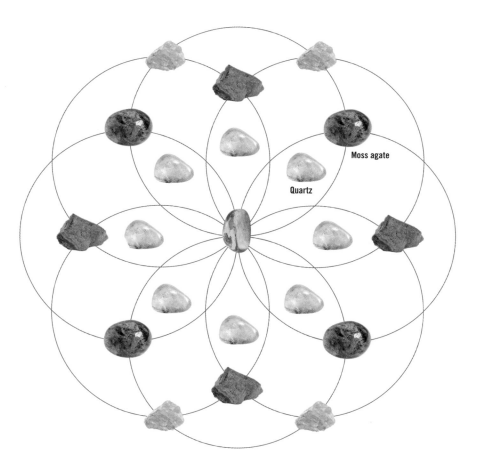

Moss agate

Quartz

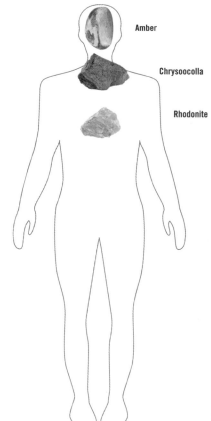

Amber

Chrysoocolla

Rhodonite

HYPERVENTILATION

Hyperventilation occurs when you breathe very fast and exhale more than you inhale. As you breathe faster, your levels of carbon dioxide rapidly decrease, leading to a narrowing of the blood vessels that supply blood to your brain. This can result in symptoms such as feeling faint or lightheaded, tingling sensations in your fingers, sweating, feeling sick, or passing out. Hyperventilation is most commonly triggered by stress, panic attacks, anxiety, or nervousness. It can be scary, especially if it happens for the first time and you don't know why; trying to calm yourself and slowing your breathing can help. Sometimes it can be caused by a lung infection, lung disorder, heart attack, asthma, or other medical condition, so seek advice from a medical practitioner to check the cause.

KEY CRYSTALS
—

Kunzite—Place a piece of kunzite on the solar plexus chakra, to help relieve emotional stress and feelings of panic.

Rhodonite—The calming energies of rhodonite make it a good first aid crystal. Hold it in your hand to encourage calm breathing, release of panic and emotional stress. Use the indirect method to make a gem elixir and sip slowly to aid recovery from the shock of hyperventilating.

Pyrite—Hold in your hand, or place on the throat chakra, to help get breathing under control.

OTHER GRID AND LAYOUT CRYSTALS

- Rose quartz (for keeping calm when breathing is labored)
- Zoisite (to aid feelings of faintness)
- Green calcite (to absorb negativity; particularly useful in grids)
- Epidote (for emotional trauma)

ADDITIONAL THERAPIES
—

Learn self-help breathing methods to help you stay calm, as panicking can make hyperventilation worse. Try breathing through pursed lips, breathing slowly into a paper bag or into cupped hands and breathe from your stomach rather than your chest. Meditation may help with relaxation if stress is an issue, and acupuncture may also be beneficial.

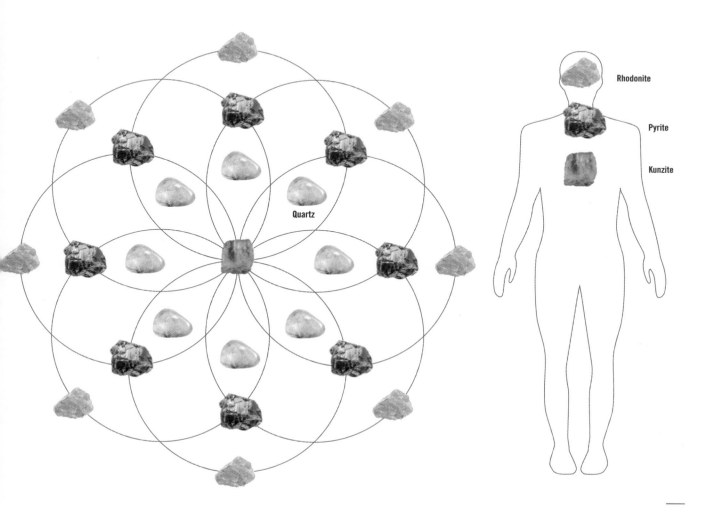

Quartz

Rhodonite

Pyrite

Kunzite

HICCUPS

Hiccups occur when the diaphragm muscle just below your lungs starts to contract. Normally your diaphragm helps regulate your breathing, but when it contracts, a sudden rush of air will go into your lungs, causing the hiccup and related noise. Sometimes hiccups start and stop suddenly, for no apparent reason. On other occasions, there could be a cause, such as eating too much, eating spicy foods, experiencing a change in air temperature, being overexcited, being stressed, accidentally swallowing too much air, or drinking alcohol or fizzy drinks. If you have regular bouts of hiccups, or they don't stop, always see a medical practitioner for advice.

KEY CRYSTALS

—

Peridot—Place on the diaphragm to ease unwanted muscle contractions.

Leopard jasper—Hold leopard jasper, as this crystal can help relax the body, reduce tension, and ease hiccups.

OTHER GRID AND LAYOUT CRYSTALS

—

• Rose quartz (to calm and relax the body)
• Ametrine (to cleanse the aura and reenergize the body)

ADDITIONAL THERAPIES

—

Holding your breath, breathing into a paper bag, drinking cold water, and relaxing may all help stop hiccups. If hiccups seemed to be caused by food or drink, eat slowly and avoid potential triggers, such as alcohol, fizzy drinks, or spicy foods.

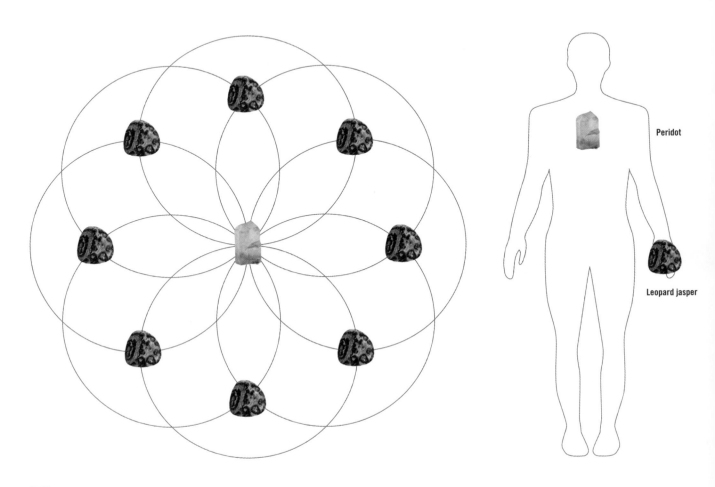

Peridot

Leopard jasper

COLDS AND FLU

Colds and flu are respiratory infections that are both caused by viruses. With a cold, you're likely to have symptoms such as a sore throat, sneezing, cough, runny nose, stuffy nose, and a headache. Colds tend to come on gradually and are normally mild, clearing up within ten days. Sometimes colds are mistaken for flu, but with real flu you'll also have symptoms such as a fever, chills, severe muscle aches, a hacking cough, severe fatigue, and sometimes nausea and vomiting. Flu tends to come on much more rapidly, and the symptoms can be severe, lasting for up to two weeks. If you have a sudden severe cough, a very high fever that won't subside, or your symptoms don't improve, seek advice from a medical practitioner.

KEY CRYSTALS
—

Carnelian—Hold a tumbled carnelian gemstone in both hands or place around your body, to help give strength to the immune system in fighting a cold or flu.

Larimar—Place larimar on your third eye chakra, or around your head, to soothe, calm, and cool a flu fever.

Fluorite—Place fluorite stones around your body to tackle toxins, cleanse, and purify. Alternatively, make a gem elixir and spray around your aura.

Green aventurine—Place on your body in areas where muscles ache, to help ease the aches and pains of flu.

Blue lace agate—Gently rub a piece of tumbled blue lace agate on your forehead and temples. It is soothing and can help ease a headache or blocked sinuses caused by a cold or flu.

OTHER GRID AND LAYOUT CRYSTALS
—

• Emerald (for a blocked and stuffy nose and head cold)
• Green opal (to strengthen the immune system)
• Lapis lazuli (to help with flu headaches)
• Bloodstone (to balance and cleanse the bloodstream and fight infection)
• Moss agate (to aid recovery)
• Citrine (for energy as you recover from flu)

ADDITIONAL THERAPIES
—

Stay warm, rest, and drink plenty of fluids; fluids will help loosen mucus and rehydrate your body if you have a fever. Make a warm honey and lemon drink to sip—it can soothe an irritated throat—or try eating a traditional chicken soup. Pop a few drops of eucalyptus essential oil into a warm bath and inhale the steam as you relax. Take echinacea or goldenseal drops or capsules to help boost your immunity. Add extra vitamin C to your diet, by eating oranges, strawberries, and broccoli.

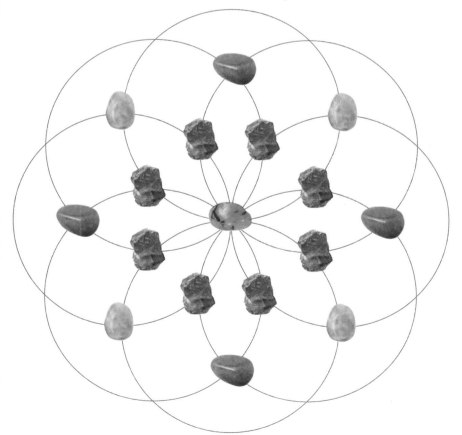

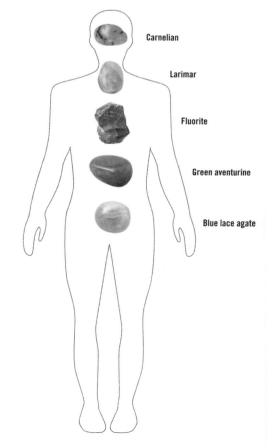

Carnelian

Larimar

Fluorite

Green aventurine

Blue lace agate

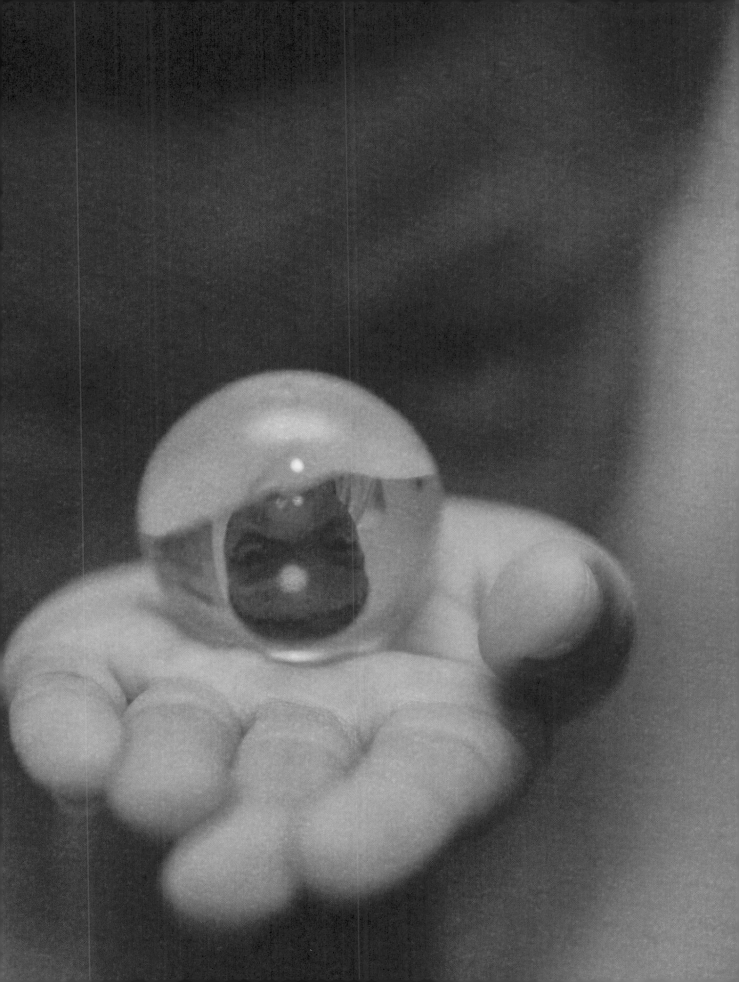

HIGH BLOOD PRESSURE

High blood pressure, also known as hypertension, puts you at a greater risk of other health conditions, including developing heart disease or having a stroke. It's often a silent condition, so you may be unaware that you have high blood pressure until you have your blood pressure taken. If you have severe hypertension, then you may experience symptoms such as headaches, shortness of breath, dizziness, chest pain, and nosebleeds. In the United States, blood pressure is considered as being high if you have a reading of 130/80mmHg or above. Find out your blood pressure by having an annual check at your medical practice. If you have a family history of hypertension or heart disease, you may need more regular blood pressure checks.

KEY CRYSTALS
—

Chrome diopside—Place a green chrome diopside on the heart chakra, to help unblock the flow of energy and rebalance the chakras. This may assist in regulating blood pressure.

Amethyst—Hold amethyst crystals in both hands, or place one piece on the heart chakra. The soothing energy may help calm and stabilize high blood pressure, plus it could calm stress.

Tugtupite—Place on the heart chakra to help stabilize high blood pressure.

OTHER GRID AND LAYOUT CRYSTALS
—

• Lapis lazuli (for cardiac rhythm and circulation)
• Labradorite (for reducing stress and anxiety, which can exacerbate blood pressure)
• Ussingite (for stabilizing blood pressure)
• Charoite (to regulate blood pressure and pulse rate)

ADDITIONAL THERAPIES
—

In addition to any prescribed medication, losing weight and doing more exercise can both help to bring down high blood pressure. Aim to eat plenty of fresh fruits and vegetables, cut down on salt, avoid smoking, and avoid drinking too much alcohol or caffeinated drinks. Focus on your sleep, too, as getting a good night's sleep can help bring down blood pressure.

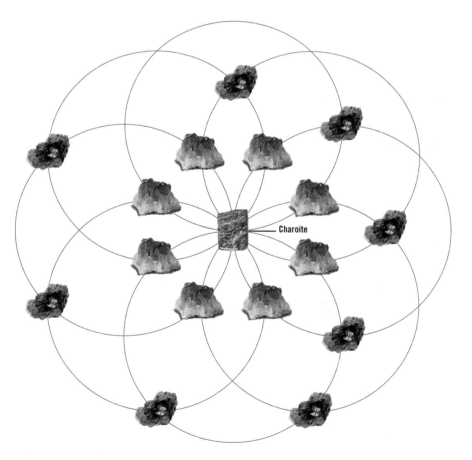

Charoite

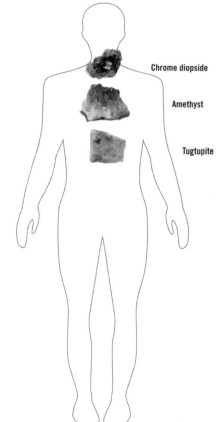

Chrome diopside

Amethyst

Tugtupite

LOW BLOOD PRESSURE

Low blood pressure is known as hypotension. Your blood pressure can lower due to certain medical conditions, such as diabetes, or when you take some medications. It can also be inherited, or occur as you get older or as a result of being pregnant. Often it doesn't cause any symptoms and you may only become aware of it when you have a routine blood pressure check. Sometimes low blood pressure causes symptoms such as lightheadedness, feeling dizzy, nausea, blurred vision, confusion, or fainting. If you're concerned you could have low blood pressure, see a medical practitioner for a blood pressure check.

KEY CRYSTALS
—

Green aventurine—Place on the heart chakra to help balance blood pressure to a normal level. The soothing energies of green aventurine will also comfort and protect you and help release negative energy blockages.

Kyanite—Hold kyanite to help balance and regulate your blood pressure. Alternatively, make a crystal gem elixir using the indirect method and spray it around your aura to cleanse and purify.

OTHER GRID AND LAYOUT CRYSTALS
—

• Chrysocolla (to strengthen weak blood vessels)
• Black tourmaline (for vitality)
• Lapis lazuli (for circulation)
• Greenlandite (to balance blood pressure)

ADDITIONAL THERAPIES
—

In addition to any medication prescribed by a medical practitioner, there are some self-help measures you can take to ease low blood pressure symptoms. If you feel faint or lightheaded when moving from a sitting to standing position, aim to get up slowly. Drink more water to ensure you're fully hydrated. Cut down on alcohol and caffeinated drinks, especially at night, and avoid sitting or standing in the same position for long periods of time.

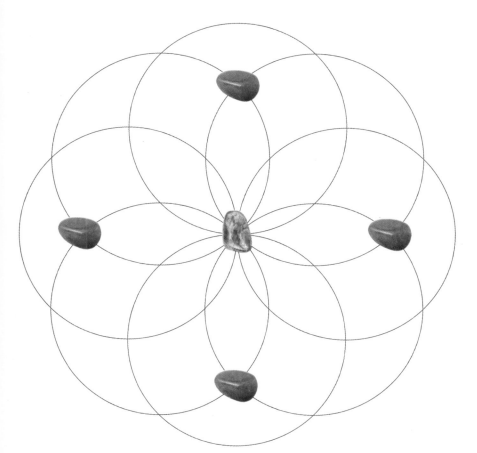

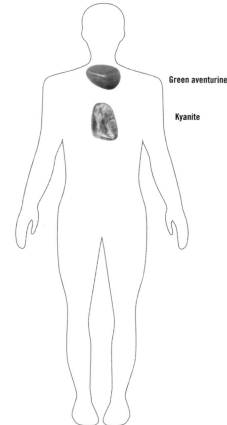

Green aventurine

Kyanite

ANEMIA

Anemia occurs when you're deficient in iron. Symptoms include being tired and lacking in energy, having pale skin, experiencing shortness of breath and heart palpitations. It can occur if you don't have enough iron in your diet, due to blood loss from heavy periods, pregnancy, bleeding in the stomach or the intestines (such as due to piles). If it's left untreated, it can make you more at risk of developing infections and illnesses, or in pregnancy it can increase the risk of complications. A simple blood test can diagnose anemia.

KEY CRYSTALS
—

Bloodstone—Bloodstone lives up to its name by being great to use with blood-related conditions, including anemia. Hold or place around your upper body to encourage the purification of the blood and to support and regulate blood flow. To stimulate the immune system, place on the thymus gland (in the upper part of your chest, just above the heart).

Citrine—Utilize the sunny disposition of citrine to reenergize your body when you're feeling tired and sluggish from low iron levels. Wear a citrine point on a necklace to draw the energy down into your body, reenergizing you and supporting blood circulation. It's especially useful to wear during a heavy period to aid energy levels and fatigue.

Carnelian—Place on the root chakra to energize and rejuvenate the body. Carnelian is often known as the life force crystal, and it may help improve your energy levels when iron is lacking.

OTHER GRID AND LAYOUT CRYSTALS
—

• Ruby (for energy and overcoming lethargy)
• Black tourmaline (to ground and stabilize energy; good to use on the root chakra)
• Garnet (to purify and reenergize the blood)
• Kunzite (to stimulate the immune system)

ADDITIONAL THERAPIES
—

In addition to taking any prescribed medication, you can improve your iron levels by eating dark green leafy vegetables such as kale or watercress, fortified cereals, and bread. Meat provides iron, too, as do pulses and dried fruits such as prunes and apricots.

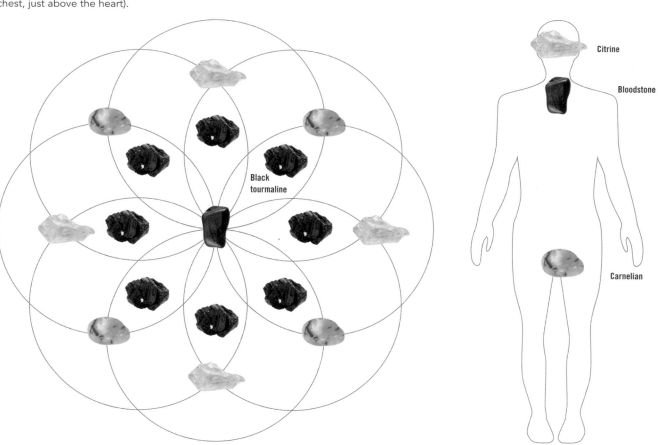

Black tourmaline

Citrine

Bloodstone

Carnelian

PALPITATIONS

Palpitations is the name given to the feeling that your heart is beating faster, missing a beat, or fluttering, often suddenly and for a few seconds or minutes at a time. You may feel it in your chest, as well as in your neck or throat. It can be scary, especially the first time it happens, but in many cases it's not serious. Palpitations can commonly be triggered by stress and anxiety, by drinking too much caffeine or alcohol, or as a result of being pregnant or perimenopausal. If you are concerned, have regular palpitations, or experience shortness of breath, dizziness, fainting, or bad chest pain, seek medical help.

KEY CRYSTALS
—

Garnet—If you keep having palpitations, wear garnet on a necklace, so that it's close to your heart chakra.

Chryosprase—Place chrysoprase on the heart chakra to encourage the flow of qi energy and release any blockages.

Lepidolite—Hold lepidolite and breathe slowly, to calm nerves and anxiety and instill a sense of peace.

OTHER GRID AND LAYOUT CRYSTALS

- Rose quartz (to calm anxiety from emotional trauma)
- Rhodonite (to ease panic or shock)
- Tree agate (to help the flow of qi energy around the body)

ADDITIONAL THERAPIES
—

Mindfulness, meditation, tai chi, and yoga can help you relax and ease stress and anxiety, as can learning breathing techniques. Some people find aromatherapy helpful. Cut down on the amount of alcohol and caffeine you consume and avoid smoking.

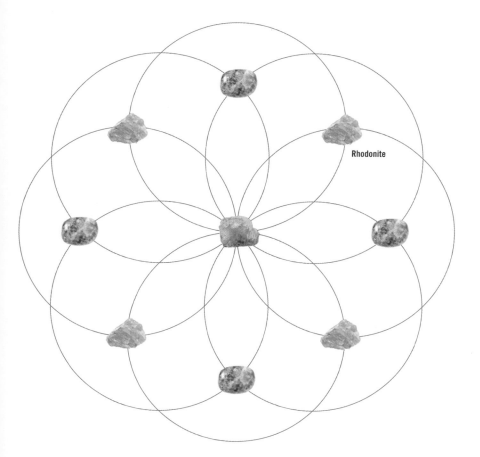

Rhodonite

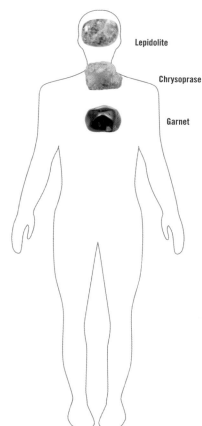

Lepidolite

Chrysoprase

Garnet

NAUSEA

Nausea is the sensation of feeling sick. It's a common condition and can go away on its own without you actually being sick. A variety of different things can bring on feelings of nausea, including strong food smells, perfumes, traveling (motion sickness), an infection, migraine, vertigo, acid reflux, being pregnant (morning sickness), anxiety, medications, alcohol, or having had a surgical operation.

KEY CRYSTALS

—

Red jasper—Place on the root chakra to help ground your energy, and clean and stabilize your aura. If you experience motion sickness, pop a piece of tumbled red jasper in your pocket and hold and play with it like a worry bead when you're traveling to ease feelings of, and distract from, nausea.

Brown agate—Place on the abdomen to balance negative energies and relieve feelings of nausea.

Gaspéite—If you feel nauseous as a result of anger, hurt, or distress, use gaspéite to ground you and calm your emotions. Keep a piece in your pocket and carry it with you.

Dumortierite—Holding dumortierite in your hand may help feelings of nausea and sickness. It's also a useful stone to use if you feel sick due to overexcitement, stress, or anxiety.

OTHER GRID AND LAYOUT CRYSTALS

—

• Dioptase (to reduce nausea)
• Emerald (for nausea related to infections)
• Blue sapphire (to ease sickness; use on throat chakra)

ADDITIONAL THERAPIES

—

In traditional Chinese medicine, ginger is used for nausea. Try sipping ginger tea, eating a ginger biscuit, or sucking a piece of crystallized ginger when you feel nauseous. Acupuncture can help, too. For sea, travel, or pregnancy sickness look out for special acupressure bands that you wear on your wrists on the nausea points. Fresh air can help, too, as can eating smaller meals.

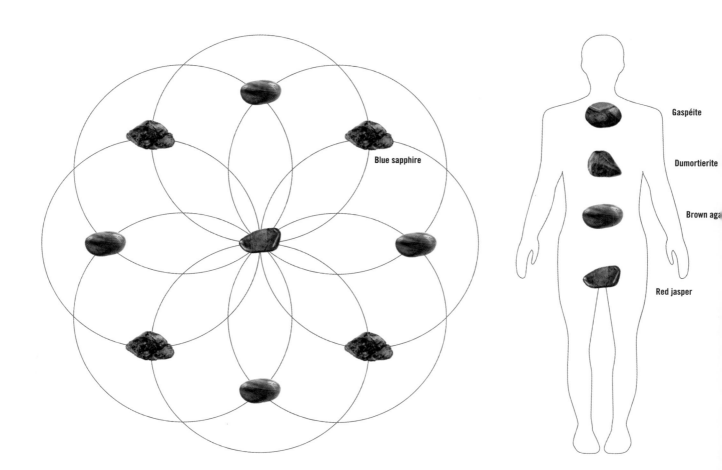

Blue sapphire

Gaspéite

Dumortierite

Brown aga[te]

Red jasper

GASTROENTERITIS

Gastroenteritis is a common form of stomach bug that causes vomiting and diarrhea. It's normally caused by a virus or a bacterial infection. The main symptoms are having sudden, watery diarrhea, feeling sick, vomiting, and a mild fever. Sometimes you may have aching limbs and a loss of appetite too. It's important to rest and sip water, as it's easy to get dehydrated through fluid loss. Be aware that the bug can spread, so take care to clean surfaces, avoid sharing towels, and avoid preparing food for other people while you're unwell.

KEY CRYSTALS
—

Carnelian—Hold a tumbled carnelian gemstone in both hands or place around your body, to help give strength to the immune system in fighting a cold or flu.

Larimar—Place larimar on your third eye chakra, or around your head, to soothe, calm, and cool a flu fever.

Fluorite—Place fluorite stones around your body to tackle toxins, cleanse, and purify. Alternatively, make a gem elixir and spray around your aura.

Green aventurine—Known as the "life force" crystal, green aventurine could help boost your energy when you're feeling wiped out by gastroenteritis. Place it on the root chakra to stimulate and unblock energy centers.

Jasper—Utilize the nurturing energies of jasper to realign your chakras and support your body's natural healing process. It could help reenergize and aid your recovery from gastro illness. Make a crystal gem elixir and spray around your aura, and keep a piece of jasper by your bed as you recover.

Brown agate—Place on the abdomen to calm and soothe an irritated stomach and relieve feelings of nausea.

Shungite—Hold or place on the solar plexus to boost physical and emotional well-being and clear the body of negative toxins.

OTHER GRID AND LAYOUT CRYSTALS
—
• Peridot (for the intestines)
• Thulite (good all-rounder for gastric upsets)
• Dumortierite (for nausea)

ADDITIONAL THERAPIES
—
Sip water or suck on an ice cube to replace lost fluids and ensure you remain hydrated. Eat small portions of foods when you feel able to. Taking a probiotic supplement after your illness might help restore a good balance of healthy flora (bacteria) in your gut.

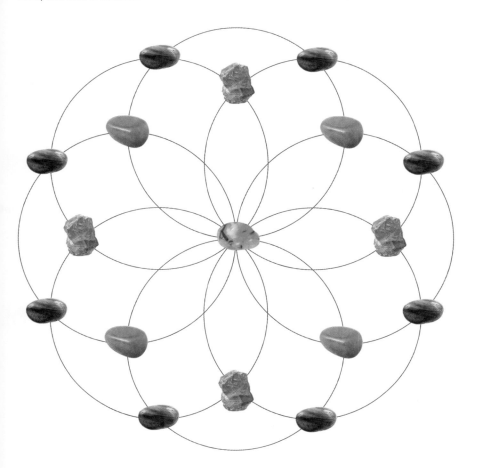

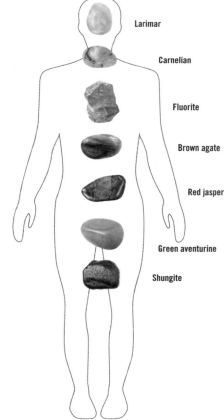

Larimar

Carnelian

Fluorite

Brown agate

Red jasper

Green aventurine

Shungite

INDIGESTION

Indigestion is a feeling of discomfort in your upper abdomen. Mild indigestion is common and may occur after you've eaten a big meal, eaten fatty foods, or rushed through eating a meal. Symptoms of indigestion include bloating, a warm or burning sensation in your upper abdomen, burping, flatulence, and nausea. Sometimes indigestion can be linked to other health conditions. If you have regular bouts of indigestion, or it's severe, consult your health practitioner.

KEY CRYSTALS
—

Citrine—Hold, wear, or place on your body to detoxify, balance, and reenergize the digestive system.

Jasper—Jasper may help support the digestive system, so pop a piece in your pocket, or place on your stomach, to help aid digestive problems.

Peridot—Place on the throat chakra to relieve hiccups, burping, or general indigestion problems. Wear on a necklace to aid ongoing issues.

Tourmaline—Place tourmaline on the solar plexus chakra to cleanse and purify the body and remove blockages, helping energy to follow through in a normal manner.

OTHER GRID AND LAYOUT CRYSTALS
—

• Candle quartz (to help you feel positive that you'll conquer your indigestion)
• Pyrophyllite (for indigestion, heartburn, and acid)
• Montebrasite (for heartburn)
• Moonstone (to help the digestive system)

ADDITIONAL THERAPIES
—

Take care of what you eat and drink and watch out for spicy, greasy, or fatty foods that may trigger symptoms. If you rush food, try to slow down and become more mindful about slowly chewing each mouthful. Cut down on sparkling drinks, caffeine, and alcohol, and avoid smoking. Peppermint can ease digestive complaints, so drink a cup of peppermint tea after eating.

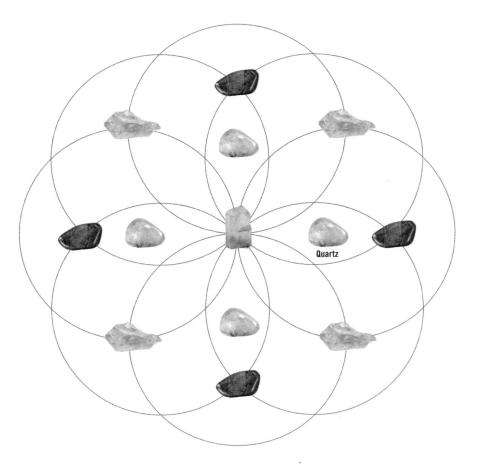

Quartz

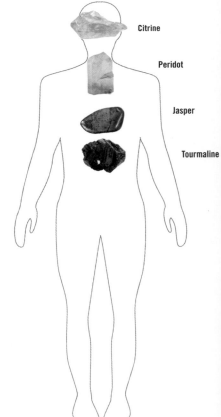

Citrine

Peridot

Jasper

Tourmaline

FLATULENCE

Flatulence or wind is a normal way of releasing gas from your body. On average, people break wind about five to 15 times a day, but it's different for everyone. On some occasions you may find yourself with more flatulence than is normal for you. This can be caused by swallowing too much air or eating foods that your body finds hard to digest properly. Some other health conditions can also cause flatulence, including irritable bowel syndrome, constipation, food allergies, or celiac disease. You may also experience changes in your flatulence habits while taking certain medications, such as antibiotics, statins, or non-steroidal inflammatory drugs (NSAIDs).

KEY CRYSTALS

—

Green garnet—Place green garnet on the root chakra to energize your body, clear out blockages, and rebalance the chakras. It may also help you to digest vitamins and minerals in foods better.

Diamond—Wear a diamond to cleanse and purify your body and help balance your metabolism.

Carnelian—Place on the root chakra, or around the body, to help calm the digestive system and reduce flatulence.

OTHER GRID AND LAYOUT CRYSTALS

—

• Emerald (for detoxification)
• Peridot (to aid digestion)
• Amethyst (for bloating)

ADDITIONAL THERAPIES

—

Try to identify if certain foods or drinks trigger symptoms and, if so, avoid them where possible. Drinking ginger or peppermint tea might help your digestive system. Aim to eat smaller meals and exercise regularly to improve your digestion.

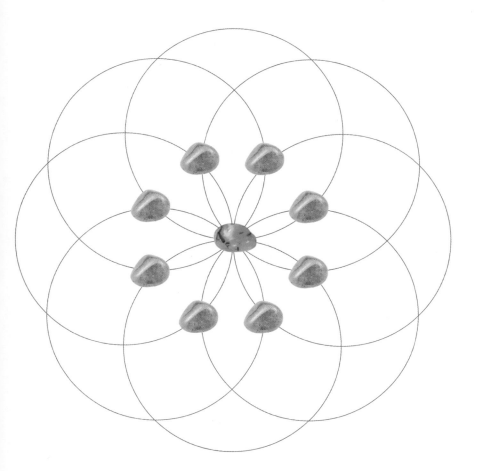

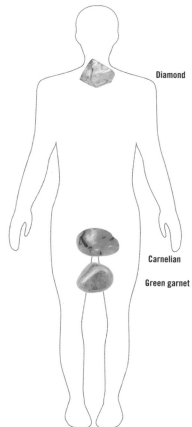

Diamond

Carnelian

Green garnet

STOMACH ULCERS

Stomach ulcers, also sometimes called gastric or peptic ulcers, are open sores that develop on the lining of your stomach. Ulcers that occur in your intestine are called duodenal ulcers. Symptoms of a stomach ulcer include pain in your stomach that can extend up to your neck or through to your back and last from minutes to hours, indigestion, heartburn, nausea, vomiting, loss of appetite, burping, bloating, and weight loss. Stomach ulcers can be caused by taking non-steroidal anti-inflammatory drugs or by *Helicobacter pylori (H. pylori)* infections. It's also likely that drinking alcohol, eating spicy foods, and smoking might play a part. If you think you could have a stomach ulcer or you have blood in your stools or vomit, see a medical practitioner.

KEY CRYSTALS
—

Rhodonite—Place rhodonite on your stomach and let its gentle healing energies soothe the discomfort of a stomach ulcer.

Pyrophyllite—Place on the solar plexus, as this crystal could help reduce the amount of acid in your body.

Montebrasite—Make a crystal gem elixir and spray around your aura to aid healing.

Blue lace agate—Make a crystal gem elixir and spray on and around your body for a calming and soothing effect.

OTHER GRID AND LAYOUT CRYSTALS
—

- Obsidian (to detoxify and dissolve blockages)
- Bloodstone (to boost the immune system)
- Green aventurine (to purify the stomach)
- Calcite (for cleansing)

ADDITIONAL THERAPIES

In addition to any prescribed medical treatments, adjusting your lifestyle habits may be beneficial, such as exercising, cutting back on alcohol, and quitting smoking. If you're stressed, learn to relax more by practicing meditation or doing qigong exercises. Take probiotics to improve the levels of healthy bacteria in your gut. Some research suggests cranberry extract may help with *H. pylori* infections and that eating honey could reduce the growth of *H. pylori*.

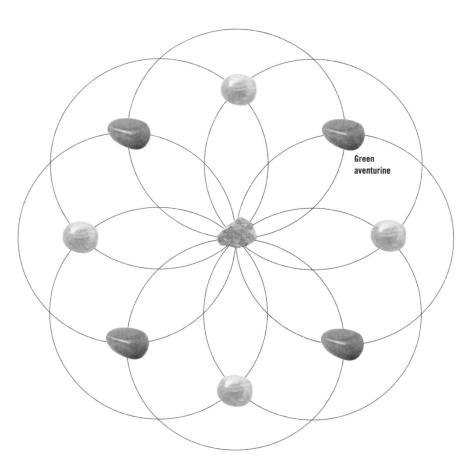

Green aventurine

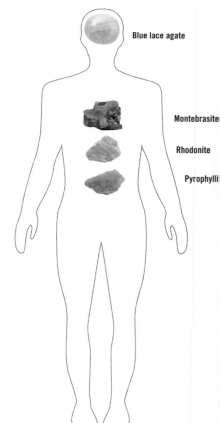

Blue lace agate

Montebrasite

Rhodonite

Pyrophylli

CONSTIPATION

Constipation is a bowel condition where you have infrequent bowel movements of three or less per week or find it difficult to pass stools. Symptoms include having hard or lumpy stools, straining to open your bowels, feeling that you can't completely empty your bowels, and the sensation of a bowel blockage. Constipation is common and it's not unusual to experience it at some point in your life, but for some people the symptoms can be chronic and ongoing. The most common causes of constipation include not eating enough fiber in your diet, not drinking enough water, taking prescribed medications that change your bowel movements, spending long periods sitting or lying down, not exercising enough, stress, or ignoring the urge to go to the toilet. It's also common to experience constipation when pregnant or in the weeks after you've given birth. If you frequently have constipation, see a medical practitioner.

KEY CRYSTALS
—

Amber—Amber is a good crystal to use to help support a healthy colon and digestive system.

Calcite—Place a piece of calcite on your stomach or solar plexus chakra to encourage the bowel movements.

Sodalite—Place sodalite on or around your abdomen to help ease stomach cramps associated with bad constipation. Make a crystal gem elixir and add it to a spray bottle. Spray it onto your abdomen and massage it in.

OTHER GRID AND LAYOUT CRYSTALS
—

• Ruby (to energize the colon)
• Sapphire (for nausea)
• Fluorite (to cleanse the bowel, detox, and reduce inflammation)
• Citrine (to improve digestion)

ADDITIONAL THERAPIES
—

Regular exercise can help the digestive system and reduce the risk of constipation. Diet can play a big role in constipation, particularly if you don't eat enough fiber. Aim to include more fruits, vegetables, and healthy wholegrains in your diet and drink plenty of water to aid digestion. Massaging your stomach might help get things moving, as can having regular exercise. If you're stressed, try meditation or yoga to aid relaxation.

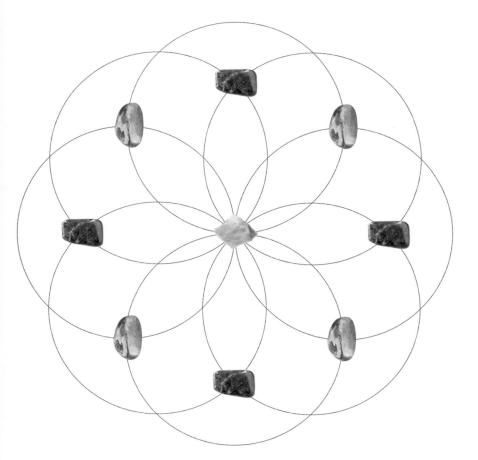

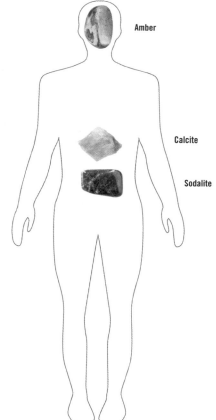

Amber

Calcite

Sodalite

DIARRHEA

If you have diarrhea, you'll have loose, watery bowel movements, sometimes accompanied by a sense of urgency to go to the toilet. Sudden diarrhea can be caused by a stomach bug or food poisoning, but other conditions, such as irritable bowel syndrome, food allergies, inflammatory bowel disease, or celiac disease, can also cause diarrhea. If you have diarrhea that continues for longer than five to seven days, and it's accompanied by sickness, consult a medical practitioner for advice.

KEY CRYSTALS
—

Smoky quartz—Place on the root chakra with the point facing away from the body to draw out negative energies and ease bowel cramps.

Orange calcite—Place orange calcite around the body to let its energies calm and ease colonic cramps.

Hematite—Place on your root chakra to encourage the easing of stomach cramps and diarrhea.

Rhodonite—The gentle energies of rhodonite may help calm and soothe an inflamed colon after a bout of diarrhea.

Yellow jasper—Place several pieces of yellow jasper on or around the body to help ease symptoms of diarrhea.

OTHER GRID AND LAYOUT CRYSTALS
—

• Pyrophyllite (for digestion and diarrhea)
• Sodalite (for stomach cramps)
• Orange calcite (to calm colonic cramps)

ADDITIONAL THERAPIES
—

If you have a bout of diarrhea, sip slowly on water to replace lost fluids and rehydrate your body. Avoid fruit juice or carbonated drinks, as they can make diarrhea symptoms worse. Eat small amounts of food when you feel able to. Be aware that diarrhea stomach bugs can spread, so take steps to avoid infecting others by cleaning surfaces, door handles, toilet seats, and flushes daily, and avoid sharing towels or cutlery and preparing food for other people.

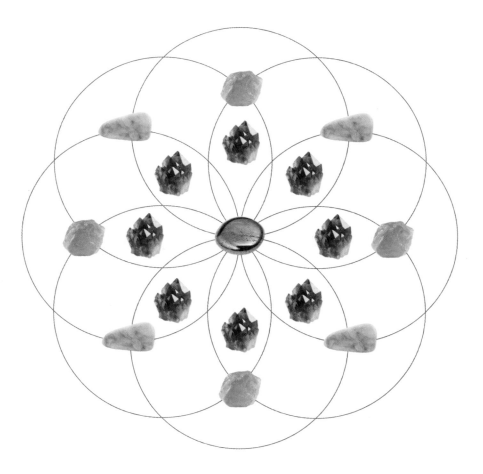

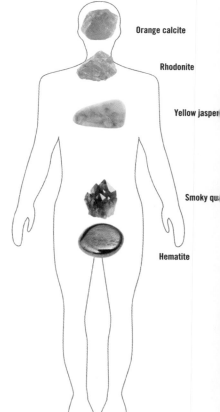

Orange calcite

Rhodonite

Yellow jasper

Smoky qua[rtz]

Hematite

IRRITABLE BOWEL SYNDROME

Irritable bowel syndrome (IBS) is a common digestive condition that causes symptoms such as constipation, bloating, stomach cramps, and diarrhea. Other associated symptoms include passing mucus with bowel movements, nausea, tiredness, and flatulence. People living with IBS may find that some days are better than others and symptoms may be triggered by diet. The exact cause of IBS is unknown, but it's linked to factors such as stress, an oversensitive gut, a family history of digestive issues, and food passing through your body too quickly. If you have symptoms that could be caused by IBS, see a medical practitioner for diagnosis.

KEY CRYSTALS
—

Sodalite—Place sodalite on or around your abdomen to help ease stomach cramps. Make a crystal gem elixir and add it to a spray bottle. Spray it onto your abdomen and gently massage it in.

Orange calcite—Orange calcite can help calm the colonic cramps often associated with irritable bowel syndrome. Place on the abdomen or directly on the area of pain.

Citrine—If irritable bowel syndrome is causing problems with digestion, place citrine on the solar plexus chakra to aid the digestive process.

Rhodonite—Irritable bowel syndrome can leave your body feeling inflamed and sore, so place rhodonite around your body, or pop a piece into your pocket and carry it with you, to ease inflammation.

OTHER GRID AND LAYOUT CRYSTALS
—

• Yellow jasper (for diarrhea)
• Hematite (for cramps and spasms)
• Citrine (for digestion and colon healing)
• Carnelian (for flatulence)
• Dalmation jasper (to soothe irritated bowels)

• Ocean jasper (to cleanse and detoxify the bowels)
• Amethyst (for stomach bloating)

ADDITIONAL THERAPIES
—

Probiotic supplements could help restore healthy flora in the gut. Yoga and Pilates may help to ease pain or discomfort and meditation could aid relaxation. It may help to avoid hot, spicy, and fatty foods and cut down on alcohol, fizzy drinks, and caffeine. Eat slowly and chew every mouthful. Keep a food diary and record symptoms. See a qualified nutritionist for advice.

Taking probiotics may help by restoring the right levels of healthy bacteria into your body, and acupuncture could help restore balance. Bathing in magnesium salts may help cleanse your body and adding buckwheat to your diet may offer some benefits.

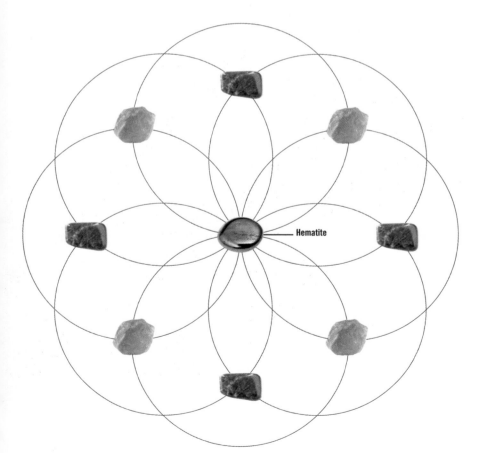

Hematite

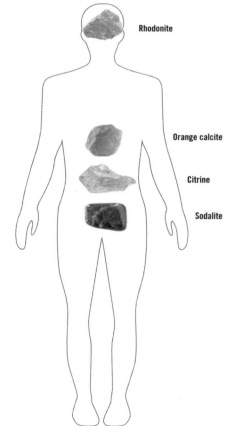

Rhodonite

Orange calcite

Citrine

Sodalite

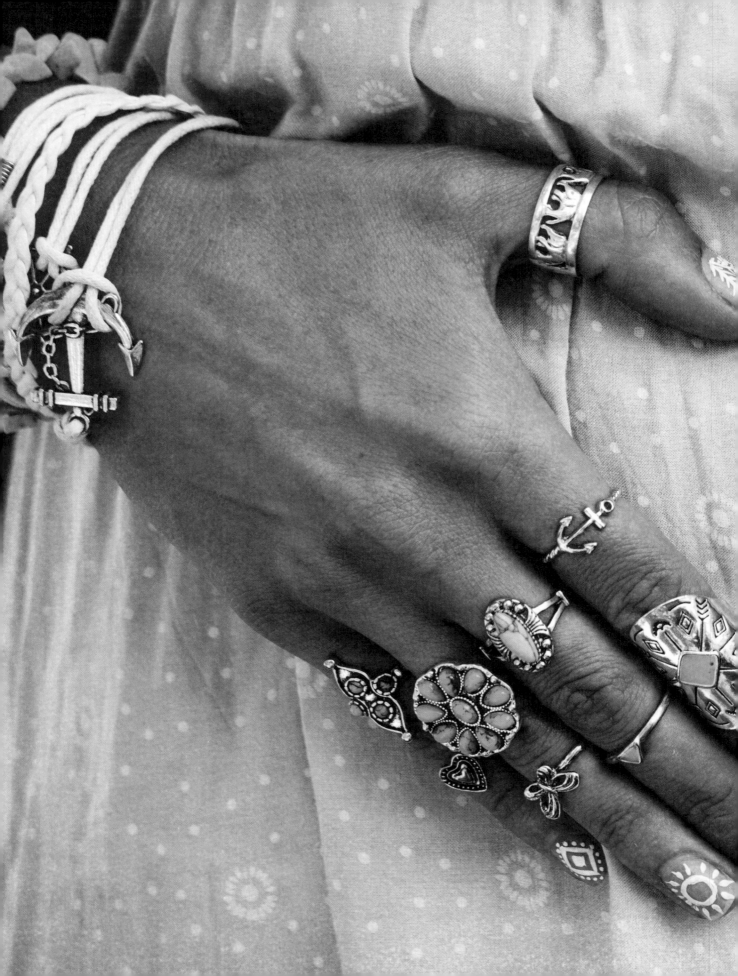

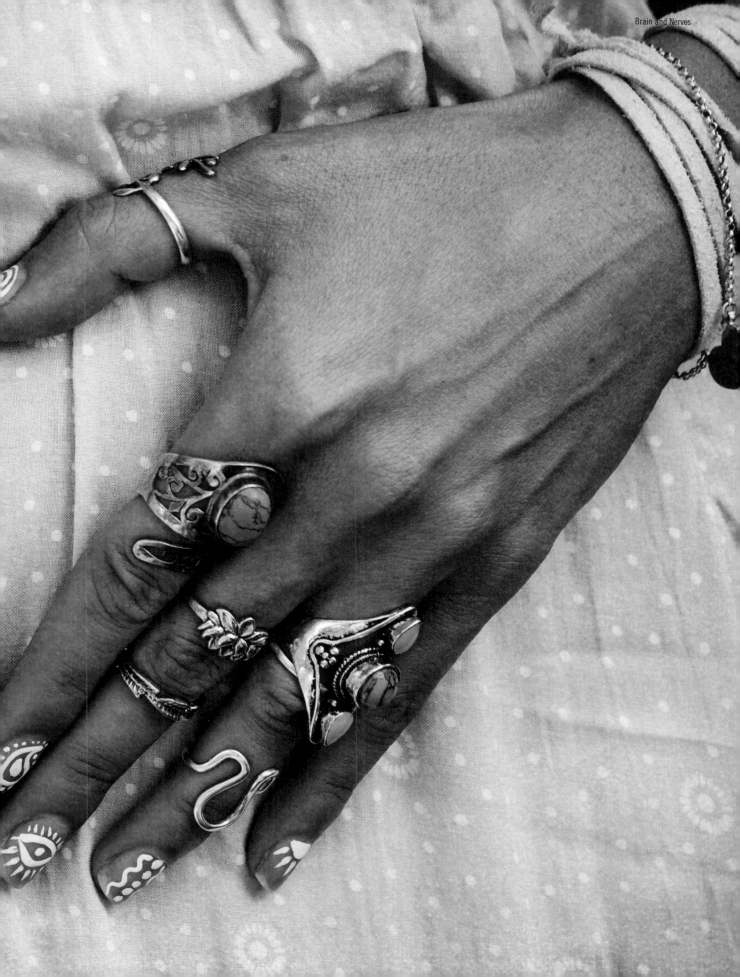

HEMORRHOIDS

Hemorrhoids, also known as piles, are swollen blood vessels that form into lumps inside and around your bottom. Piles are often associated with pregnancy, constipation, pushing too hard when having a bowel movement, and heavy lifting. They can cause symptoms such as an itchy bottom, pain around your bottom, mucus, or bright red blood when emptying your bowels and lumps. In many cases hemorrhoids clear up on their own, but sometimes you may need prescribed creams or other treatments to help. Always consult a medical practitioner if you have unexplained bleeding from your bottom.

KEY CRYSTALS
—

Amethyst—Make a crystal gem elixir and dab it gently around your bottom (externally only) to relieve itchiness. Place a piece of amethyst near your bed, so its gentle energies will surround you as you sleep.

Rhodonite—Place on the root chakra to encourage reduction of inflammation, healing, and hemorrhoid shrinkage. If you have a small piece of tumbled rhodonite, you could tape it in place for a short while.

OTHER GRID AND LAYOUT CRYSTALS
—

- Agate (to ease discomfort)
- Bloodstone (for inflammation and bleeding)
- Citrine (for the intestines)

ADDITIONAL THERAPIES
—

Have warm baths to ease the pain and itching of hemorrhoids. Exercise regularly, drink lots of fluids, and eat plenty of fiber to keep stools soft and avoid constipation. Some people find draping a cold flannel or ice pack on their bottom while lying down can ease some pain and itching.

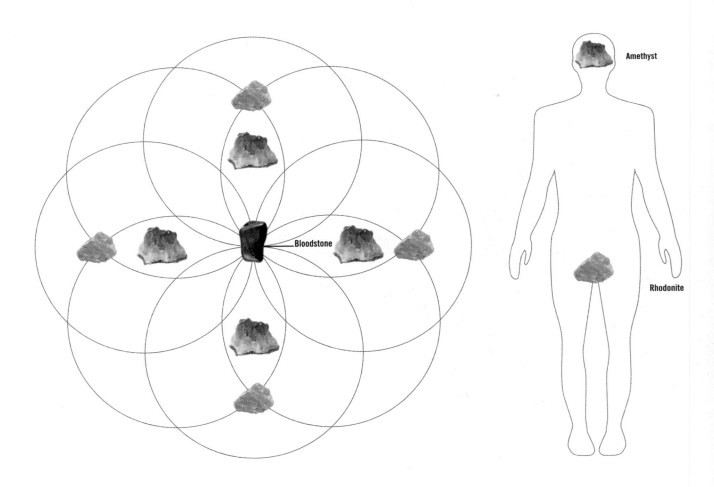

Bloodstone

Amethyst

Rhodonite

GASTROESOPHAGEAL REFLUX DISEASE

Gastroesophageal reflux disease, also known as GERD, is a digestive condition caused by stomach acid flowing back up your esophagus from your stomach and into your mouth. When this happens regularly, the stomach acid irritates the lining of your esophagus. Symptoms include a burning feeling in your chest (heartburn), problems swallowing, a lump-like feeling in your throat, chest pain, a chronic cough, and sour liquid in your mouth. Chronic inflammation can cause serious problems over time, so don't delay seeing a medical practitioner if you think you could have GERD.

KEY CRYSTALS
—

Citrine—Place on the solar plexus chakra to calm the esophagus and aid digestion.

Peridot—Place on the throat chakra to relieve burping and indigestion problems. Wear on a necklace to aid ongoing issues.

Apatite—Apatite can be used in conjunction with either the throat or solar plexus chakras, to help break down food, improve digestion, and eliminate toxins.

OTHER GRID AND LAYOUT CRYSTALS
—

• Pyrophyllite (for acid)
• Amazonite (to calm the digestive system)
• Lapis lazuli (for digestive pain)
• Carnelian (to stimulate digestion)
• Smoky quartz (to ground you)

ADDITIONAL THERAPIES
—

In addition to any prescribed medications, acupuncture may help to relieve some symptoms, and learning to relax—by practicing mindfulness, tai chi, or qigong—could be beneficial if stress is an issue. If you are prone to GERD, avoid eating big meals late at night and keep a food diary to detect which foods or drinks might trigger your symptoms. Eating an anti-inflammatory diet may help—see a qualified nutritionist for advice.

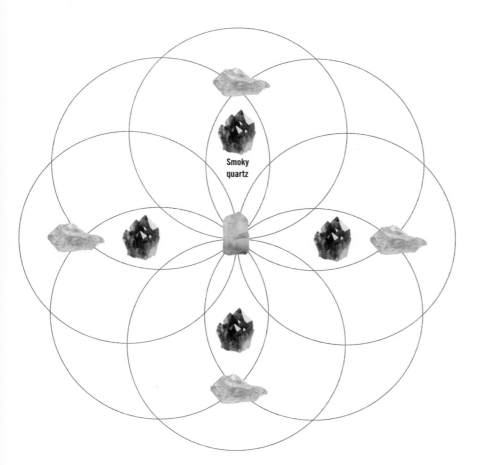

Smoky quartz

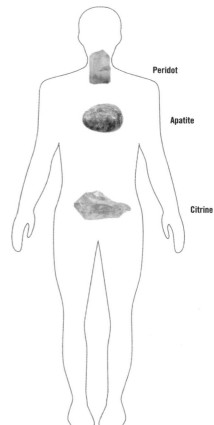

Peridot

Apatite

Citrine

KIDNEY AND BLADDER STONES

Kidney stones occur in one or both kidneys, or in the tube connecting the bladder to the kidneys. They can be severely painful, especially if large, causing pain in your abdomen, nausea, and vomiting. If not treated, they can lead to kidney infections. Kidney stones form from waste products in the blood that build up into hard crystal-like lumps. Stones can also form inside the bladder, normally as a result of not being able to empty your bladder properly. Symptoms include frequent urination, lower abdominal pain, and blood in the urine. Small kidney and bladder stones may be passed without knowing, but larger ones may need to be properly treated and broken down by laser treatment or surgery. Always see a medical practitioner for diagnosis.

KEY CRYSTALS
—

Bloodstone—Wear a bloodstone crystal when you have bladder or kidney stones, as it can be beneficial for cleansing and reenergizing when you're feeling drained by pain and discomfort. If you have an infection alongside your kidney or bladder stones, bloodstone may also help with detoxifying your body and aiding your immune system.

Carnelian—Place carnelian on the sacral chakra to release blockages and help regulate the kidneys.

Magnesite—Place on the sacral chakra, or directly over the area of pain, as magnesite may help with kidney and bladder stone pain relief. It can help balance body temperature, too, which can be useful if the pain is making you feel feverish.

Rhyolite—Place directly over the kidney, as rhyolite may be able to help dissolve kidney stones.

OTHER GRID AND LAYOUT CRYSTALS
—

• Honey calcite (for bladder and kidney function)
• Actinolite (for blockages)
• Amber (for calming and healing)
• Citrine (to support the kidneys and bladder)
• Sunstone (for healing and pain relief)
• Jade (for kidney support)
• Cavansite (to support kidney function)

ADDITIONAL THERAPIES
—

Drink plenty of water daily and at least one glass of lemon in water as this may help in passing stones. Avoid fizzy drinks and salt. Depending on what type of stones you have, your doctor may suggest avoiding certain foods, like spinach or strawberries. Acupuncture treatments may help with pain.

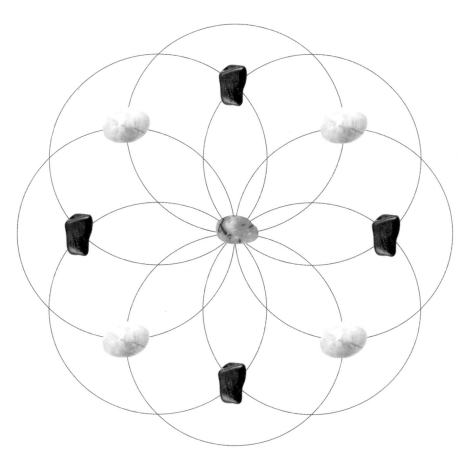

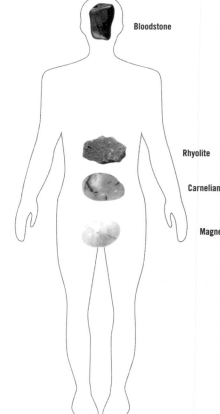

Bloodstone

Rhyolite

Carnelian

Magne[

CYSTITIS

Cystitis is a common form of urinary tract infection (UTI) that affects the bladder. Symptoms include pain, burning, or stinging when urinating, frequent and urgent urination, dark or cloudy urine, lower abdominal pain, and feeling unwell and tired. Mild cases may get better on their own within a few days, but recurrent bouts may need antibiotic treatment. If recurrent cystitis isn't treated, it could lead to more serious kidney infections. Women are often more prone to cystitis due to having a shorter urethra than men.

KEY CRYSTALS
—

Fluorite—Fluorite that's predominantly blue-green in color can be placed on the bladder to support healing and ease discomfort when you have an infection.

Carnelian—Place on the root chakra to rebalance and energize your body, which is especially helpful when you're trying to fight an infection.

Citrine—The sunny energies of citrine can be uplifting and may help reduce bladder infections and cystitis. Place around the body or wear as jewelry while you're recovering from cystitis.

OTHER GRID AND LAYOUT CRYSTALS
—

• Bloodstone (to cleanse and detoxify)
• Amber (for healing)
• Aquamarine (for bladder healing)
• Dalmation jasper (to support the urinary system)
• Jade (to cleanse the kidneys and urinary system)

ADDITIONAL THERAPIES
—

There is some evidence that cranberry extract could help reduce the risk of cystitis, so taking cranberry supplements may be beneficial. Drink plenty of water to keep the bladder and kidneys well flushed. Avoid having sex while you have symptoms and use a hot water bottle to aid pain relief.

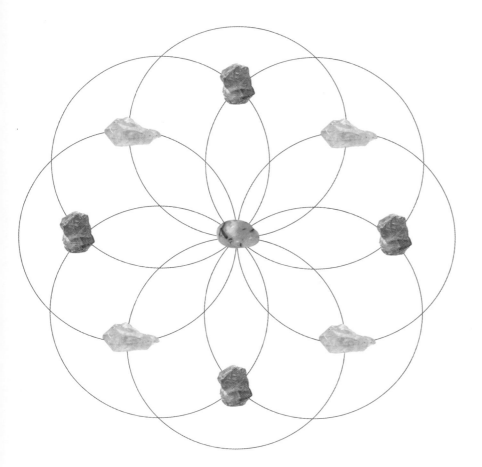

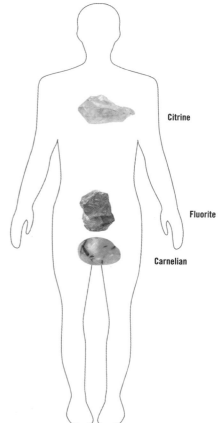

Citrine

Fluorite

Carnelian

INCONTINENCE

Urinary incontinence occurs when the bladder is unable to help passing urine. There are various different types of incontinence and some people have a mix of one or more types. Stress incontinence happens due to the bladder being under pressure, such as when you laugh or cough. Urge incontinence is when you get a sudden urgent need to pass urine and can't control it. Overflow incontinence is due to being unable to fully empty your bladder, so it causes leaks. If you're totally incontinent, you're unable to store any urine in your bladder. Incontinence is common and can be caused by weakened muscles, bladder blockages, spinal injuries, age, pregnancy, and obesity. Speak to your medical practitioner for advice if you have concerns.

KEY CRYSTALS
—

Amber—Place on the sacral chakra to cleanse and heal. The sunny outlook of this gemstone can also help lift the spirits and improve positivity if you're feeling down about having incontinence.

Fluorite—Place blue-green-colored fluorite on the bladder to get the energies moving as they should and encourage the removal of stagnant blocks.

Scapolite—Carry or wear scapolite to help strengthen the bladder muscles and reduce instances of incontinence.

OTHER GRID AND LAYOUT CRYSTALS
—

• Topaz (for emotional support)
• Citrine (to support the bladder)
• Petrified wood (to help incontinence)
• Jade (if there are related kidney problems)
• Prehnite (for the bladder)

ADDITIONAL THERAPIES
—

Pelvic floor exercises and kegel balls can be used by women to help strengthen pelvic muscles that may have become weaker after pregnancy or as a result of hormone changes during menopause. Losing weight may help reduce incontinence issues and cutting down on alcohol and caffeinated drinks may help your bladder.

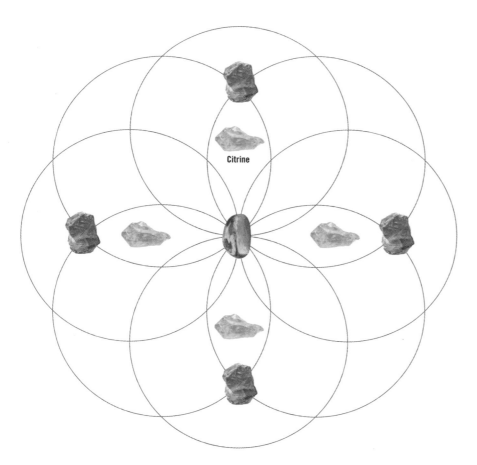

Citrine

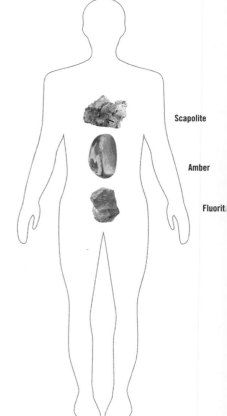

Scapolite

Amber

Fluorit

BED-WETTING

Bed-wetting is being unable to control your bladder at night and waking up to find you've wet the bed. It's common in young children but can occur in older people, too. It can happen as a one-off, or regularly. Sometimes it can be linked to underlying stress or emotional issues, or it could be connected to a bladder or kidney issue, such as a urinary tract infection (UTI). In many cases it's a temporary situation and gets better over time, but if you have any concerns, consult a medical practitioner.

KEY CRYSTALS
—

Amber—Place amber around the bed at night to create a positive and healing atmosphere. The energies of amber can help lift the spirits, which is beneficial if bed-wetting is linked to stress or underlying emotional issues.

Jade—Make a crystal gem elixir with jade and spray it around the aura to stabilize the body, remove negative energies, and help cleanse the urinary system.

Jasper—Place on the bladder to gently calm and provide stability. Brown jasper can be placed in the room to help remove negative energies.

Rose quartz—Place rose quartz under the pillow, or wear on a necklace during the day, to boost feelings of self-esteem.

OTHER GRID AND LAYOUT CRYSTALS
—

• Scapolite (to strengthen bladder muscles)
• Topaz (for emotional support)
• Prehnite (to support the kidneys and bladder)
• Tiger's eye (if bed-wetting is linked to bad dreams or nightmares)
• Carnelian (to regulate the kidneys)

ADDITIONAL THERAPIES
—

In addition to any prescribed medications or treatments, it may be useful to limit the consumption of liquids before bedtime, especially any containing caffeine, or you could try setting an alarm for the middle of the night as a reminder to go to the toilet before an accident occurs.

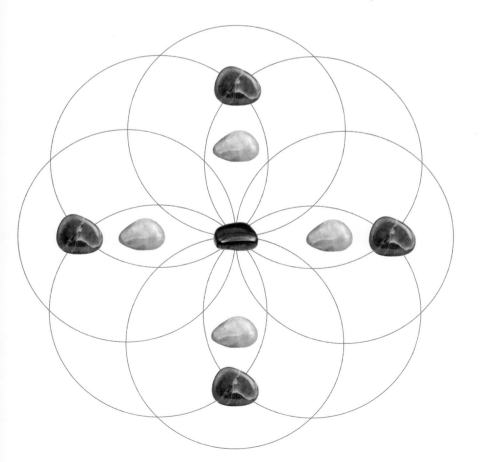

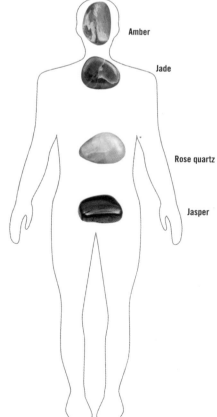

Amber

Jade

Rose quartz

Jasper

MENSTRUAL PROBLEMS

Menstrual problems are common in women and relate to the menstrual cycle. There are different types of menstrual problems, including dysmenorrhea (painful periods), menorrhagia (heavy periods), amenorrhea (no periods), and oligomenorrhea (light or infrequent periods). They can be caused by fibroids, hormonal imbalances, polycystic ovary syndrome (PCOS), genetics, and endometriosis. Menstrual problems can vary in severity, with some women being mildly affected and others severely. If you have any concerns about menstrual issues, see a medical practitioner for diagnosis or treatment. It may help to keep a record of your symptoms and when they occur in your cycle.

KEY CRYSTALS
—

Moonstone—Wear moonstone jewelry in the run up to, and during, your period. Moonstone has a calming energy and may help to regulate your periods and reduce water retention and bloating.

Citrine—Make a crystal gem elixir with citrine and add it to bathwater or put it in a spray bottle and apply regularly to your skin. It can help to balance hormones and alleviate the tiredness and fatigue you can feel during a period.

Chrysoprase—Place on the sacral chakra and let its gentle energies calm and soothe menstrual stomach cramps and balance the hormones.

Malachite—Put a piece of malachite by the side of the bed to help absorb negative emotions. The energies of malachite may also help reduce stomach cramps and bloating, detoxify, and ease feelings of nausea.

OTHER GRID AND LAYOUT CRYSTALS
—

• Magnesite (for stomach cramps)
• Serpentine (for emotional imbalances and grounding)
• Rose quartz (to calm the mind and ease pain)
• Bloodstone (for heavy periods)
• Amethyst (for menstrual headaches and bloating)
• Carnelian (to regulate menstrual flow, ease cramps, and calm emotions)

ADDITIONAL THERAPIES
—

Dietary changes, such as reducing sugar, salt, caffeine, and alcohol, may help some menstrual problems. Ginger tea can help ease nausea and evening primrose oil may be beneficial. Therapies such as acupuncture and reflexology could help with pain and discomfort.

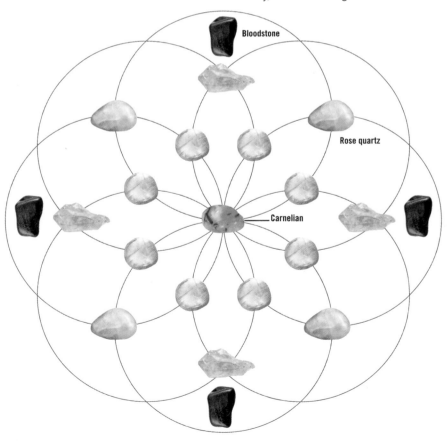

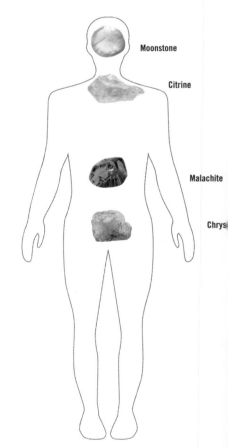

PREMENSTRUAL SYNDROME

Premenstrual syndrome, or PMS, occurs when fluctuating hormone levels before your monthly period cause physical and emotional symptoms. Some of the symptoms may include headaches, feeling irritable, bloating, breast tenderness, mood swings, fatigue, anxiety, backache, cramps, spots, and loss of interest in sex. Not every woman experiences premenstrual syndrome and it can vary in severity. Symptoms tend to ease when a period starts.

KEY CRYSTALS
—

Moonstone—Place moonstone on the solar plexus or heart chakras. It's a powerful crystal for helping to soothe emotional instability and stabilize fluctuating feelings.

Chrysoprase—Use on the sacral chakra to help balance premenstrual hormones.

Jet—Place on the root chakra to help stabilize and ground. It can also help aid mood swings and low feelings, bringing more balance to your emotions.

Rose quartz—Wear rose quartz jewelry or keep a piece of rose quartz close to you, to help clear the mind, calm tension, and relieve pain. Let its gentle energies ease the discomfort and frustration of PMS.

Carnelian—Carry carnelian crystals in your pocket to help regulate menstrual flow, ease period cramps, and calm emotions.

OTHER GRID AND LAYOUT CRYSTALS
—

• Citrine (to combat fatigue and stabilize emotions)
• Magnesite (for stomach cramps)
• Malachite (for negative emotions)
• Amethyst (for bloating and headaches)

ADDITIONAL THERAPIES
—

Lack of sleep can make PMS symptoms worse, so try to get eight hours a night. Eat healthy foods and cut down on caffeine—try chamomile tea instead. For symptoms such as stress and anxiety, try yoga, massage, or meditation. Some studies suggest that taking calcium and vitamin B6 supplements may help, plus magnesium supplements may ease PMS-related headaches. Evening primrose oil supplements might also help PMS symptoms, but research is inconclusive.

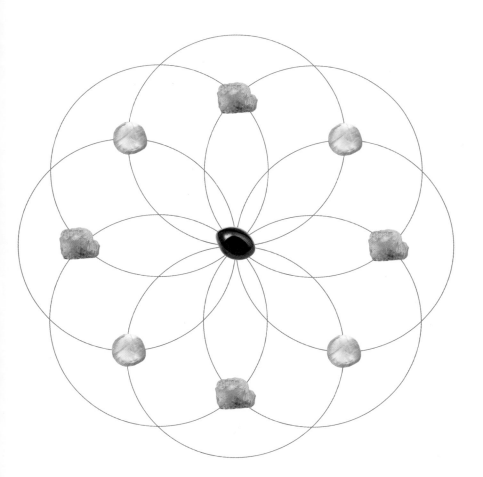

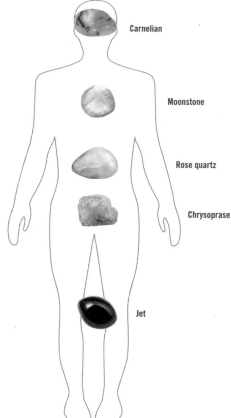

Carnelian

Moonstone

Rose quartz

Chrysoprase

Jet

INFERTILITY

Infertility is the inability to conceive, even after frequent sex, for at least a year. About one-third of all cases in couples is due to female infertility (and one-third to male infertility). Infertility can be caused by a range of factors, including ovarian disorders, damage to fallopian tubes, endometriosis, polyps, or fibroids, or it may be unexplained. Depending on the cause, some treatments are available, including medication, surgery, and assisted conception, but dealing with infertility can be emotionally and physically draining. If you have concerns about infertility, seek advice from a medical practitioner.

KEY CRYSTALS

—

Rutilated quartz—The vitality of rutilated quartz can help soothe the trauma of infertility and promote feelings of forgiveness. Make a crystal gem elixir and spray over the aura to reduce negativity, or keep rutilated quartz in the bedroom to facilitate change and adjustments.

Moonstone—Keep a piece of moonstone by your bed, or under your pillow, as it may help to promote conception. Its calming energies may also help to soothe worries and insecurities about your fertility.

Rose quartz—Wear rose quartz to soothe and calm worries about infertility and to boost feelings of love. Also place a piece in the relationship corner of your home (the far right corner of the house) to promote love in your relationship.

OTHER GRID AND LAYOUT CRYSTALS

- Chrysoprase (for the fallopian tubes and infertility caused by infections)
- Thulite (for diseases of the reproductive organs)
- Carnelian (to stimulate hormone production)
- Molvadite (to boost fertility)
- Scepter quartz (for infertility)
- Zincite (for purification)
- Tiger's eye (to promote hormonal balance)
- Zoisite (for ovarian problems)

ADDITIONAL THERAPIES

—

A healthy diet and nutritional approach, especially from a nutritional therapist, may be worth trying. Therapies such as acupuncture, reflexology, or Bowen therapy may offer some help, but there's no strong evidence. It's important to look after yourself and focus on self-care, relieving stress, sleeping well, and exercising.

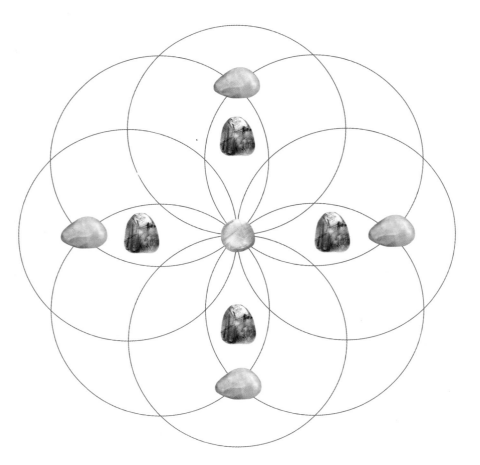

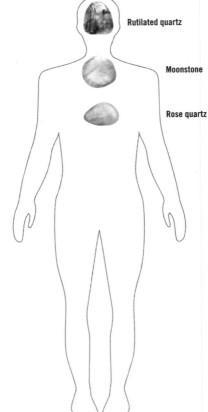

Rutilated quartz

Moonstone

Rose quartz

MISCARRIAGE

A miscarriage is defined as losing a baby during the first 23 weeks of pregnancy. They are relatively common, affecting approximately one in eight women. The majority of miscarriages aren't caused by anything the mother has done, but it inevitably feels like it to those who lose a pregnancy in this way. It can be highly traumatic, at whatever stage of pregnancy a loss is experienced, and it can be emotionally and physically draining. It's normal to experience feelings of anger, shock, and guilt and go through stages of grief. Always see a medical practitioner if you suspect you could be having a miscarriage, as you may need medical treatment.

KEY CRYSTALS
—

Rose quartz—The gentle energies of rose quartz can have a comforting presence and help to promote self-compassion when you are dealing with grief. Place pieces of rose quartz in the rooms of your home and wear a piece on a necklace to keep it near your heart chakra and remind you to be kind to yourself.

Rhodonite—Place rhodonite on your heart chakra to help promote gentle acceptance as you deal with the grief and trauma of a miscarriage.

Lepidolite—Hold lepidolite to help with the release of suffering. The calming vibrations will support you as you face trauma and cope with healing.

OTHER GRID AND LAYOUT CRYSTALS
—

• Moonstone (for coping with change and different stages of grief)
• Smoky quartz (to help keep you grounded when your emotions are all over the place)
• Pyrite (for emotional exhaustion)
• Amethyst (for emotional comfort when you feel overwhelmed)
• Obsidian (for protection against negative energies)

ADDITIONAL THERAPIES
—

Couples counseling may be helpful. If you find it hard to talk about how you feel, write it down instead. Honor and remember your baby by having some form of memorial, as this could help you grieve. Take time to look after yourself, practice self-care, and fully recover from a miscarriage.

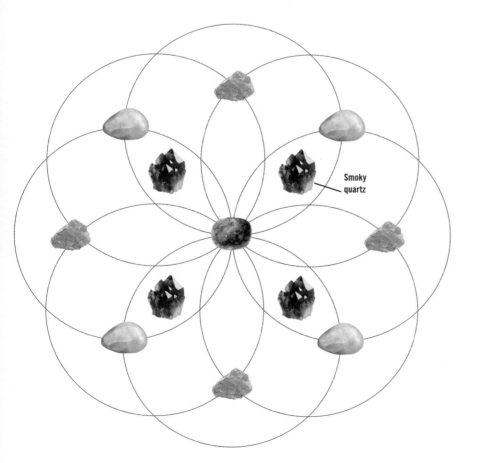

Smoky quartz

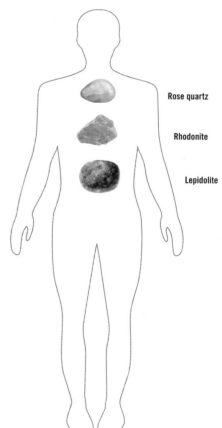

Rose quartz

Rhodonite

Lepidolite

PREGNANCY

During pregnancy your body goes through a number of changes and you can experience physical and emotional symptoms. Some of the common symptoms you may experience include nausea and morning sickness (particularly in the first three months), heartburn and digestive issues caused by changing hormones, high blood pressure, cramps as the muscles in your uterus stretch, back pain (especially in early pregnancy), acne due to hormones, changes to your breasts (such as feeling tender, swollen, heavy or full), and hip pain (particularly in later pregnancy as you cope with changes in your posture and uterus). You may also feel stressed and anxious about your forthcoming new role as a mom. Medical monitoring is essential during pregnancy to ensure everything is going smoothly and your baby is healthy and developing well.

KEY CRYSTALS

—

Lepidolite—Place lepidolite on the sacral chakra. Its soothing energies may help to relieve anxiety about pregnancy and promote a sense of happiness and confidence as you go through your pregnancy journey.

Aquamarine—The soothing energy of aquamarine may help to ease worries, fears, and anxiety about pregnancy. Keep a piece in your pocket and hold it whenever you need to.

Leopard skin jasper—Place on the root or sacral chakras to promote strength and stability during pregnancy and a safe birth.

OTHER GRID AND LAYOUT CRYSTALS

—

• Unakite (for a healthy pregnancy)
• Tiger's eye (for hormonal balance and courage to face change)
• Black onyx (for stamina and strength)
• Amethyst (for protection and stability)
• Moonstone (for balancing hormones)
• White agate (to protect mother and baby and for morning sickness)

ADDITIONAL THERAPIES

—

Drinking ginger tea, eating ginger biscuits, or having acupressure may help to ease symptoms of nausea and morning sickness. Massage and aromatherapy may help anxiety, as could relaxation and breathing techniques.

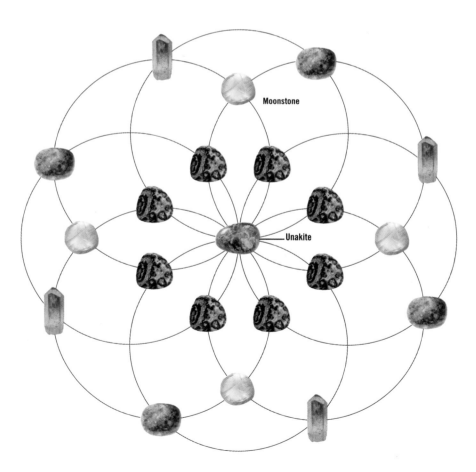

Moonstone

Unakite

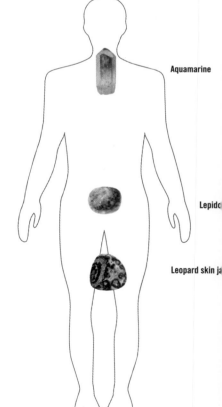

Aquamarine

Lepido

Leopard skin ja

LABOR

The experience of labor is different for every woman. Some sail through it with ease, while for others it can be lengthy, painful, or emotional. You can tell labor is starting or is on its way when you begin to feel an increased pressure in your uterus and your waters break. You may start to feel some contractions, but they'll get much stronger and more intense as your labor progresses. You won't know exactly how your labor will progress, or how it will make you feel, until it actually happens, but if you're well prepared, have attended all your medical checks, and are equipped with the support you need, you'll be in a good position.

KEY CRYSTALS

—

Unakite—Hold a piece of tumbled unakite when labor first starts. This gentle stone promotes feelings of nurturing and caring and can aid patience and persistence as labor gets underway.

Emerald—Keep an emerald crystal near you to promote patience, compassion, and unconditional love, and to aid in bonding with your baby.

Black onyx—Hold black onyx to help promote feelings of stamina and strength to get you through labor.

OTHER GRID AND LAYOUT CRYSTALS

—

• Red tiger's eye (for confidence)
• Malachite (for contractions and labor pains)
• Orange calcite (to promote positive thinking)
• Rose quartz (for protection during labor)
• White agate (for labor pains and encouraging milk flow)
• Moss agate (to encourage a successful birth)

ADDITIONAL THERAPIES

—

A TENS machine may be helpful during labor to ease pain and discomfort, and some women find hypnotherapy techniques useful. Other remedies and therapies that may be helpful include acupuncture, acupressure, shiatsu massage, aromatherapy massage, and reflexology. Hydrotherapy, or water birthing, could be beneficial, too.

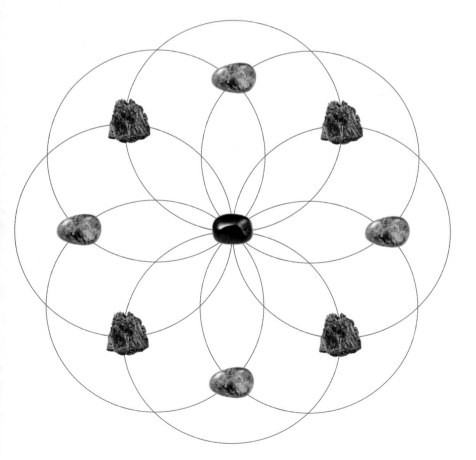

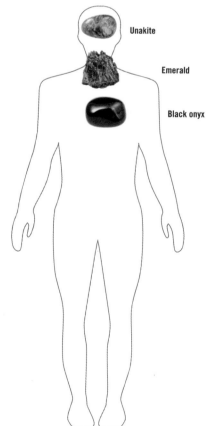

Unakite

Emerald

Black onyx

BREASTFEEDING

Breastfeeding gives your baby the best start in life. Breast milk can help boost your baby's immune system, helping to protect them from infections, plus breastfeeding can also help you lose weight faster after giving birth. Emotionally, it's a great way to connect with your baby through skin-to-skin contact and it can enhance your bond. Although it's the most natural way of feeding a baby, it's not always a skill that comes naturally to everyone and it can take practice to get your baby latching on comfortably and find the best positions that work for you both. If you're struggling with breastfeeding, speak to your obstetrician or midwife for advice and guidance.

KEY CRYSTALS
—

White agate—Keep white agate near you while breastfeeding to help promote a healthy flow of milk.

Rose quartz—Wear a rose quartz necklace to promote unconditional love and compassion and strengthen the connection with your baby as you breastfeed.

Moonstone—Place moonstone on the heart chakra to help balance your hormones, stabilize emotions, and adjust to the demands of nursing your baby.

OTHER GRID AND LAYOUT CRYSTALS
—

• Selenite (to create a safe, sacred space as you breastfeed)
• Aquamarine (for inner strength and courage if you feel overwhelmed by responsibility for your baby)
• Chalcedony (for lactation)
• Hematite (for grounding)
• Rhodonite (to help you stay calm if breastfeeding is hard)

ADDITIONAL THERAPIES
—

Being stressed won't help you or your baby, so try therapies such as meditation or mindfulness, or relaxation techniques to help you unwind. Burning aromatherapy essential oils such as lavender, bergamot, or neroli may help to promote relaxation, too.

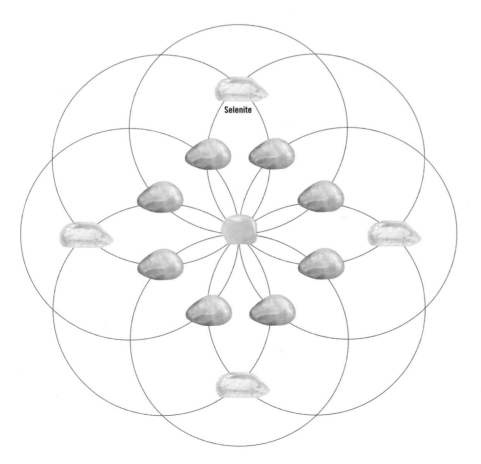

Selenite

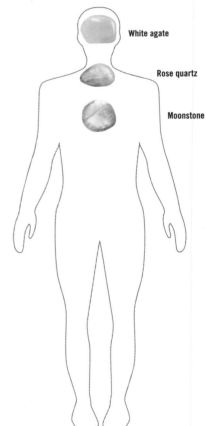

White agate

Rose quartz

Moonstone

POSTNATAL ILLNESS

Postnatal depression is a form of postnatal illness that occurs after having a baby. It's not uncommon to feel low, tearful, or anxious after giving birth, but if it lasts for more than two weeks, it could be postnatal depression. Signs and symptoms of postnatal depression include a low mood, loss of interest in anything, trouble sleeping at night, difficulty bonding with your baby, feeling tired in the day, not wanting contact with other people, difficulties making decisions, concentration issues, and negative thoughts about your baby. Postnatal depression can creep up on you slowly, and not just immediately after giving birth—it can happen at any time within the first year. It's essential to get help from a medical practitioner. Treatments are available depending on your individual symptoms and needs. Don't suffer alone.

KEY CRYSTALS
—

Aquamarine—If you feel overwhelmed by your new role as a mother, holding aquamarine may help to reduce stress, promote inner strength, and aid courage.

Celestite—If you are feeling anxious or overwhelmed, hold a celestite crystal. It can help promote restfulness and may help both you and your baby sleep soundly.

Brecciated jasper—If you experience postnatal depression, use brecciated jasper on the root chakra to help to ground you, reduce fear, and aid in the battle against negativity.

Chrysocolla—Place chrysocolla on the heart chakra to soothe and calm your body and mind when you're feeling stressed or fearful.

OTHER GRID AND LAYOUT CRYSTALS
—

• Red tiger's eye (for confidence as a new mother)
• Clear quartz (to dispel negativity)
• White jade (for support)
• Sodalite (to calm the mind if you have self-doubt)
• Amethyst (for peace)
• Citrine (for positive, supportive energy)

ADDITIONAL THERAPIES
—

Good support is essential to help you deal with postnatal illness, so accept help from friends or family. Talking about your feelings may be beneficial and it's important to practice self-care and look after yourself. Try to get sleep when you can, eat healthily, and have some exercise. Therapies such as counseling or cognitive behavioral therapy (CBT) may be beneficial.

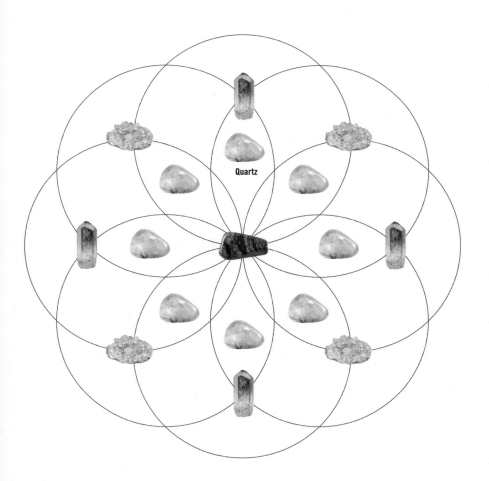

Quartz

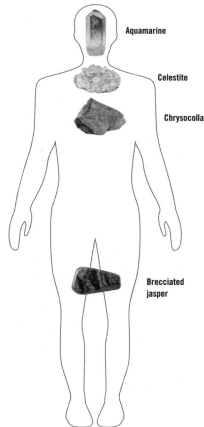

Aquamarine

Celestite

Chrysocolla

Brecciated jasper

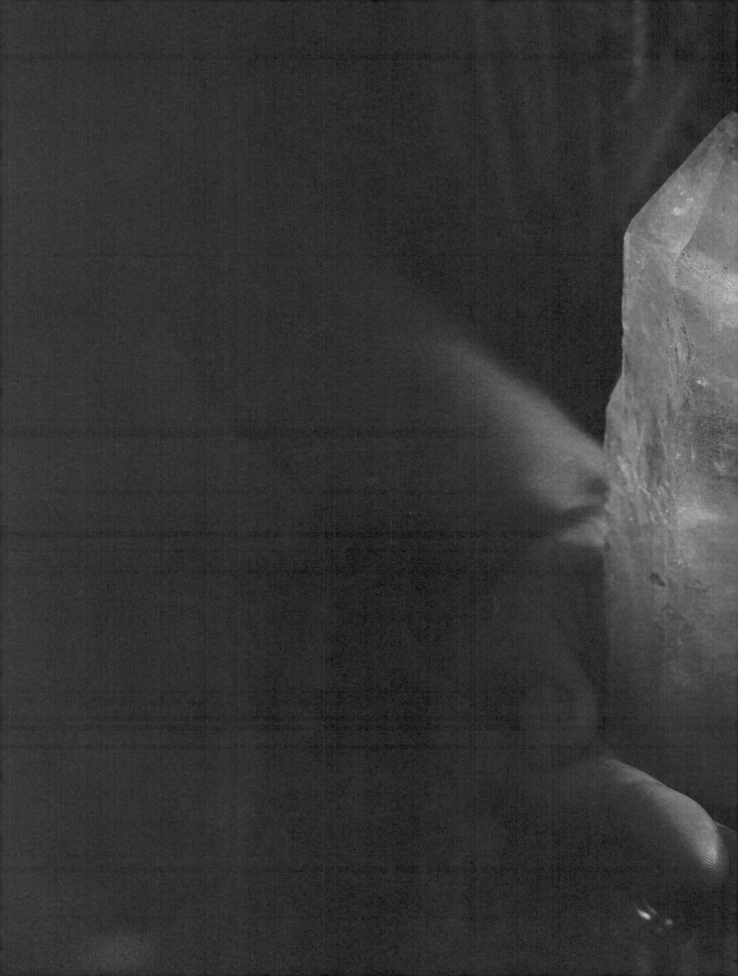

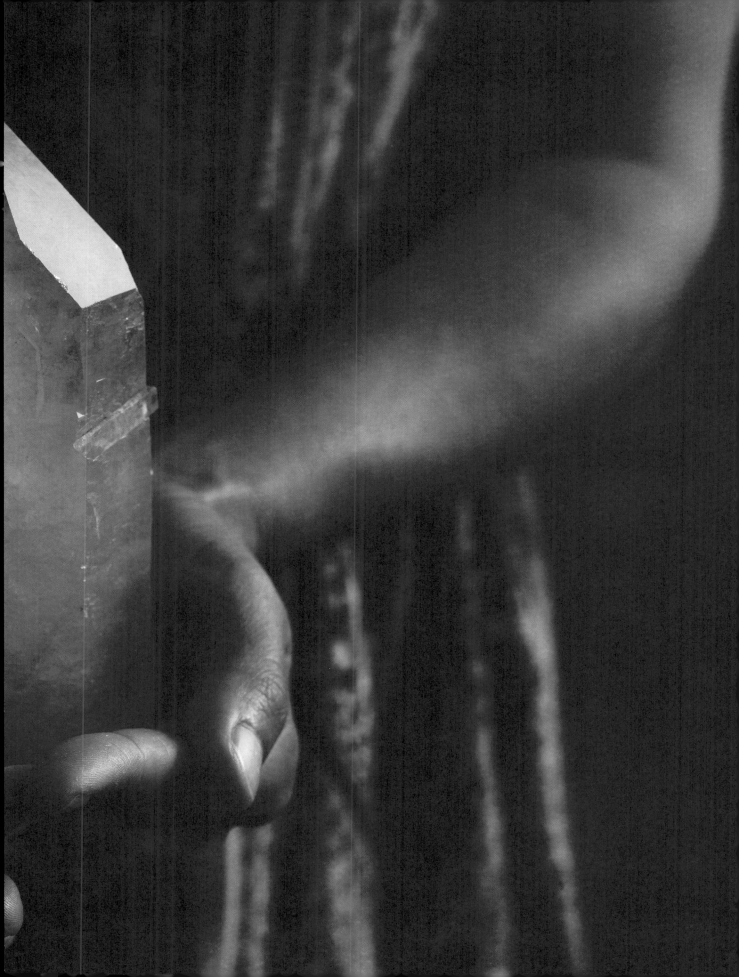

MENOPAUSE

Menopause typically occurs between the ages of 45 and 55 years old and is characterized by the decline of estrogen levels and periods that begin to become infrequent and gradually stop. The change in hormone levels can cause a range of symptoms, including hot flashes, night sweats, sleeping problems, low mood, anxiety, loss of libido, concentration and memory issues, and vaginal dryness. Not all women are affected in the same way and for some it's more severe than others. If you think you could be entering menopause, see a medical practitioner as a blood test could confirm it. Treatments such as hormone replacement therapy (HRT) are available.

KEY CRYSTALS
—

Citrine—Wear jewelry with citrine, as it can help with balancing the hormones, reduce the severity of hot flashes, and ease feelings of fatigue.

Rose quartz—Keep a piece of rose quartz close to you at home and in your pocket or bag when you're out and about. The gentle energies of rose quartz can help clear the mind, calm the emotions, and generally help you feel better about yourself and the changes you're going through.

Chrysoprase—If you're struggling to sleep through the night, put chrysoprase under your pillow or beside your bed. It can help promote sleep and may reduce restless leg syndrome, too.

Hematite—Place hematite on your wrist to help ease night sweats and hot flashes, as it can help regulate temperature. As a bonus, it's good for grounding, too.

OTHER GRID AND LAYOUT CRYSTALS
—

• Zincite (to balance hormones and release blockages)
• Emerald (to soothe emotions and help with changes)
• Amethyst (to relieve stress, soothe irritability, and balance mood swings)
• Fluorite (for concentration and easing self-doubt)
• Lapis lazuli (for depression and insomnia)
• Lepidolite (to stabilize hormonal mood swings)
• Moonstone (for hormonal stages of life and to balance fluctuating emotions)
• Orange calcite (for bones and joints)

ADDITIONAL THERAPIES
—

The herbal remedy, black cohosh, may be helpful for dealing with hot flashes, as could acupuncture, and vitamin D could help promote bone renewal, as bone density loss is associated with menopause. Exercises such as yoga could help body and mind.

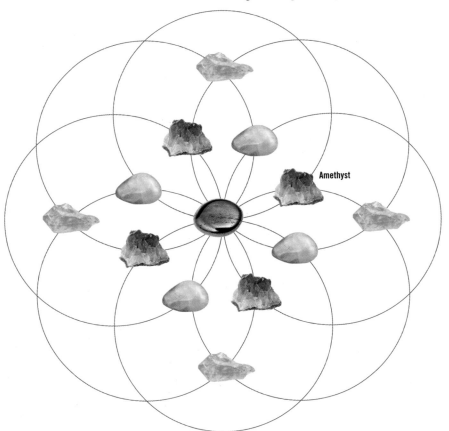

Amethyst

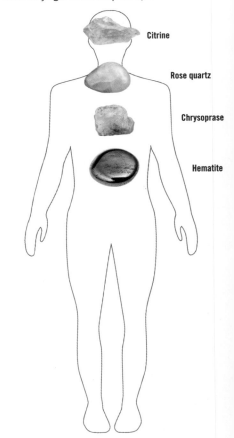

Citrine

Rose quartz

Chrysoprase

Hematite

ENDOMETRIOSIS

The gynecological condition endometriosis affects up to ten percent of women and is a long-term condition. With endometriosis, tissue from the lining of the uterus grows in other places outside of the womb, such as the ovaries, fallopian tubes, pelvis, and in the abdomen. When a monthly period occurs, this tissue responds to the hormone changes and bleeds, but unlike a period, it has nowhere to go. This leads to inflammation, swelling, and scarring. Endometriosis varies in severity, from mild to severe, and it can cause symptoms such as extremely painful periods, heavy bleeding, pain during intercourse, pelvic pain, nausea, and infertility. Endometriosis often takes a while to get diagnosed, so it's important to seek advice from a medical practitioner if you suspect you could have symptoms.

KEY CRYSTALS
—

Smoky quartz—Place smoky quartz on areas of pain, as it could help reduce discomfort and inflammation.

Jade—Wear or hold jade, as it could help to deal with stomach cramps and feelings of nausea.

Magnesite—Magnesite can be used to help with pain relief and fatigue when dealing with an endometriosis flare-up. Make a crystal gem elixir and spray it on or around your body when needed. Add it to a warm bath and soak in it to help ease aches and pains.

OTHER GRID AND LAYOUT CRYSTALS
—

• Moonstone (for womb healing and balancing your cycle)
• Citrine (to energize when you're feeling fatigued)

• Clear quartz (to cleanse and rebalance the chakras; to calm and relax)
• Bloodstone (to strengthen the immune system)
• Emerald (for healing)
• Tiger's eye (to aid sleep)
• Onyx (for headaches)
• Amethyst (to relieve stress and aid relaxation)

ADDITIONAL THERAPIES
—

In addition to any prescribed medication, acupuncture treatments may help take the edge off some symptoms and turmeric capsules could help. Heat pads may be beneficial for severe pain, ginger tea for nausea, and chamomile tea for general period aches and pains. A gentle massage with lavender essential oil may reduce menstrual cramps.

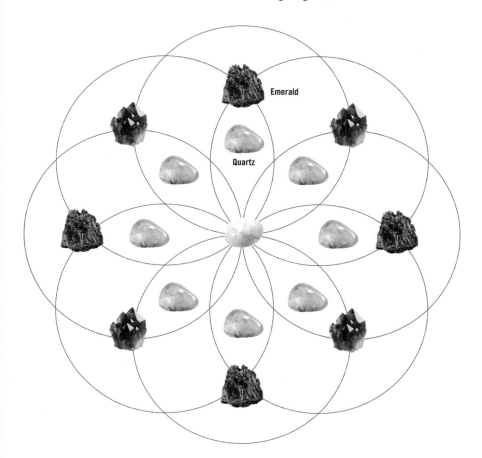

Emerald

Quartz

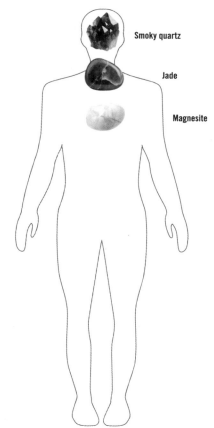

Smoky quartz

Jade

Magnesite

PAINFUL INTERCOURSE

Painful intercourse is also known as dyspareunia and it refers to experiencing genital pain before, during, or after having intercourse. The pain can be superficial or deep and symptoms can include burning, throbbing, or aching sensations during sex, pain after having sex, and pain having an orgasm. Physical causes can include illness, surgery, or infections, but emotional causes, such as stress, anxiety, fear of intimacy, or past trauma, can play a part, too. Don't be afraid or embarrassed to ask for help if you experience painful intercourse, as treatments are available.

KEY CRYSTALS
—

Rhodochrosite—Place on the solar plexus or root chakra to help ground you and give you the strength to deal with emotional causes related to painful intercourse.

Pink tourmaline—Place pink tourmaline on your heart chakra, as its gentle healing energies could help you open up emotional blockages.

Celestite—For strength, inner peace, and balance, place celestite beside your bed.

OTHER GRID AND LAYOUT CRYSTALS
—

• Fire agate (for protection)
• Carnelian (for negativity)
• Fluorite (to bring repressed feelings to the surface)
• Ametrine (for healing)

ADDITIONAL THERAPIES
—

Counseling and talking therapies could help with emotional causes of painful intercourse, particularly if past trauma is an issue, as could hypnotherapy treatments. If stress is involved, yoga, tai chi, mindfulness, and meditation could all be beneficial to help relax your body and mind.

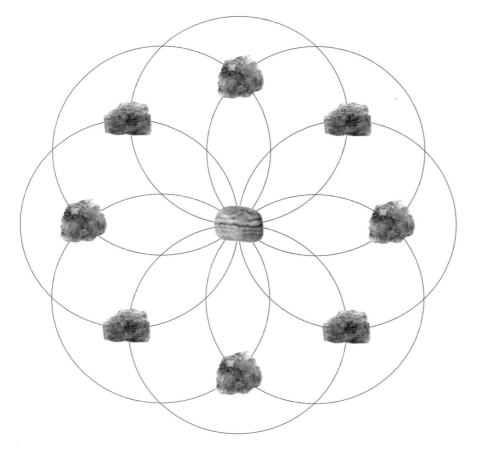

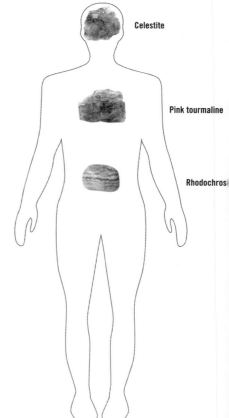

Celestite

Pink tourmaline

Rhodochros

LOSS OF LIBIDO

Loss of libido, or sex drive, can occur at any point in life. It can be caused by medical conditions such as diabetes, an underactive thyroid, heart disease, surgery, menopause, during pregnancy or when you've given birth, or due to taking certain medications. It can also be related to issues such as stress, anxiety, exhaustion, or relationship problems. It's not something to be embarrassed or ashamed about and if you're concerned that a loss of libido could be related to a medical condition, speak to your health practitioner.

KEY CRYSTALS
—

Zincite—Use zincite to clear blockages in chakras, reenergize your entire body, and increase passion. It's a powerful crystal, so use it in moderation. Make an elixir and spray it around your aura and on your body.

Red tiger's eye—Use the passionate energies of red tiger's eye to boost a lacking libido and deepen connections with your partner. Place it on the root chakra.

Carnelian—Place on the root chakra to open up kundalini and reenergize sexual desire.

Red jasper—Carry red jasper tumbled gemstones in your pocket to keep them close to your body. The vibrational energy of the crystal may help energize sexual desire and boost the libido.

OTHER GRID AND LAYOUT CRYSTALS
—

• Hessonite (to reenergize and spark sexual desire)
• Red spinel (to arouse desire)
• Fire opal (to enhance libido)
• Unakite (to release emotional blocks and trauma)
• Serpentine (to activate kundalini and sexual energy)
• Yellow jasper (to boost physical energy and drive)

ADDITIONAL THERAPIES
—

If stress or anxiety is likely to be an underlying cause, make an effort to relax and unwind more—try an aromatherapy massage, meditation, relaxation exercise, yoga, or mindfulness. If relationship issues could be the cause, consider couples counseling or simply opening up and talking more with your partner. Eat healthily, exercise regularly, and get plenty of sleep to restore energy.

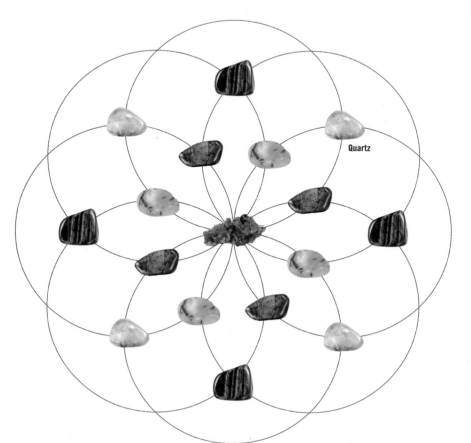

Quartz

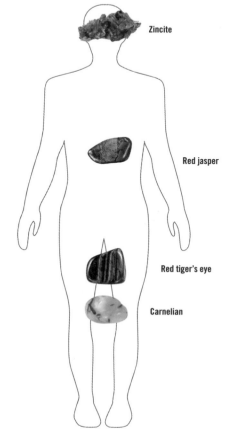

Zincite

Red jasper

Red tiger's eye

Carnelian

ERECTION PROBLEMS

It's not uncommon to have erection problems, or to experience the failure to be able to get and maintain an erection firm enough for many forms of sexual activity. Many men experience it at some point and it becomes more common in later years. In many cases, it's not a major cause for concern and could be due to stress, anxiety, tiredness, or drinking too much alcohol. Sometimes it can be due to emotional issues. If it happens frequently, there may be an underlying physical cause, such as high blood pressure, high cholesterol, or hormone issues, which would need investigation. Speak to a medical professional for advice if you're concerned about erection problems.

KEY CRYSTALS
—

Carnelian—Place on the sacral chakra to cleanse your sexual centers, promote vitality, and enhance sexual desire.

Amber—Use amber on the sacral chakra to help clear emotional blockages, reduce negative energy, and aid stress, which can cause erection problems.

Smoky quartz—Carry smoky quartz in your pockets, or place some in your bedroom to promote virility and healthy, enjoyable sex.

OTHER GRID AND LAYOUT CRYSTALS
—

• Hessonite garnet (for virility, libido, and sexual courage)
• Zoisite (for testicle problems)
• Goldstone (to reawaken sexual energy and desire, and boost performance confidence)
• Red jasper (to remove energy blocks and inhibitions, to enjoy sex without shame)

ADDITIONAL THERAPIES
—

Try exercise to stimulate blood flow to the penis, such as running, jogging, or a gym workout. Relaxation, such as meditation, yoga, or Pilates, can help reduce stress and anxiety.

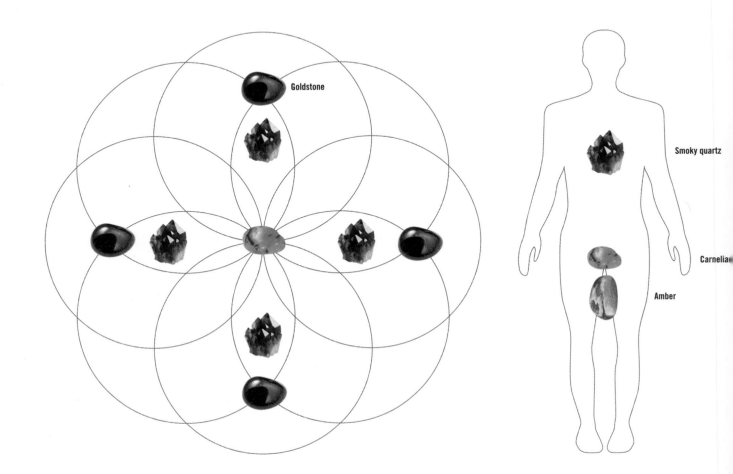

Goldstone

Smoky quartz

Carnelian

Amber

EJACULATION PROBLEMS

The most common form of ejaculation problem is premature ejaculation. It can be caused by physical, mental, or emotional issues, or a mix of factors, including prostate, diabetes, or thyroid problems; the use of recreational drugs; prescribed medications such as antidepressants; depression, stress, anxiety, or relationship issues; conditioning beliefs about sex; or traumatic experiences in the past. It's also possible to have delayed ejaculation or, more rarely, retrograde ejaculation, where semen goes back into the bladder rather than out of the urethra. Occasional ejaculation problems may be nothing to worry about, especially as you get older, but if you have frequent issues, do consult a medical practitioner.

KEY CRYSTALS
—

Carnelian—Place a red- or orange-colored carnelian crystal on the sacral chakra to strengthen sexual dysfunction. Its energies may enhance sexual confidence and make sex more fulfilling.

Orange calcite—Keep orange calcite in your pockets, or place under your pillow or near your bed. The vibrational energy of orange calcite may offer help to relax and release blockages associated with ejaculation problems, and restore passion, confidence, and enthusiasm for sex.

Black onyx—Place on the sacral chakra, or carry with your in your pocket, to boost positivity and aid in overcoming ejaculation issues.

OTHER GRID AND LAYOUT CRYSTALS

• Red jasper (to remove guilt or shame about sex)
• Shiva lingam (to release blockages and inhibitions)

ADDITIONAL THERAPIES
—

In addition to any medical treatments, you may benefit from trying couples therapy to talk through any issues. Holistic therapies such as energy healing, reflexology, or acupuncture may be beneficial, and in order to relax and relieve stress, try yoga and meditation.

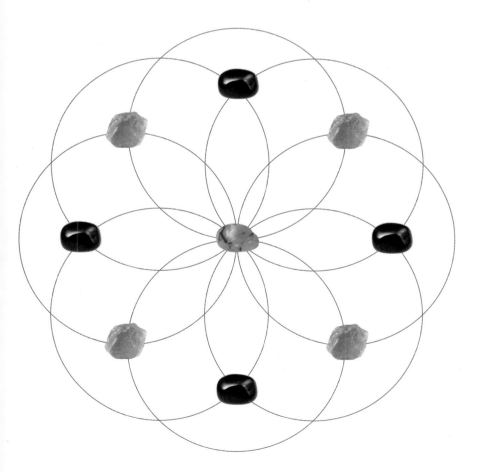

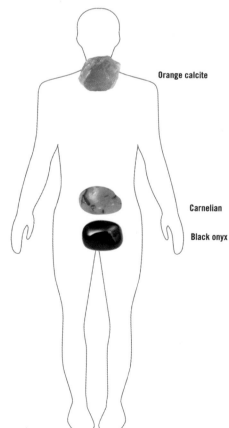

Orange calcite

Carnelian

Black onyx

INFERTILITY

Infertility is the inability to conceive a baby with a partner, even after having regular sex. Some of the common reasons for infertility in males include a low sperm count, ejaculation disorders, and abnormal sperm function. Past illnesses, injuries, health conditions, and lifestyle choices (such as alcohol consumption, recreational drug use, weight, and smoking) may be linked to infertility. If you've not conceived after a year of conscious attempts to achieve pregnancy, it's worth seeing a medical practitioner for advice, as various treatments are available.

KEY CRYSTALS
—

Garnet—Place garnet on your sacral chakra, as it may help to dissolve blockages and promote healthy intimate relationships.

Rose quartz—Place rose quartz beside your bed, as its gentle energies may help you feel more positive about fertility issues, promote feelings of self-love, and improve communication between partners.

Goldstone—If you are feeling down or depressed about infertility and have lost interest in sex as a result, use goldstone to reawaken sexual energy. Place goldstone on your sacral chakra or meditate with it.

OTHER GRID AND LAYOUT CRYSTALS
—

• Smoky quartz (for virility)
• Cinnabar (for low sperm count)
• Shiva lingam (to release blockages and balance the sexual energy)

ADDITIONAL THERAPIES
—

In addition to any prescribed medical treatments, it may be beneficial to find ways to manage stress and anxiety, such as relaxation exercises or breathing techniques. Couples therapy may be helpful, to enable both partners to express their thoughts and feelings, as infertility can be hard to come to terms with.

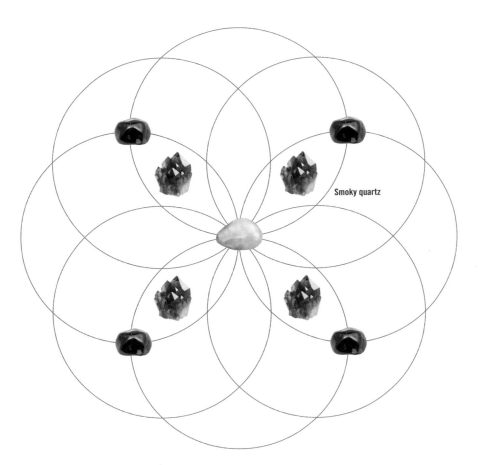

Smoky quartz

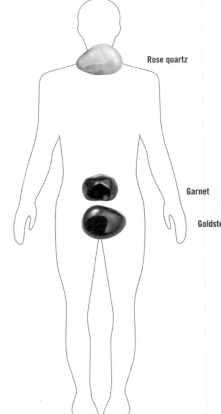

Rose quartz

Garnet

Goldst●

PROSTATE PROBLEMS

The prostate gland in men starts off about the size and shape of a walnut, but it can get bigger as you age, particularly post 50 years old. Sometimes it can also become swollen due to prostate problems such as prostate enlargement, prostate inflammation (prostatitis), or prostate cancer. Depending on the prostate problem in question, some of the symptoms may include needing to go to the toilet more often, straining to empty your bladder, waking up during the night to go, pain when urinating, pain in the pelvis, genitals, or lower back, and a weak flow of urine. It's always advisable to see a medical practitioner to check symptoms and rule out more serious causes, especially as they can be similar to prostate cancer.

KEY CRYSTALS
—

Obsidian—Obsidian can be used to help release negative energy and blockages in the meridians and to detoxify the chakras, which could help with the discomfort of an enlarged prostate. Place on the root chakra, have pieces by the bed, or meditate with them.

Chrysoprase—Place on the sacral chakra to help unblock chakras and balance hormones.

Zincite—Zincite is a powerful crystal that's often small in size, but more than makes up for it in healing actions. It can help deal with issues related to the prostate gland and is ideal to use to help clear energy blocks in the chakra system, helping to get a better flow of energy throughout your body. For the best effects, use it in moderation.

OTHER GRID AND LAYOUT CRYSTALS
—

• Malachite (to remove obstacles and energy blocks)
• Moonstone (to cool male energy and balance feminine energies)
• Amethyst (to clear negativity)
• Red jasper (to remove guilt and shame)
• Smoky quartz (for strength)

ADDITIONAL THERAPIES
—

In addition to any prescribed medical treatment, self-help measures such as cutting down on alcohol and drinking less before going to bed may help to control some of the symptoms, such as frequency and urgency to go to the toilet during the night. Acupuncture may provide some pain relief, and therapies such as massage, aromatherapy, hypnotherapy, or reflexology may help relieve stress and aid relaxation.

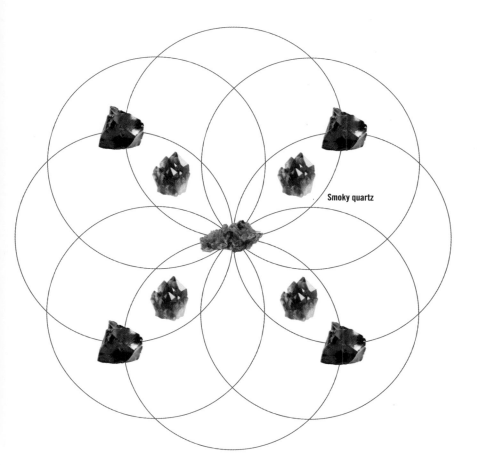

Smoky quartz

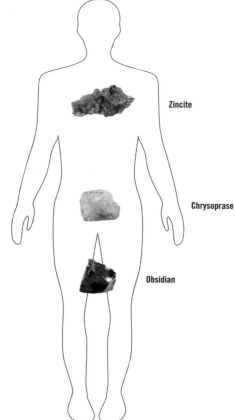

Zincite

Chrysoprase

Obsidian

THYROID PROBLEMS

The thyroid gland is located in the neck and is responsible for producing hormones that help regulate metabolism. The most common thyroid problems involve the abnormal production of thyroid hormones. When too many thyroid hormones are produced, it results in hyperthyroidism, an overactive thyroid. When too few hormones are produced, it causes hypothyroidism, or an underactive thyroid. Symptoms of an overactive thyroid include difficulty sleeping, palpitations, swelling in the neck from an enlarged thyroid gland, anxiety, irritability, and tiredness. Symptoms of an underactive thyroid include tiredness, muscle aches, and cramps, weight gain, sensitivity to cold, and depression. If you think you could have a thyroid problem, always seek advice from a medical practitioner. If thyroid issues aren't dealt with, they can lead to other medical problems.

KEY CRYSTALS
—

Kyanite—Place a kyanite crystal on the throat chakra, as it may help to stimulate a sluggish thyroid.

Rutilated quartz—Make a crystal gem elixir with rutilated quartz and add it to bathwater. This crystal may help with strength and vitality when you're feeling run down and exhausted by thyroid issues.

Aquamarine—Use aquamarine on the throat chakra, or wear as a pendant, to help balance the thyroid gland.

OTHER GRID AND LAYOUT CRYSTALS
—

• Atacamite (for hypothyroidism)
• Citrine (for energy)
• Rhodochrosite (to balance the thyroid)
• Azurite (for cleansing)
• Chrysocolla (to strengthen the thyroid)

ADDITIONAL THERAPIES
—

In addition to medical treatment, body—mind exercises such as yoga, Pilates, tai chi, and qigong may help with endocrine balance, and acupuncture treatments might help some symptoms. Some research shows that taking selenium could help to balance thyroxine or T4 levels, but it's important to check with your medical practitioner to see how much you need, as everyone is different. B12 may help with hypothyroidism and there's some evidence that probiotics might be beneficial, too.

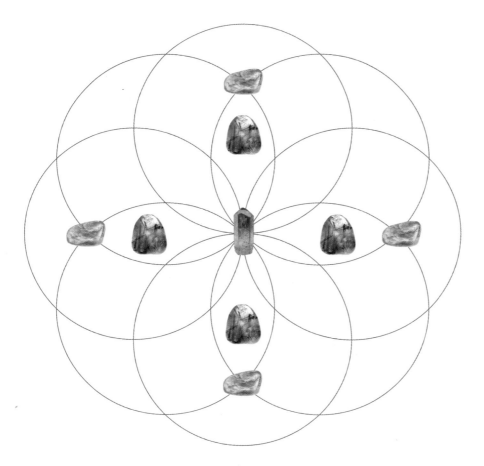

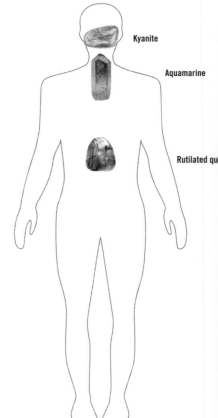

Kyanite

Aquamarine

Rutilated qu

DIABETES

Diabetes is a chronic health condition that occurs when your body doesn't make enough insulin or isn't able to make insulin properly. Normally, when you eat food it's broken down into sugar and released into your bloodstream, and as sugar levels go up, the pancreas releases insulin. With Type 1 diabetes, an autoimmune response occurs that stops your body from making insulin. Type 1 develops suddenly and you'll need to take insulin daily to survive. With Type 2 diabetes, your body doesn't produce enough insulin or it doesn't react properly to insulin. Type 2 develops over years and can be prevented or delayed by healthy lifestyle changes. Symptoms of undiagnosed diabetes including extreme thirst, tiredness, thrush, blurred vision, frequent urination, and weight loss. Diabetes is serious, so see a medical practitioner if you have potential symptoms.

KEY CRYSTALS
—

Serpentine—Hold a piece of serpentine to access its cleansing and detoxifying energy, as it may be of support to diabetics.

Citrine—The sunny disposition of citrine can have an reenergize effect on a sluggish system. Place on the throat chakra to reenergize your body.

Red jasper—Use red jasper to gently stimulate your body and unblock chakras. It can cleanse and stabilize the aura and dissolve blockages.

OTHER GRID AND LAYOUT CRYSTALS

- Malachite (for pancreatic support)
- Sodalite (to balance the endocrine system)
- Emerald (for regulating insulin)
- Pink opal (to calm the metabolic system)

ADDITIONAL THERAPIES
—

Aromatherapy can be calming and may help emotionally to improve the management of diabetes. Massage therapy and reflexology may be beneficial for stimulating blood flow and circulation, which can be affected by diabetes. Guided meditations or visualizations could be helpful to create a positive mental image. There is some evidence that herbal remedies may be helpful, but more research is needed, as some could interact with diabetes medication such as insulin.

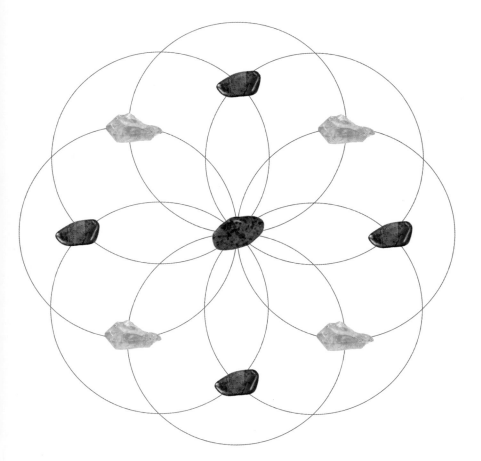

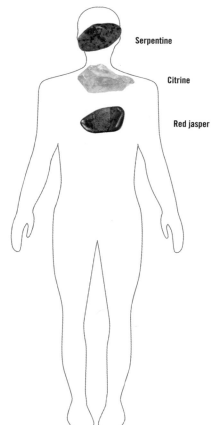

Serpentine

Citrine

Red jasper

HYPOGLYCEMIA

Hypoglycemia is a medical condition where your blood sugar level, or glucose, drops too low. It is related to diabetes, but it's also possible to just have issues with low blood sugar levels. Signs of hypoglycemia include tiredness, dizziness, shaking, trembling, sweating, turning pale, palpitations, tingling lips, and feeling hungry. If it's not treated, symptoms can worsen and you may experience weakness, blurred vision, confusion, slurred speech, extreme drowsiness, or passing out. With diabetes, a hypo—a sudden drop in blood sugar level—can occur if you don't eat enough carbohydrates, if you skip or delay eating, after drinking alcohol, or as the result of taking too much insulin or other medications. Eating a sugary drink or snack could help boost blood sugar levels, but if you have any concerns or don't feel better, always seek medical help.

KEY CRYSTALS
—

Serpentine—Hold a piece of serpentine, as its energies may help to ground and balance your body.

Pink opal—Wear pink opal on a necklace and its energies will calm and soothe your chakras and meridians.

Sodalite—Place sodalite on the heart or throat chakra, as it could help to cleanse your body of toxins and level your metabolic rate.

OTHER GRID AND LAYOUT CRYSTALS
—

- Rhodonite (to soothe and balance)
- Citrine (to energize and boost stamina)
- Emerald (for regulating insulin)

ADDITIONAL THERAPIES
—

In addition to any prescribed medication, there's some evidence to suggest that taking vitamin D supplements may help to balance blood sugar levels. Some herbal remedies may be beneficial, but more research is needed, as they could interact with other medication.

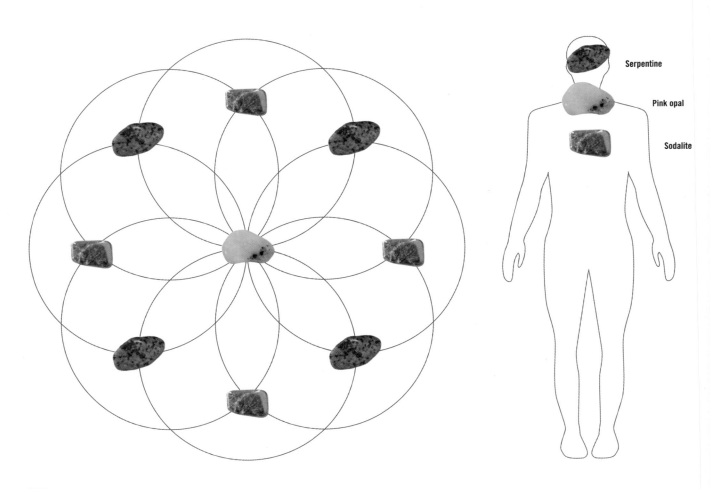

Serpentine

Pink opal

Sodalite

OBESITY

Obesity is a complex medical disease that occurs when you're carrying too much body fat and when your body mass index (BMI) is 30 or higher. Being obese increases the risk of other major health problems including diabetes, high blood pressure, heart disease, and cancer. Obesity occurs due to a combination of factors, including genetics, hormones, metabolic issues, and behavioral factors, such as diet and exercise choices. Put simply, though, it's primarily caused by eating more calories than you burn off. Obesity can be tackled on a personal level by making changes to your diet and exercise regimes. Sometimes medications and surgical procedures are needed. If you have concerns about obesity, see a medical practitioner for advice.

KEY CRYSTALS

—

Black onyx—If you are embarking on a new diet and exercise plan, wear black onyx to help boost your mental and physical strength and determination to succeed.

Citrine—Place citrine on the throat chakra to energize and revitalize your body. It can be useful if you feel fatigued due to excess body weight, plus it can help raise your self-esteem and self-confidence and aid in the battle against destructive tendencies.

Yellow apatite—Make a crystal gem elixir using the indirect method and drink during the day. Yellow apatite could have the ability to help suppress the appetite.

OTHER GRID AND LAYOUT CRYSTALS

—

• Smithsonite (for comfort eating)
• Iolite (if food is an addiction)
• Kyanite (to help reduce excess weight)
• Blue apatite (to facilitate results; effective when used with other crystals)
• Green tourmaline (to detoxify)
• Magnetite (to help speed up fat metabolism)
• Moonstone (for emotional and stress-related eating patterns)

ADDITIONAL THERAPIES

—

A healthy diet and exercise regime are two of the best ways of beating obesity. If you struggle with motivation or doing it alone, join a group or hire a personal trainer.

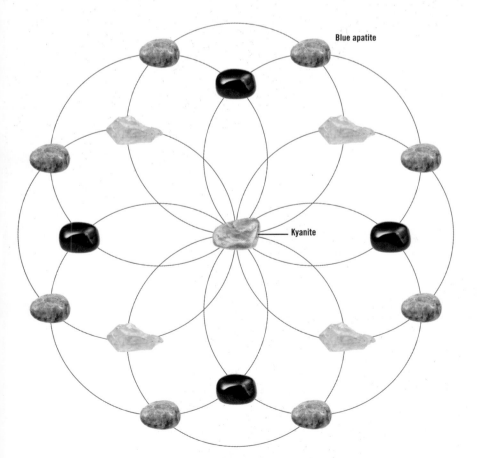

Blue apatite

Kyanite

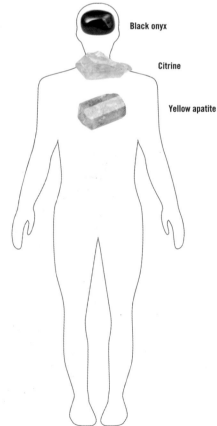

Black onyx

Citrine

Yellow apatite

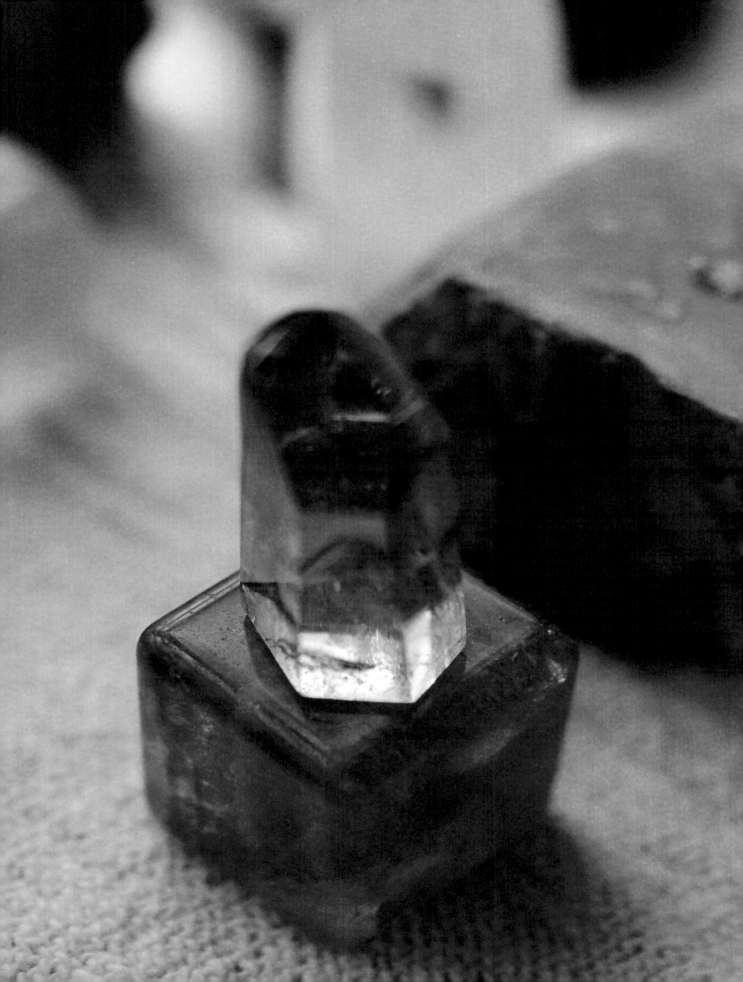

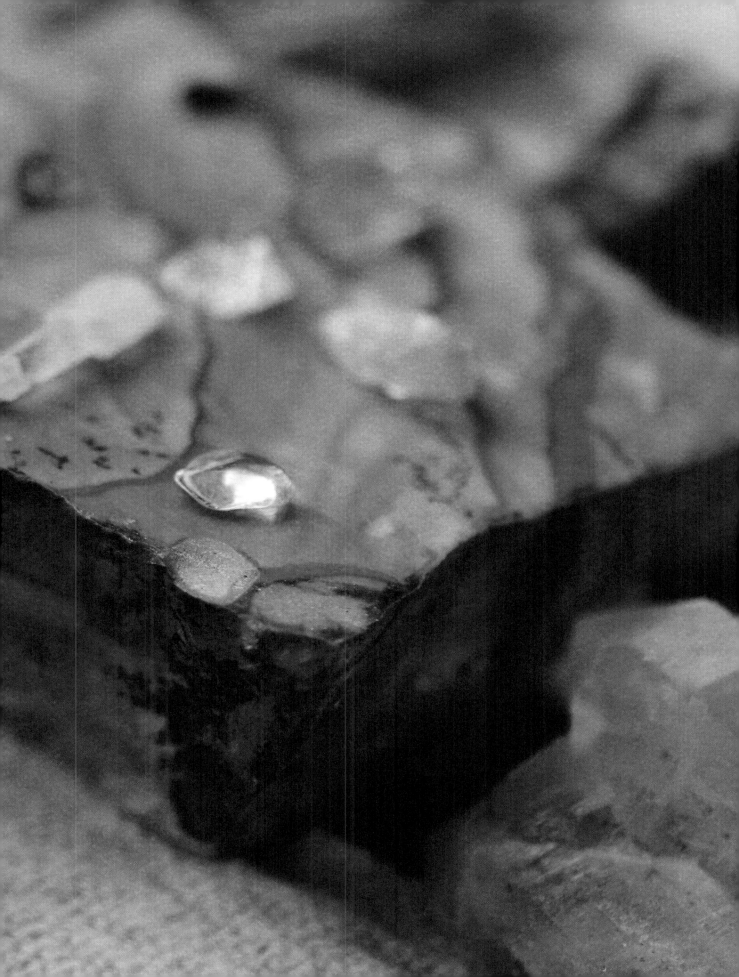

GOUT

Gout is a form of arthritis that causes joints to become hot, red, swollen, and intensely painful very suddenly. Gout can be triggered by having high levels of uric acid in your body. Urate crystals form in a joint and build up, causing pain, swelling, and inflammation. An attack of gout typically lasts for up to a week before getting better and tends to be treated with non-steroidal inflammatory medications or steroid tablets or injections. Diet can increase your risk of gout if you eat a lot of red meat or shellfish and have drinks sweetened with fructose. Drinking a lot of alcohol, especially beer, can also increase the risk. If you have symptoms of gout, always get a proper diagnosis from a medical practitioner.

KEY CRYSTALS
—

Chiastolite—The crystal chiastolite may be helpful for reducing acid and easing the pain and discomfort of gout. Place on the affected area.

Chrysoprase—Make a crystal gem elixir using the indirect method. Use the elixir in a bath to ease swelling or spray directly onto the affected area.

Labradorite—Place on the heart chakra, or directly onto gout, and let the calming energy of labradorite infuse a sense of balance and health.

OTHER GRID AND LAYOUT CRYSTALS
—

• Turquoise (to purify and balance the chakras)
• Variscite (to neutralize overacidity)
• Prehnite (to ease gout)
• Amazonite (for pain)

ADDITIONAL THERAPIES
—

Acupuncture could help relieve the pain of gout. Hot and cold compresses may help with the pain and swelling. Vitamin C supplements may help to reduce the risk of gout recurring by lowering uric acid levels, but you need to be careful to get the right amount, as too much can be counterproductive. Losing weight, eating a healthy diet, and cutting down on alcohol can all be beneficial.

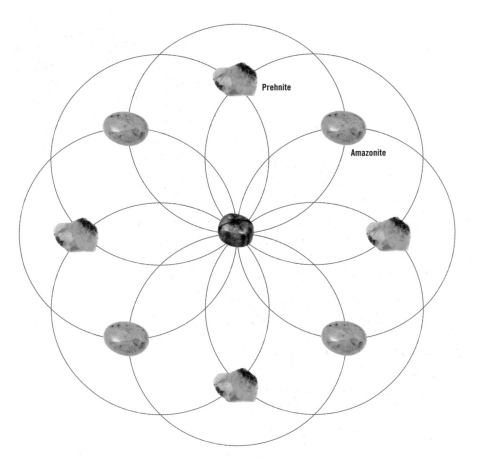

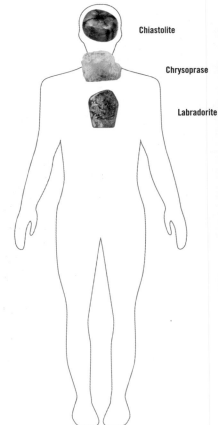

ALLERGIES

An allergy occurs when your immune system reacts unexpectedly to a substance or food. Common allergies include particular foods (such as nuts, shellfish, eggs, or milk), insect stings, prescribed drugs, latex, mold, dust mites, animal fur, household chemicals, and pollen, such as grass and tree pollen. An allergic reaction usually happens very quickly, within minutes of exposure. Symptoms depend on the allergen and can be mild or severe. Examples of symptoms include wheezing, coughing, a red itchy rash, swelling, tingling, sneezing, a runny nose and red, itchy, and watery eyes. In severe cases, anaphylaxis or anaphylactic shock can occur, which can be life-threatening. Allergies can run in families and are often linked to other conditions, such as asthma and eczema. See a medical practitioner for a suspected allergy diagnosis.

KEY CRYSTALS
—

Apophyllite—Place on the chest area, as it could help ease wheezing and coughing caused by allergies.

Aventurine—If you have a skin allergic reaction, it may be beneficial to hold aventurine, or place it on the affected area, as it may have anti-inflammatory properties.

Lepidolite—Make a crystal gem elixir using the indirect method and sip the water slowly. Its soothing energies could have a beneficial effect on the immune system and relieve allergies.

OTHER GRID AND LAYOUT CRYSTALS
—

• Danburite (to detoxify and ease allergy symptoms)
• Diamond (for allergic reactions)
• Muscovite (to aid healing)
• Aquamarine (for hay fever)
• Carnelian (for reenergizing the body after an allergic reaction)

ADDITIONAL THERAPIES
—

In addition to any prescribed treatments, acupuncture could help to reduce the severity of allergies. Spirulina blue-green algae may have anti-allergic properties and help hay fever. Quercetin could help stabilize the release of histamine and help allergy symptoms, and increasing vitamin C could be beneficial, too. Allergy testing may help to identify potential allergens.

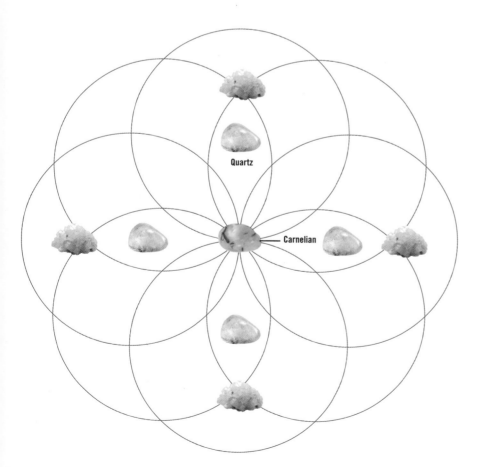

Quartz

Carnelian

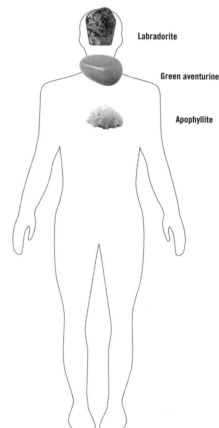

Labradorite

Green aventurine

Apophyllite

RHEUMATISM

Rheumatism is a form of musculoskeletal disease that affects the bones, muscles, ligaments, and joint tendons. There are a number of different types of rheumatic diseases, including rheumatoid arthritis, scleroderma, lupus, polymyalgia, osteoporosis, osteoarthritis, and ankylosing spondylitis. Depending on the exact type of rheumatic disorder you have, symptoms may include joint pain, swelling in joints, fatigue, joint stiffness, and loss of motion in joints. Seek advice from a medical practitioner if you have ongoing joint problems, as a proper diagnosis will help enable you to get the best treatments.

KEY CRYSTALS

—

Chrysoprase—Place chrysoprase on the affected area or pop it under your pillow at night. The calming energies bring a sense of security and could help you get a better night's sleep if you've been struggling due to rheumatism pain.

Labradorite—Wear over the heart chakra, or place directly onto the affected area. The energy of labradorite could help to ease some of the discomfort of rheumatism.

Sunstone—Use the uplifting energies of sunstone to help clear blockages from your chakras, lift your mood and stimulate self-healing of aches and pains. Make a crystal gem elixir and spray it on your aura.

OTHER GRID AND LAYOUT CRYSTALS

—

- Chiastolite (for strength)
- Emerald (for easing rheumatism discomfort)
- Fuchsite (for flexibility)
- Turquoise (to strengthen and regenerate tissue)
- Kunzite (for joint pain)
- Carnelian (for lower back problems)

ADDITIONAL THERAPIES

—

In addition to any medical treatments and therapies, acupuncture may help to reduce joint swelling and massage could be helpful when you're stiff and achy. Gentle exercises such as tai chi, yoga, or Pilates may be kinder on your joints and help you move more easily. Cold and heat compresses could be helpful for pain. The supplement turmeric may also be beneficial, but check with your doctor first to ensure it won't adversely interact with any prescribed drugs you're taking.

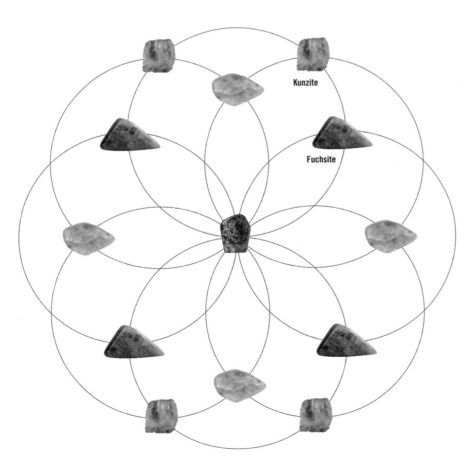

Kunzite

Fuchsite

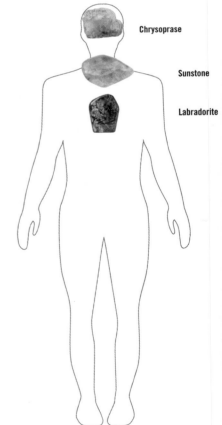

Chrysoprase

Sunstone

Labradorite

SPRAINS AND STRAINS

Sprains and strains are common—they can affect the muscles and ligaments, and can occur as the result of exercises such as running, sports, tennis, football, or rugby. Some sprains and strains can occur when you're doing activities around the house or garden, often as the result of moving awkwardly, overstretching, or not warming up properly before exercising, or due to tired muscles, or lifting and moving heavy items. Although painful initially and an inconvenience, most sprains and strains will improve within two weeks. If the injury doesn't get better, the pain or swelling gets worse, or you develop a high temperature, visit a doctor.

KEY CRYSTALS

—

Magnetite—Place on the muscle that is sprained or strained. Its anti-inflammatory energies could help with healing.

Sunstone—Place sunstone directly onto the area you've sprained or strained. This cheery stone may help to stimulate self-healing and uplift your mood.

Serpentine—Hold light-green-colored serpentine or place it onto the area of discomfort. This crystal could help to relieve aches and pains.

OTHER GRID AND LAYOUT CRYSTALS

—

• Carnelian (to boost energy after a sprain or strain)
• Chrysocolla (to strengthen muscles)
• Kyanite (for natural pain relief)
• Turquoise (for anti-inflammatory benefits and tissue healing)
• Green calcite (for the ligaments and muscles)

ADDITIONAL THERAPIES

—

Depending on your individual injury, a course of physiotherapy or osteopathy might help relieve the pain and discomfort of a muscle sprain or strain. Hot and cold compresses can help reduce swelling, too, as can keeping the affected limb raised where possible. The homeopathic remedy arnica can help with bruising and can be taken as tablets or used as a cream rubbed into the skin. Supplements such as vitamin C, vitamin E, and beta-carotene may help to repair damaged tissue, reduce swelling, and aid pain relief.

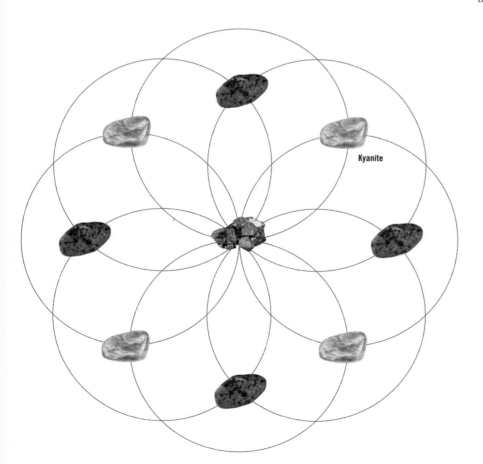

Kyanite

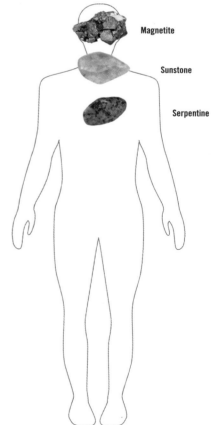

Magnetite

Sunstone

Serpentine

NECK PROBLEMS

Neck problems can be caused by various factors, including bad posture, a pinched nerve, an injury such as whiplash, a fall, or accident, or be due to conditions such as osteoarthritis, joint issues, or as the result of referred pain from your shoulders or back. Neck problems can cause symptoms such as pain, stiffness, difficulty moving your neck in the usual way, muscle spasms, or headaches. Minor neck problems can be uncomfortable but tend to resolve relatively quickly. If, however, your neck pain is severe, persists for several days and doesn't get better, spreads down your arms or legs, or if you have numbness, weakness, or tingling sensations, see a medical expert immediately.

KEY CRYSTALS
—

Alexandrite—If you have issues with your neck muscles, place alexandrite on the area of your neck that is causing problems. The soothing energies may help to relieve tensions in your neck muscles.

Blue lace agate—Place on the throat chakra to clear blockages, and to strengthen and aid the healing of neck complaints.

Larimar—Place larimar on the area of discomfort or pain in your neck. It may help to dissolve energy blockages and draw out the pain.

OTHER GRID AND LAYOUT CRYSTALS

• Siberian blue quartz (to ease inflammation, stiffness, and muscles)
• Seraphinite (to release muscle tension)
• Kunzite (for joint pain)
• Moss agate (to reduce swelling)
• Fuchsite (to aid flexibility)
• Green calcite (to ease neck muscle discomfort)
• Kyanite (for pain relief)

ADDITIONAL THERAPIES
—

A heat pad can help ease muscle aches and pains. Depending on your diagnosis, therapies such as acupuncture, massage, Bowen therapy, chiropractic, and osteopathy treatments may help to relieve neck discomfort and improve movement.

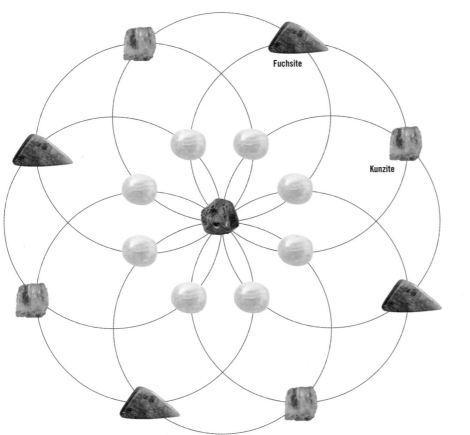

Fuchsite

Kunzite

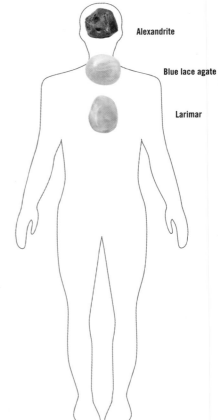

Alexandrite

Blue lace agate

Larimar

BACK PROBLEMS

Back problems can be caused by various different factors and medical conditions, including slipped and herniated disks, muscle injury, pinched nerves, spinal stenosis, vertebral fractures, osteoporosis, osteoarthritis, muscle strains, or simply as a result of aging. Back problems can vary in severity—from mild to severe—and cause different types of pain. For example, back pain can be sharp, dull, constant, throbbing, or electric shock-like, and it can be confined to one area (such as a muscle strain or disk problem) or move around (known as referred pain). Sometimes back pain can travel into the legs, as is the case with sciatica. Back problems are complicated and need to be properly diagnosed by a doctor.

KEY CRYSTALS
—

Aragonite—Place aragonite on the area of your back that is painful or uncomfortable. This crystal can stabilize and calm muscle spasms and be useful for disk-related problems.

Carnelian—Place on the root chakra or directly onto the area of your back causing issues to ease lower back pain and aid the healing of ligaments and bones.

Lepidolite—If your back pain is caused by sciatica, hold lepidolite or put it in your pocket and carry it with you. It may help to numb the pain and symptoms caused by the sciatic nerve.

OTHER GRID AND LAYOUT CRYSTALS
—

• Mahogany obsidian (for pain)
• Fire opal (for lower back pain)
• Fuchsite (for flexibility)
• Hematite (for spinal alignment)
• Kunzite (to soothe joint pain)
• Moss agate (for swelling and anti-inflammatory relief)
• Selenite (for alignment and joint pain)

ADDITIONAL THERAPIES
—

Depending on the cause and nature of your back problems, therapies such as acupuncture, Bowen therapy, massage, chiropractic, or osteopathy treatments may be beneficial. A TENS machine could help provide some relief from back pain, as could using a heat pad. Exercises such as yoga, Pilates, and swimming can be gentle on the back and improve flexibility and movement.

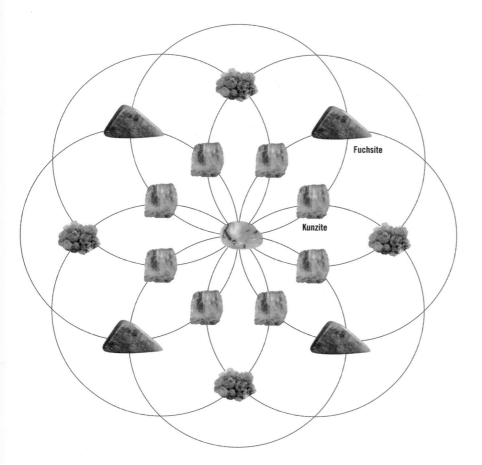

Fuchsite

Kunzite

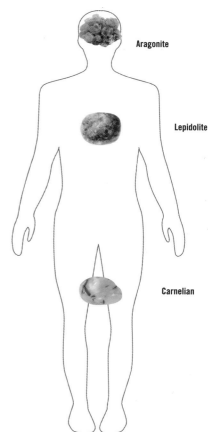

Aragonite

Lepidolite

Carnelian

ARTHRITIS

Arthritis is a condition that causes inflammation and pain in joints. There are various types of arthritis, but the two most common forms are osteoarthritis and rheumatoid arthritis. With osteoarthritis the joint cartilage breaks down and the bones change, causing symptoms such as stiffness, pain, aching, and swelling. It can lead to a reduced range of motion and functionality and, in some cases, disability. Rheumatoid arthritis is an immune disorder, where the immune system targets joints, causing swelling and pain. It can eventually cause the bone and cartilage to break down and change the shape of the joint. It's important to have a formal arthritis diagnosis, so you know what type you have and can access the best treatment regime.

KEY CRYSTALS

—

Blue lace agate—Utilize the gentle and calming energies of blue lace agate to ease the pain and discomfort of arthritis. Make a crystal gem elixir and add it to your bathwater or spray it on the affected area.

Amethyst—Wear over the heart chakra, or place directly onto areas of discomfort to help swelling and pain. It may also be beneficial to have under your pillow at night, as it could help you sleep more comfortably.

Chrysocolla—Place this calming and cleansing crystal on the area of discomfort to help ease arthritic pain.

OTHER GRID AND LAYOUT CRYSTALS

—

- Apatite (to ease joint problems)
- Azurite (for osteoarthritis in the back)
- Green calcite (for the ligaments and muscles)
- Carnelian (for rheumatoid arthritis)
- Fluorite (to help mobilize joints)
- Rhodonite (for joint inflammation)
- Black tourmaline (for arthritis pain relief)

ADDITIONAL THERAPIES

—

In addition to any prescribed drugs or treatments, exercise may help to treat osteoarthritis, as could physical therapy with muscle-strengthening exercises. Losing excess weight could help to reduce the strain put on joints. The supplements glucosamine and chondroitin may help to rebuild connective tissue, but you should check with your doctor first before taking them.

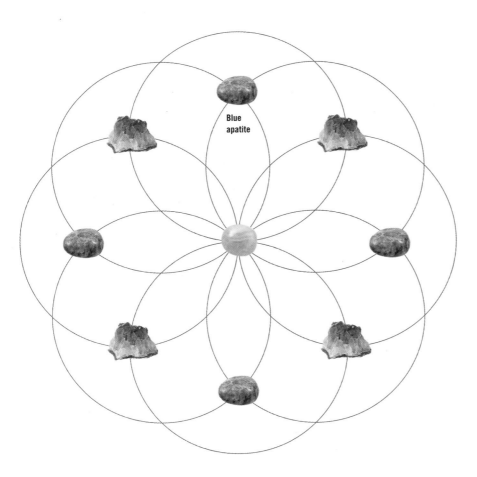

Blue apatite

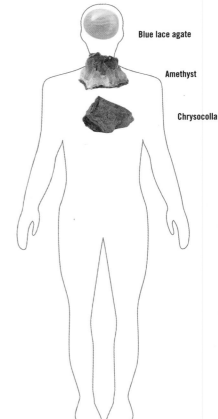

Blue lace agate

Amethyst

Chrysocolla

CRAMP

Cramp is a sudden pain that occurs due to a muscle contracting and making it hard to move. Cramp commonly occurs in the legs and feet (and often at night) but it can happen in any muscle. Cramp is really painful and makes it difficult to use the affected muscle, but it tends to last for a few seconds or minutes before easing. Afterward the muscle can feel sore and uncomfortable for a while. Muscle cramps can be caused by periods of inactivity, overuse of a muscle, dehydration, or muscle strain. Sometimes an underlying medical condition may be to blame, such as nerve compression; a lack of the minerals potassium, calcium, or magnesium; or an inadequate supply of blood. If you get cramp frequently, or it's accompanied by muscle weakness, swelling, or skin changes, see a medical practitioner.

KEY CRYSTALS

—

Magnetite—Place magnetite around the end of your bed to reduce the risk of developing cramp in your feet or legs during the night.

Chrysocolla—Hold chrysocolla if you get muscle cramps, as this crystal could ease the spasms and pain of cramp.

Turquoise—Turquoise has anti-inflammatory properties and can help reduce the discomfort of muscle cramps. Make a crystal gem elixir and pop it in a spray bottle, so you can spray it on the affected area.

OTHER GRID AND LAYOUT CRYSTALS

- Amazonite (to soothe muscle cramps)
- Smoky quartz (for leg cramp)
- Rhyolite (to help improve muscle tone)
- Serpentine (for aches and pains post-cramp)

ADDITIONAL THERAPIES

—

Dehydration is linked to cramp, so drink plenty of water daily, especially if the weather is hot and you're exercising in warm temperatures. If you're prone to getting cramp in your feet or legs during the night, try doing light exercise before bed to help prevent this. Putting hot or cold compresses on a muscle cramp could help ease it and gentle massage could relieve some of the discomfort, especially just after the cramp has gone away.

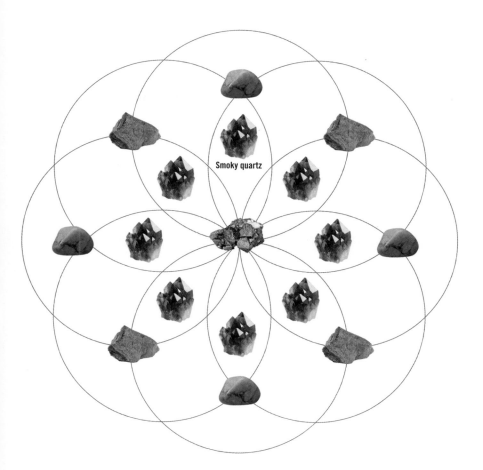

Smoky quartz

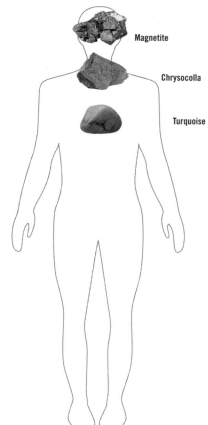

Magnetite

Chrysocolla

Turquoise

LIVING WITH HIV / AIDS

If you're living with HIV (human immunodeficiency virus) or AIDS (acquired immune deficiency syndrome), your immune system will be affected and your ability to fight off common infections such as flu will be severely hampered. They are both long-term conditions and there's no cure for HIV, but the symptoms can be effectively managed with drug treatments. HIV and AIDS can affect you physically, mentally, and emotionally. Physical symptoms may include fatigue, joint pain, muscle pain, weight loss, night sweats, skin problems, and diarrhea. Mental and emotional symptoms may include anxiety, depression, and low moods.

KEY CRYSTALS
—

Petalite—This high-vibrational crystal has a very calming energy, which can calm both the physical body and your aura and help fill you with a sense of inner peace. Its energy may also help to activate energy systems in your body, potentially benefiting the endocrine system and issues with the eyes, lungs, and muscles. Keep a piece in your pocket or under your pillow.

Ametrine—Ametrine combines the properties of amethyst and citrine to produce a powerful cleansing crystal. Place ametrine on the solar plexus or wear as a pendant on jewelry to encourage the release of toxins and strengthen the immune system.

Carnelian—Carnelian has an energy of vitality, so wear this crystal to help lift your energy when you're feeling drained. It's also a good crystal for positivity. Wear it on jewelry.

OTHER GRID AND LAYOUT CRYSTALS
—

• Zincite (for the immune system and to help you deal with changes in your life)
• Rhodonite (for self-love, forgiveness, and emotional wounds)
• Dioptase (for T-cell activation)
• Clear quartz (for cleansing)
• Lapis lazuli (for protection, self-awareness, and self-expression)
• Rutilated quartz (for fear, anxiety, and low moods)
• Sugilite (for forgiveness, dealing with hostility, and emotional turmoil)

ADDITIONAL THERAPIES
—

Holistic therapies such as reflexology, aromatherapy, and acupuncture may help to ease some symptoms. Eating a healthy nutritional diet, having regular exercise, and stopping smoking are all beneficial. Good support can help, so consider finding support groups.

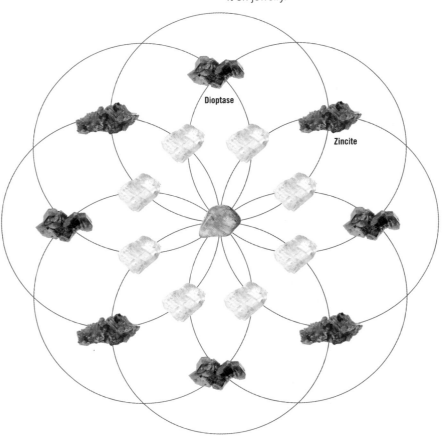

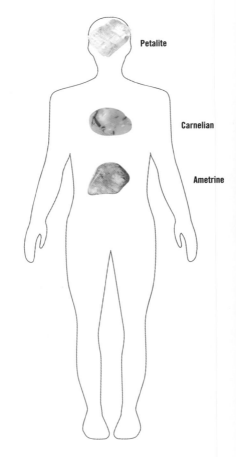

UNDERGOING CANCER TREATMENT

Undergoing cancer treatment can take its toll on your physical, mental, and emotional health. Treatments such as chemotherapy, radiation therapy, or cancer drug treatments can cause side effects such as tiredness, weakness, breathlessness, nausea, sickness, diarrhea, and changes to your hair, skin, and nails. There can also be an increased risk of getting infections. Not everyone gets every side effect and once your treatment has finished, many side effects will ease.

KEY CRYSTALS
—

Petalite—Petalite is a high-vibrational crystal that is very calming, but it also works to help activate energy centers in the body. It's a beneficial crystal to carry with you while you're at home before and after undergoing cancer treatments. If you feel you could benefit from releasing emotional baggage, try pink petalite, too. It can help release fears and worries while promoting inner strength.

Sugilite—If you're experiencing emotional turmoil dealing with your cancer, keep sugilite with you. The energies of sugilite help support you as you deal with difficult issues and cope with an array of emotions.

Dioptase—Place on the heart chakra or hold to help ease fatigue, lessen feelings of nausea, and cleanse and detoxify your body.

OTHER GRID AND LAYOUT CRYSTALS

• Clear quartz (to cleanse)
• Amethyst (for headaches, cleansing, bruising, and aiding restful sleep)
• Jade (for emotional release and irritability)
• Larimar (for calm)
• Red jasper (to calm and stabilize the aura)
• Smoky quartz (for pain and to help with chemotherapy treatment)
• Tourmaline (for mental and emotional healing)
• Unakite (for convalescence and recovery)
• Seraphinite (to cleanse the heart chakra)

ADDITIONAL THERAPIES
—

Drink ginger tea to help deal with nausea from cancer treatments. Acupuncture and reflexology may offer holistic support alongside conventional cancer treatments and relaxing aromatherapy massage may help ease stress.

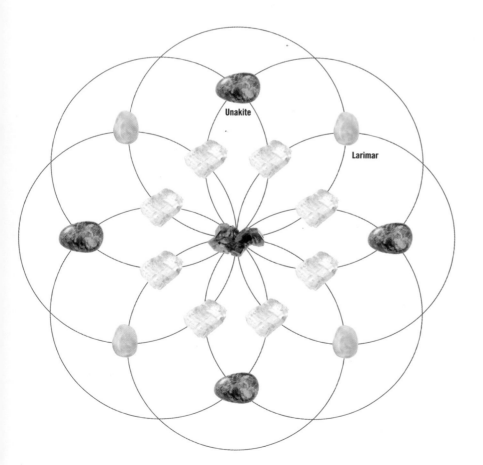

Unakite

Larimar

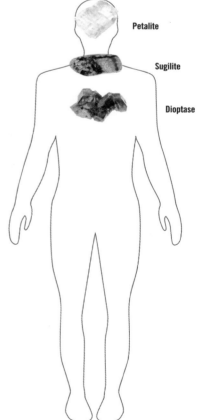

Petalite

Sugilite

Dioptase

CHRONIC FATIGUE SYNDROME

Chronic fatigue syndrome (CFS) is a long-term illness that causes a range of symptoms—much more than just fatigue. Symptoms may include muscle pain, joint pain, sleeping issues, headaches, brain fog, dizziness, nausea, palpitations, concentration and memory issues. There are different ranges of severity—from mild to severe—and the physical symptoms and fatigue can have a major effect on daily life and normal activities. Living with CFS and coping with all the symptoms can sometimes affect mental health, too.

KEY CRYSTALS
—

Ametrine—Place ametrine on the solar plexus chakra as it can help deal with the symptoms of long-term chronic fatigue syndrome. In particular it may help clear brain fog, cleanse toxins from the body, strengthen the immune system, and ease headaches, anxiety, and tiredness.

Yellow apatite—Place on the solar plexus chakra to help with fatigue, lethargy, concentration issues, and digestion.

Kunzite—Place on the heart chakra to soothe and comfort. Use green kunzite to promote the joy of life and acceptance of who you are and what you're going through.

OTHER GRID AND LAYOUT CRYSTALS
—

• Green tourmaline (for exhaustion and fatigue)
• Citrine (for energy and vitality)
• Zincite (to boost the immune system)
• Orange calcite (to stabilize and strengthen the joints)
• Carnelian (for motivation)
• Serpentine (to cleanse and detoxify)
• Sunstone (to lift low moods and improve positivity)
• Rose quartz (to boost morale when living with chronic illness)

ADDITIONAL THERAPIES
—

Ginger tea or sucking a small piece of crystallized ginger can help ease nausea. Some symptoms of pain may be relieved by holistic therapies such as acupuncture, reflexology, homeopathy, or Reiki. Exercise can be difficult with CFS, but some gentle exercise such as swimming, yoga, tai chi, or Pilates may help the muscles. Connecting with others in a similar situation is good for support.

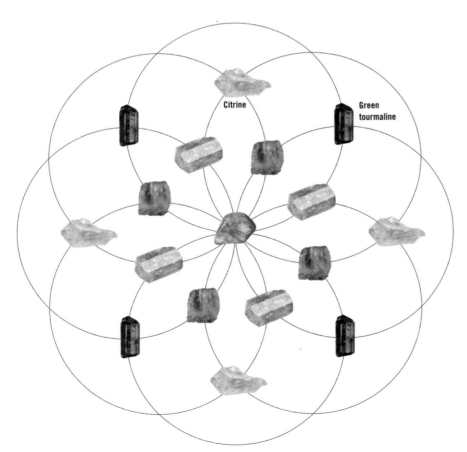

Citrine

Green tourmaline

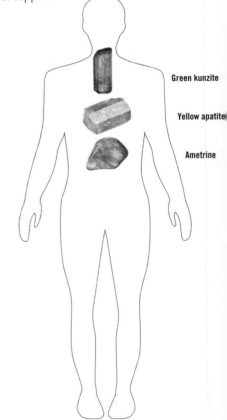

Green kunzite

Yellow apatite

Ametrine

RECUPERATION

When you've experienced chronic or serious illness, you may need time to recuperate to get you back to your normal level of physical strength. Recuperation can take many forms and depends on your individual circumstances and illness. Early recuperation after being in hospital may involve the need for bed rest, while recuperation at later stages may involve the gradual buildup of gentle exercise and movement.

KEY CRYSTALS

—

Blue calcite—Place blue calcite around your bed or hold a piece in your hand. The gentle energies of this crystal can help release physical, emotional, and mental pain, negative emotions, and anxiety about illness.

Unakite—Make an elixir using the indirect method and apply to the body or spray around the aura. The supportive energies of unakite are ideal to have around while you convalesce and recover from major illness.

Rhodonite—Place on the heart chakra to stabilize physical and emotional symptoms and promote strength for recovery.

OTHER GRID AND LAYOUT CRYSTALS

—

• Citrine (for energy)
• Amethyst (for healing, cleansing, and promoting good sleep)
• Green tourmaline (for fatigue)
• Sunstone (to uplift and energize)
• Zoisite (to help recovery after serious illness)
• Rose quartz (for its loving, soothing energy)

ADDITIONAL THERAPIES

—

Eating a healthy nutritious diet and doing appropriate exercise will be beneficial. Extra vitamins and minerals may help, depending on the illness in question. Holistic therapies such as reflexology, Reiki, aromatherapy, and acupuncture may aid ongoing symptoms. Art therapy, music therapy, and nature therapy may all be uplifting and aid recuperation.

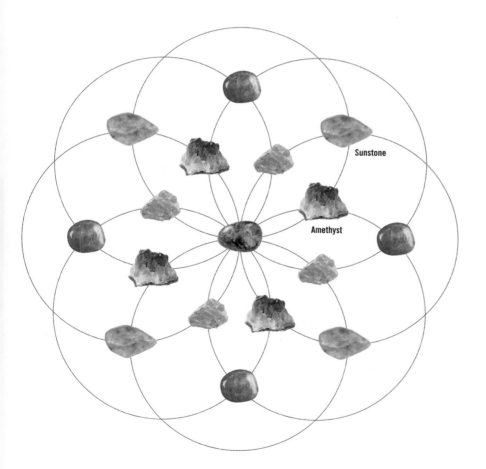

Sunstone

Amethyst

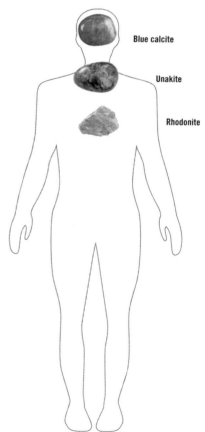

Blue calcite

Unakite

Rhodonite

ADDICTIONS

An addiction is a dependence on, or overwhelming craving for, a substance such as a drug, alcohol, or nicotine. The dependence may only be mental, but it may become physiological if body functions have been altered by prolonged use. In such cases, physical symptoms will be experienced when the user attempts to withdraw. Addictions to particular activities, such as gambling, may also be helped by the same crystals.

KEY CRYSTALS

—

Amber—Wear on the wrist or throat to cleanse and rebalance the body and the chakras. When placed on the sacral chakra, this resin also promotes emotional stability and absorbs pain and negative energy.

Amethyst—Wear on the throat or heart to strengthen the cleansing and eliminating organs, boost the immune system, and tune the metabolism. Place the crystal with the point away from you to help draw away negative energy.

OTHER GRID AND LAYOUT CRYSTALS

- Black tourmaline (for protection)
- Sodalite (for motivation)
- Lepidolite (for emotional balance)
- Rose quartz (for self-forgiveness)
- Iolite (for alcohol addiction)
- Botswana agate (for quitting smoking)
- Apatite (for food addictions)

ADDITIONAL THERAPIES

—

In addition to any medications prescribed by a specialist, you may benefit from talking therapies, meditation, and yoga. Cognitive behavioral therapy (CBT) may help you address and change addictive behavior patterns. It may be worth looking at nutrition, too, to ensure that any deficiencies (such as vitamin B in alcoholics) are addressed.

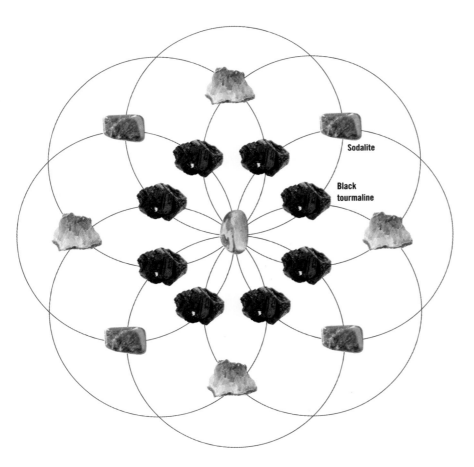

Sodalite

Black tourmaline

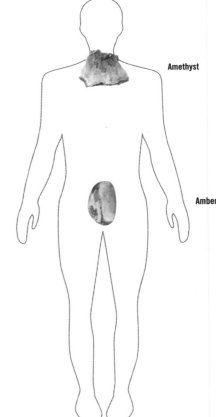

Amethyst

Amber

OBSESSIONS AND COMPULSIONS

Obsessions are unwanted thoughts that keep popping up in your mind, causing anxiety and stress; compulsions refer to the need to keep repeating certain behaviors to relieve the obsession. Common types of obsessive and compulsive behaviors include the need to clean surfaces several times in case of bacteria, switch off all the electric sockets before you go to bed "just in case," or obsessively check your doors and windows are locked before you go out. Obsessive compulsive disorder (OCD) is a known and recognized medical condition and help is available.

KEY CRYSTALS
—

Charoite—Charoite is a stone associated with transformation and can help overcome obsessive and compulsive behaviors. Place the crystal on the heart and crown chakras to help provide balance.

Chrysoprase—The calming nature of chrysoprase can help deal with impulsive actions and thoughts. It encourages positivity and can also help with getting a good night's sleep. Place or wear on the solar plexus. Alternatively, hold the stone in your hands, carry it with you in your pockets or pop it under your pillow at night.

Peridot—Peridot is a cleansing crystal and as such it can help cleanse the burden and guilt of obsessions and compulsions. It helps to release negative behaviors and encourages motivation and growth to move forward from old patterns. Use it in conjunction with the heart and solar plexus chakras.

OTHER GRID AND LAYOUT CRYSTALS
—

• Blue agate (to calm, relieve stress, and encourage positivity)
• Bloodstone (for courage)
• Green jasper (for balance and dealing with obsessive behavior)

ADDITIONAL THERAPIES
—

In addition to any medication prescribed by a specialist, anyone with obsessions and compulsions may benefit from therapies such as psychotherapy, counseling, and cognitive behavior therapy. Techniques such as yoga and meditation may prove calming.

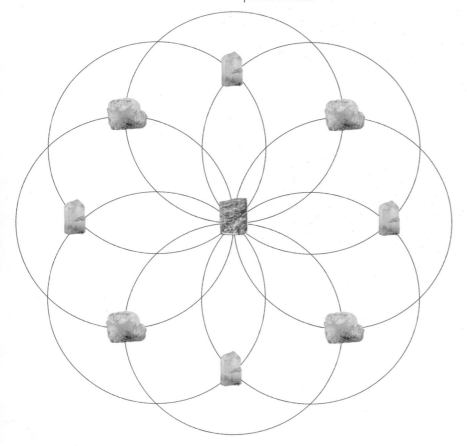

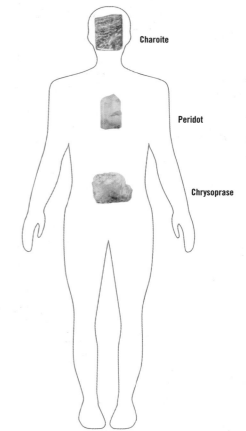

Charoite

Peridot

Chrysoprase

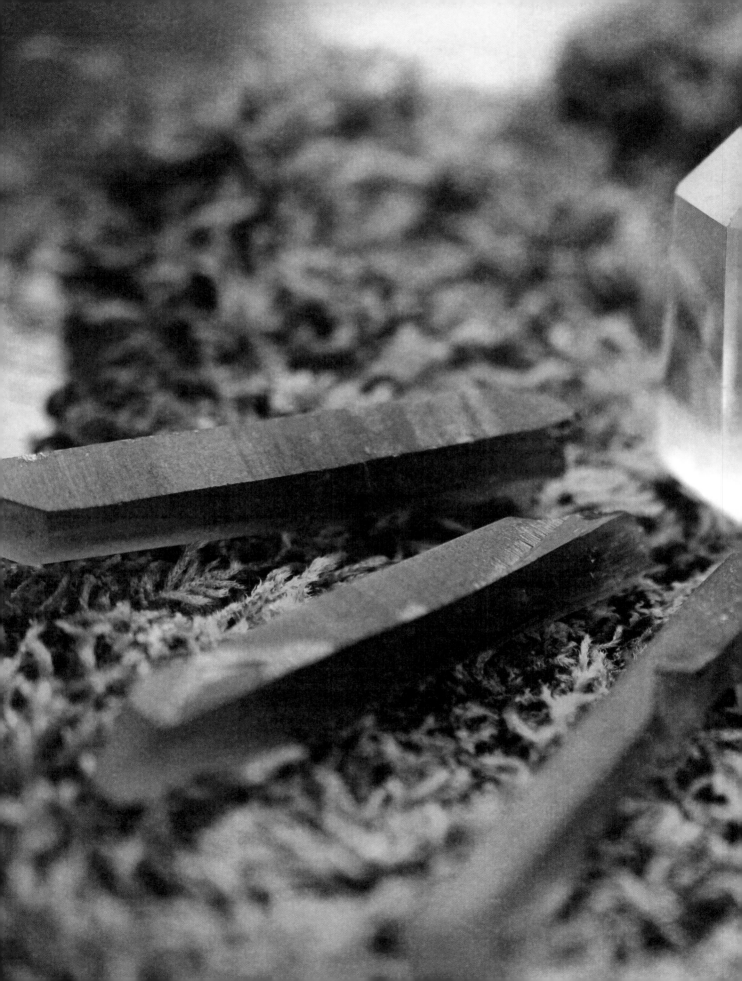

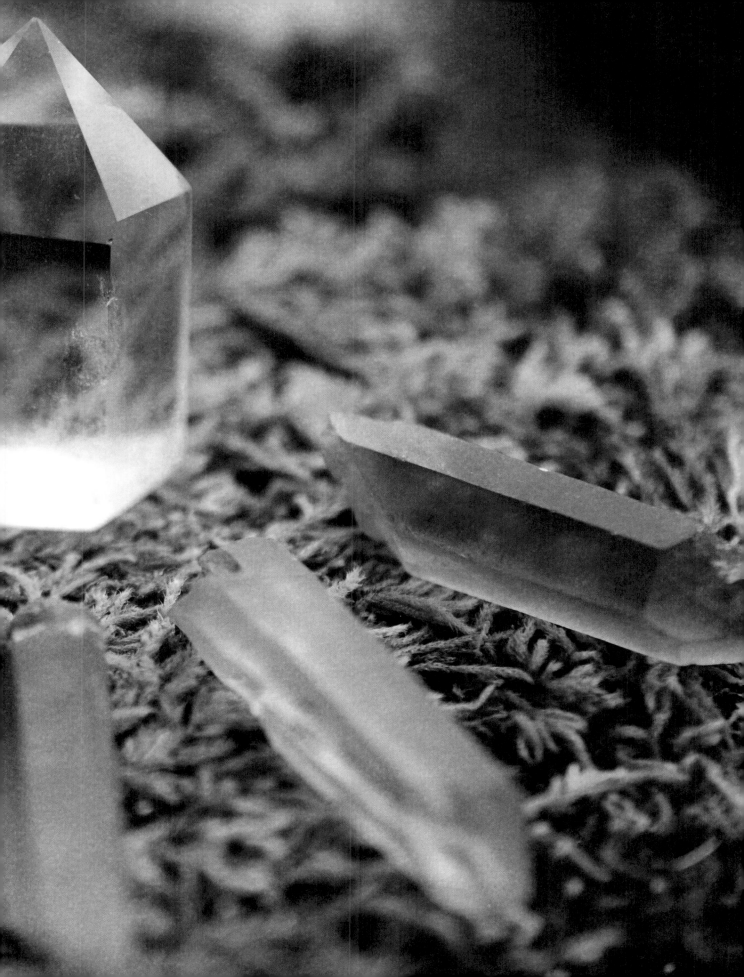

PHOBIAS

Phobias are overwhelming irrational fears of objects, events, situations, animals, or people that cause significant distress. Phobias are a form of anxiety and can develop if you have an unrealistic sense of danger or fear about something. There's no single cause for a phobia, but they can be triggered by traumatic incidents, genetics (some people are more prone to anxiety than others), and learned responses. They can be mild or severe, and symptoms include sweating, shaking, palpitations, feeling dizzy, nausea, shortness of breath, and an upset stomach.

KEY CRYSTALS
—

Aquamarine—Hold or wear aquamarine to boost your sense of courage. Its calming energies may help you focus and look closer at the cause of your phobias. Place on the throat chakra to encourage confidence at speaking up about your true feelings and sharing details of phobias with a therapist.

Rutilated quartz—Wear or place on the solar plexus chakra to help deal with negative energy and facilitate transition. It can help balance the energy field when confronting emotional issues, which can be at the root of phobias.

Citrine—This warming, energizing, and cheery crystal is a good all-rounder for balancing and boosting energy and can be helpful to use when you're coping with, or feeling drained by, emotional phobias. Wear a citrine necklace or place a stone on the throat chakra.

OTHER GRID AND LAYOUT CRYSTALS
—

- Chrysocolla (for negativity and communication)
- Opal (to aid expression of your true self)
- Blue tiger's eye (for anxiety)
- Rose quartz (for peace and inner healing when dealing with trauma)

ADDITIONAL THERAPIES
—

In addition to any medical treatment, therapies such as cognitive behavioral therapy, counseling, and psychotherapy may help. Hypnotherapy and creative visualizations may be useful to reprogram your mind and view the phobia in a more positive light. Breathing techniques and meditation could help to get fear controlled.

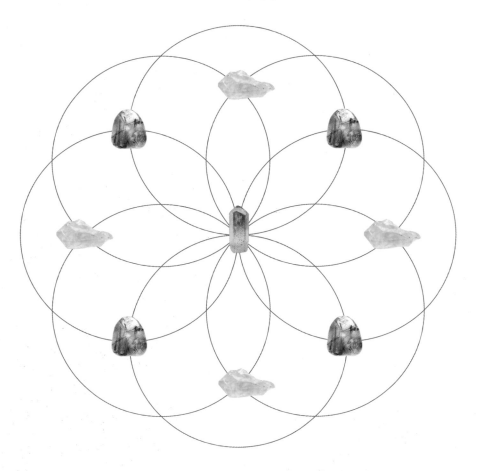

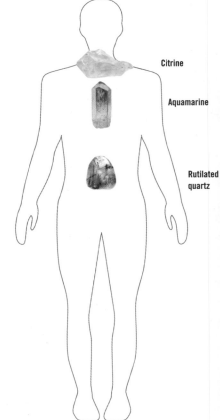

Citrine

Aquamarine

Rutilated quartz

DEPRESSION

Everyone feels down or unhappy from time to time, but depression is much more than that. Depression is a health condition where you feel constantly low for weeks or months at a time. There are physical and mental symptoms, such as anxiety, stress, feeling hopeless, being tearful, and losing interest in everything, and it can range from mild to severe. Other symptoms may include insomnia, waking up in the night, irritability, worry, low self-esteem, changes in appetite, fatigue, aches and pains, lack of energy, withdrawing from social activities, and loss of libido. See a medical practitioner for diagnosis.

KEY CRYSTALS
—

Moss agate—Hold moss agate to access the stabilizing energies of this crystal. It can help remove negativity and fear, boost self-esteem, and generally help you see things from a different perspective.

Ametrine—Place on the solar plexus chakra to help bring mental clarity and release physical, emotional, and mental blockages. It's also useful for easing headaches, tension, and stress associated with depression.

Turquoise—Place on the throat, solar plexus, or third eye chakras to relieve mental and physical exhaustion and instill a sense of inner calm.

Sunstone—Hold sunstone to help lift a dark mood. The positive energies of this crystal could help increase self-worth and enable you to see light at the end of the tunnel.

OTHER GRID AND LAYOUT CRYSTALS
—

• Lithium quartz (a natural anti-depressant to lift the mood)
• Lepidolite (for emotional stress)
• Carnelian (for energy)
• Jade (to soothe the mind and release negativity)
• Lapis lazuli (to help express feelings)
• Amethyst (to calm the mind from overthinking)

ADDITIONAL THERAPIES
—

Self-care is really important if you feel depressed. Eating a healthy diet may help boost your energy, and exercise such as walking has been found to help mild depression. Counseling, psychotherapy, or cognitive behavioral therapy may be beneficial.

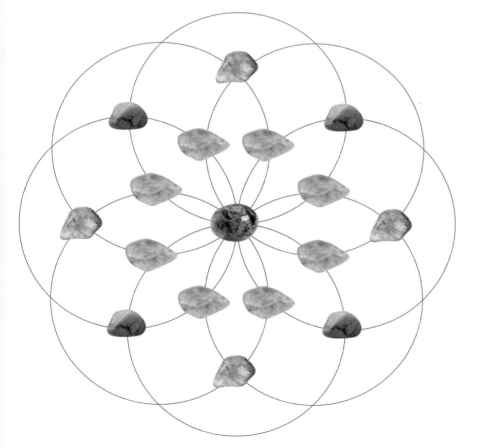

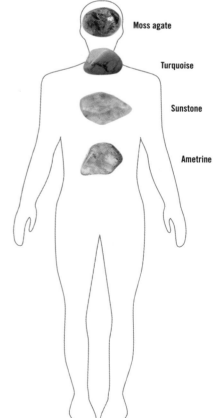

Moss agate

Turquoise

Sunstone

Ametrine

STRESS

A certain amount of stress is stimulating, but prolonged stress can cause mental and physical damage. When stress is encountered, hormones stream into the blood, the pulse quickens, the lungs take in more oxygen, blood sugar increases to supply energy, and perspiration breaks out. If the stressful situation ends, the body begins to repair the damage caused. However, if the situation does not resolve, the body runs out of energy. Common causes of stress include work issues, relationship problems, financial worries, life changes, and illness. Symptoms of long-term stress include insomnia, depression, digestive problems, ulcers, palpitations, high blood pressure, heart disease, and impotence.

KEY CRYSTALS
—

Charoite—Place on the third eye, heart, or solar plexus chakras to help with overcoming emotional turmoil, dealing with change, and living in the present moment. Charoite encourages calm and may help with short-lived obsessions and compulsions.

Green aventurine—Place on the heart or solar plexus to comfort, protect, heal the heart, and settle mild digestive disorders. It may also help to dispel negative thoughts and restore well-being.

OTHER GRID AND LAYOUT CRYSTALS

- Morganite (for casting off excess baggage)
- Lapis lazuli (for clarity of thought)
- Magnetite (for regaining a balanced perspective)
- Jasper (for resilience)
- Labradorite (for banishing insecurity)
- Dioptase (for overcoming stress)
- Black tourmaline (to ground you and release tension)

ADDITIONAL THERAPIES
—

During brief periods of stress, practicing breathing techniques and positive visualizations may help to calm the mind. In the longer term, regular exercise, meditation, yoga, and talking therapies may all be beneficial. Take a B-vitamin supplement, as this essential vitamin is often depleted by stress.

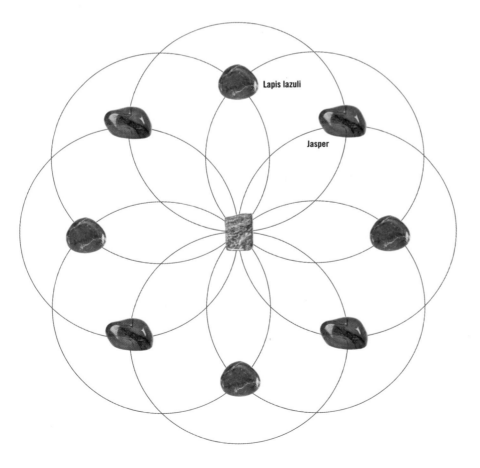

Lapis lazuli

Jasper

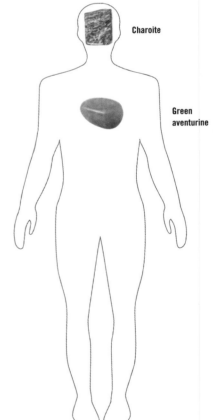

Charoite

Green aventurine

ANXIETY

It's normal to feel anxious from time to time, but some people are plagued with constant anxiety, worries, and fears. Feelings of anxiety can range in severity from mild to severe. When anxiety is constant, it can take over and affect your home, work, and social life. The symptoms may start off as psychological, but constant anxiety can lead to physical symptoms such as restlessness, insomnia, dizziness, palpitations, irritability, fatigue, and difficulty concentrating. See your doctor if you're experiencing signs of anxiety, as sometimes it can be caused by an underlying health condition.

KEY CRYSTALS

—

Green calcite—Make a crystal elixir using the indirect method and spray directly onto your body or add to bathwater when you're feeling anxious. Green calcite is a comforting crystal that could help to restore balance in your mind and help you let go of negativity and worries.

Black tourmaline—Place black tourmaline on the root chakra to help ground you and release tension. If your crystal has a point, place it with the point facing away from you, to draw off negative thoughts.

Amethyst—Wear an amethyst crystal pendant on a necklace to help calm your body and mind. It may help with decision-making if you're feeling anxious about making the right choices.

OTHER GRID AND LAYOUT CRYSTALS

—

• Black onyx (for overwhelming worry)
• Green aventurine (for comfort and calm)
• Chrysoprase (to calm and promote positivity)
• Lepidolite (for mental exhaustion)
• Lithium quartz (to lift the mood)
• Rose quartz (to calm, comfort, and heal)
• Rhodochrosite (to help encourage confrontation of fears and anxieties)
• Apophyllite (to help release suppressed emotions)

ADDITIONAL THERAPIES

—

When you're feeling anxious, breathing exercises where you simply focus on your breath, and breathing slowly on a count from one to ten, could help to calm feelings of anxiety. Flower remedies that you take under your tongue may help with mild anxiety and creative visualizations, where you mentally imagine the best outcome of a situation or event, could be useful.

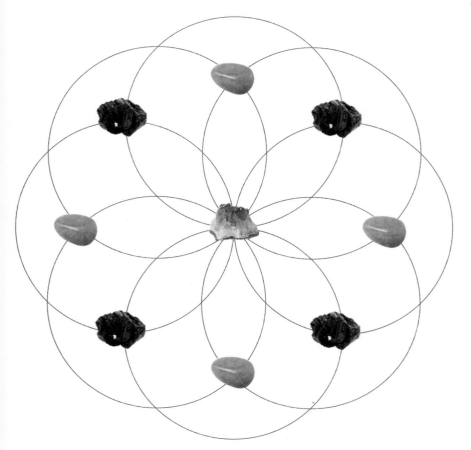

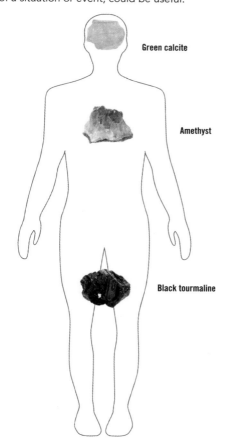

Green calcite

Amethyst

Black tourmaline

INSOMNIA

Insomnia is a sleep disorder where you find it hard to fall asleep or stay asleep, or keep waking up in the night. On average, adults need seven to eight hours of sleep a night, so disturbances to your sleep can have a significant effect. You may end up feeling tired and sleepy during the day, being irritable, find it difficult to focus and concentrate, and end up feeling anxious and worried. Insomnia can occur as the result of stress, shock, worries, or unexpected events, or it can be linked to other medical conditions or medications that you might be taking. Sometimes changing your habits can improve sleep patterns.

KEY CRYSTALS
—

Charoite—Place on the heart chakra, as its calming energies may help to promote deep sleep and overcome insomnia issues.

Howlite—Place under your pillow at night to promote calm and peaceful sleep, especially if you're prone to an overactive mind and thoughts that keep you from getting off to sleep.

Amethyst—Place amethyst around your bed to release stress, calm the mind, and provide protective energies to help you get a good night's sleep.

OTHER GRID AND LAYOUT CRYSTALS
—

- Chrysoprase (for better sleep and peaceful dreams)
- Jade (for dream-filled sleep)
- Lapis lazuli (for peaceful sleep)
- Lepidolite (for emotional healing)
- Moonstone (for emotional stability and stress)
- Muscovite (to relieve tension)
- Selenite (to balance and stabilize)

ADDITIONAL THERAPIES
—

Avoid stimulants, such as caffeine and alcohol, in the evenings and try chamomile tea instead. Melatonin may help to regulate sleep but should only be used as a temporary measure. Lavender essential oil is beneficial—spray it on your pillow or have it in a bath before bed. Regular exercise has been found to reduce insomnia. Avoid using a computer before bed and keep cellphones out of the bedroom.

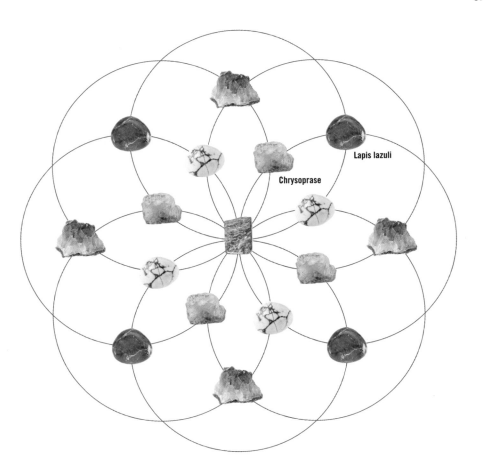

Lapis lazuli

Chrysoprase

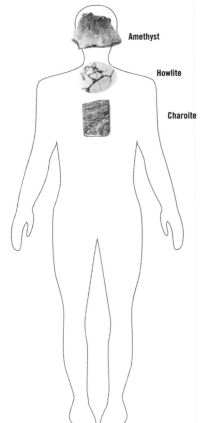

Amethyst

Howlite

Charoite

NIGHTMARES

Nightmares are vivid, scary, or disturbing dreams that wake you up feeling fearful, distressed, or terrified. They can be triggered by anxiety, worries, trauma, taking certain medications, drinking alcohol, a change in sleep patterns, or watching scary movies, or reading frightening books. In most cases, nightmares are an occasional nuisance, but if you get them frequently and they cause problems, such as fear of sleep, or have a significant impact on your ability to function, do speak to a medical practitioner for advice.

KEY CRYSTALS
—

Charoite—Place charoite on the heart chakra to promote deep sleep and peaceful dreams.

Lapis lazuli—The energy of lapis lazuli is protective, which makes it ideal to help combat nightmares. Place on the throat or third eye chakra to balance the body, mind, and spirit and promote peaceful sleep.

Celestite—Place celestite by the bed to disperse negative energies, calm mental images, ease worries, and instill a sense of inner peace.

OTHER GRID AND LAYOUT CRYSTALS
—

• Jade (for a peaceful sleep and pleasant dreams)
• Amethyst (to relax and protect you during sleep)
• Cerussite (to banish nightmares)
• Ruby (to promote positive, happy dreams)
• Smoky quartz (to ground you and dispel nightmares)
• Topaz (to stabilize emotions and bring joy)
• Chrysoprase (for nightmares in children)

ADDITIONAL THERAPIES
—

Avoid watching scary movies or reading terrifying books, especially before bed. Try to avoid drinking alcohol or caffeine or having stimulants in the evening and instead have a relaxing time in the run up to bed. Avoiding eating cheese may also reduce the risk of nightmares, but there's no major evidence to support this. Consider keeping a light on for a while if darkness spooks you.

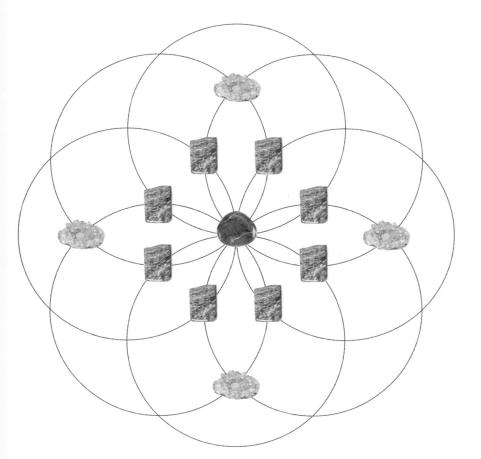

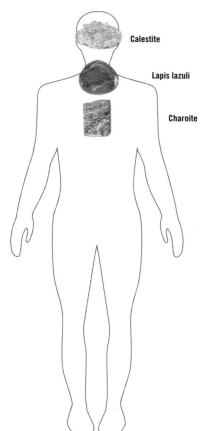

Calestite

Lapis lazuli

Charoite

PAST ABUSE

The trauma of past abuse, be it physical or emotional, can last long after the event. It's not unusual for abuse victims to repress emotions, feelings, and memories, only for them to begin surfacing many years later. They can be triggered by snippets of memories, sounds, smells, or places and can cause vivid, scary flashbacks that feel as if they're reliving the trauma. Signs and symptoms that may manifest as the result of past abuse include sleeping issues, panic attacks, anxiety, low self-esteem, fear, difficulty with relationships, alcohol or drug abuse, and eating disorders. It can be overwhelming, but help and therapies are available if you speak up and ask.

KEY CRYSTALS

—

Chrysoprase—The energies of chrysoprase are nonjudgmental, trustworthy, and secure. Hold the crystal or make a crystal gem elixir and spray it on and around your aura to soothe your inner child and reduce unpleasant flashbacks.

Amazonite—Hold amazonite to soothe and calm emotional trauma and dispel negative energy.

Kunzite—Place on the heart chakra to facilitate self-expression, release pent-up feelings, and help with panic caused by past abuse.

OTHER GRID AND LAYOUT CRYSTALS

—

• Blue lace agate (for emotional release and fear of being judged)
• Apache tear (for strength, freedom, and healing)

• Rhodochrosite (for sexual abuse)
• Rainbow aura quartz (for releasing buried hurt and grief)
• Carnelian (to calm anger of past abuse)
• Lapis lazuli (to help express feelings and emotions)
• Pink tourmaline (to cleanse, to promote feelings of self-love and self-worth, and aid in physical, mental, and emotional healing).

ADDITIONAL THERAPIES

—

Gentle healing therapies such as reflexology, Reiki, or art or music therapy may be beneficial. Nature therapy—being outside and connecting with nature—can be comforting. Gentle exercise, such as tai chi or yoga, along with breathing techniques and meditation, could help reconnect the mind to the body.

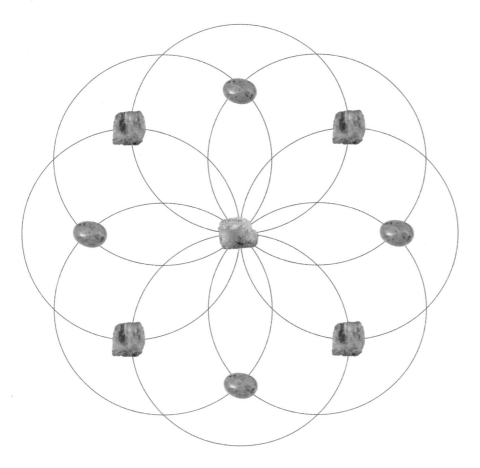

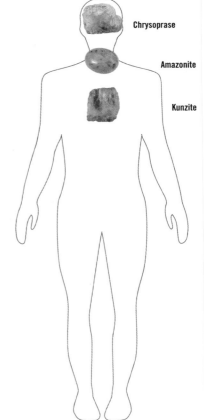

Chrysoprase

Amazonite

Kunzite

ANGER

It's normal to feel anger sometimes, but constantly feeling angry is no good for your physical or mental health. Anger can cause changes in behavior, such as shouting, being aggressive, starting fights, sulking, or ignoring people. Physically, anger can make your heart beat faster, cause tightness in your chest, make your muscles tense, and your fists clench, and mentally it can make you feel resentful, irritated, tense, nervous, or humiliated. Anger might be taken out on yourself rather than other people. It's not good for your long-term health to constantly feel angry, so speak to a medical practitioner for help and support.

KEY CRYSTALS
—

Lapis lazuli—Place on the throat chakra to help release repressed anger that's bubbling up under the surface.

Bloodstone—Place on the heart chakra to help release impatience, aggressiveness, and irritability. The energies can calm the mind and bring a better sense of logic to decisions.

Blue lace agate—Place on the throat chakra to help cool hot-headedness and neutralize feelings of anger.

OTHER GRID AND LAYOUT CRYSTALS

• Chrysoprase (to help reduce speaking out without thinking)
• Magnetite (for inner stability and to release anger)
• Amazonite (to soothe and calm)
• Celestite (to cool fiery emotions)
• Aquamarine (to calm, reduce stress, and encourage taking responsibility)
• Aragonite (to ground and center)
• Muscovite (to control anger)
• Carnelian (to protect against envy, rage, anger, and resentment)

ADDITIONAL THERAPIES
—

Learn to think before acting and do breathing exercises to calm your anger. Exercise, such as walking, running, swimming, going to the gym, or yoga are good to help relieve stress. Talking therapies can provide an outlet to express and release anger.

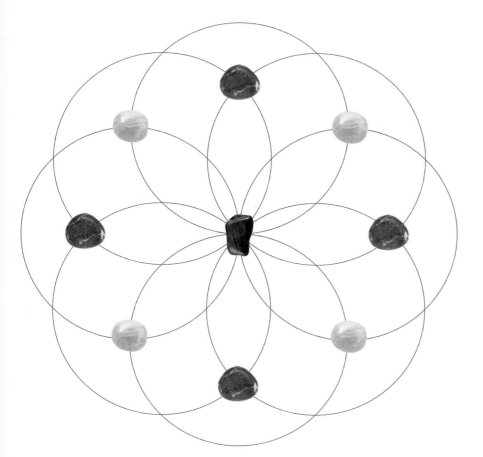

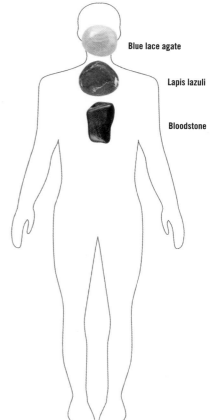

Blue lace agate

Lapis lazuli

Bloodstone

EATING DISORDERS

Eating disorders are conditions where you have disturbed or abnormal eating habits and an unhealthy relationship with food and weight. With some eating disorders you might eat too much (bulimia nervosa), with others too little (anorexia nervosa), or too much in one go (binge-eating disorder) and you're likely to use food to try to manage your feelings. Eating disorders are recognized mental health conditions and anyone of any age can develop one. Mental and physical symptoms include low self-esteem, being unable to control your eating, having a distorted view of your weight or body shape, mood swings, anxiety, depression, self-harm, weight changes, stomach pain, weakness, overexercising, and irritability.

KEY CRYSTALS
—

Carnelian—Carnelian is a crystal of vitality, which could help if you're feeling low physically or mentally due to eating disorders. It may help to promote better absorption of vitamins and minerals and ease depression and low self-worth. Place on the root chakra.

Morganite—Place on the heart chakra to encourage being loving toward yourself, in thoughts and actions, and to open up the ability to express true feelings and needs more openly.

OTHER GRID AND LAYOUT CRYSTALS
—

• Lepidolite (to help release negative behavior patterns)
• Lithium quartz (to purify and lift depression)
• Pink tourmaline (to help you love yourself)
• Praisolite (to help see the good in yourself)
• Rhodochrosite (for positivity and expression of feelings)
• Fluorite (to stabilize the mind and body)
• Apatite (to help break addictive eating patterns)
• Clear quartz (to help flush out toxic thinking)
• Topaz (to aid digestion)

ADDITIONAL THERAPIES
—

Body awareness therapy can help improve your view of yourself. Low-impact exercise, such as yoga, can help relieve stress and build self-esteem, and acupuncture could help with physical and mental health. There's also some evidence that biofeedback might be helpful.

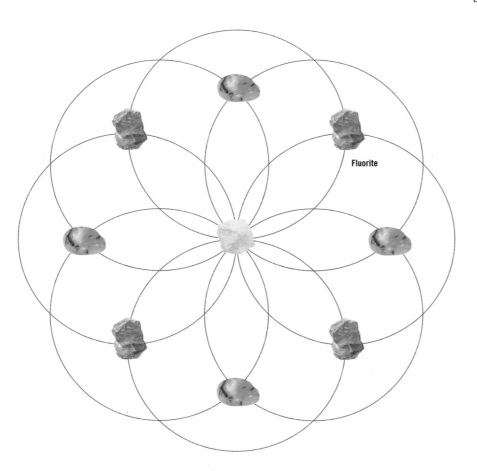

Fluorite

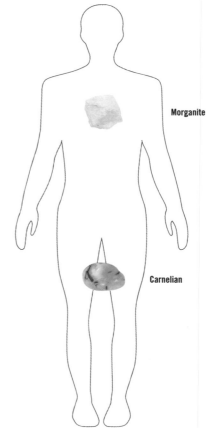

Morganite

Carnelian

CODEPENDENCY

Codependency is a condition where you become too reliant on another person, be it physically, emotionally, or mentally. It's an imbalanced and toxic form of relationship and may be formed by another person assuming responsibility for you and your needs. Codependency often involves one person being the giver and the other the taker, and can be highly complex. Being in a codependent relationship, be it with a partner, parent, friend, or child, can lead to the development of mental health symptoms such as anxiety, depression, low self-worth, and a feeling that you've lost your true sense of self.

KEY CRYSTALS
—

Sunstone—Sunstone has vibrant, uplifting energies and can help lift dark moods and discomfort in relationships. It can help you have the confidence to break free from codependency and the strength to persevere. Hold sunstone or keep a piece in your pocket at all times.

Chrysoprase—Make a crystal gem elixir using the indirect method and spray around your aura. The energy of chrysoprase gives hope, optimism, independence, self-worth, and acceptance of who you truly are.

Lepidolite—Wear or hold lepidolite to promote release from codependent situations. This crystal helps with transitions, so its energies will support you as you move to become more independent.

OTHER GRID AND LAYOUT CRYSTALS
—

• Rose quartz (to help you love yourself)
• Green aventurine (to help you cut toxic ties)
• Jasper (to dissolve negative patterns)
• Jade (to cleanse and purify)
• Selenite (for a difficult relationship with your mother)
• Pink agate (for a difficult relationship with a child)
• Carnelian (for a difficult relationship with your father)
• Rhodonite (for emotional wounds and trauma)

ADDITIONAL THERAPIES
—

Counseling, psychotherapy, and other talking therapies can help you get a better sense of perspective and be able to see the situation from another viewpoint. Holistic therapies such as aromatherapy, massage, acupuncture, reflexology, or Reiki may help to ease stress and anxiety. Cognitive behavior therapy may be useful for developing more positive behaviors and habits.

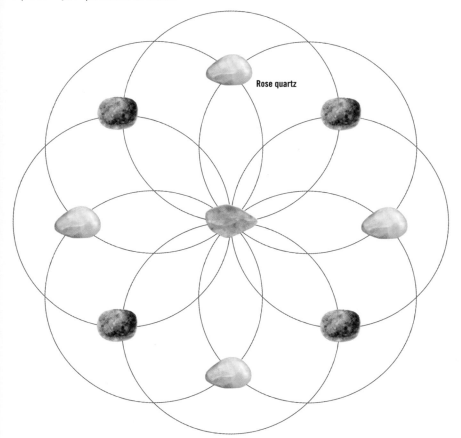

Rose quartz

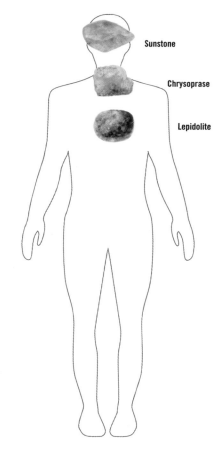

Sunstone

Chrysoprase

Lepidolite

GRIEF

Grief is the response felt—emotionally and physically—after losing someone or something important to you. It's a natural response and everyone reacts differently, and there are likely to be various stages of grief that you go through. For example, you may go through stages of denial, numbness, shock, anger, depression, sadness, panic, confusion, and eventually acceptance. Grief causes a range of physical and emotional symptoms, such as sleep issues, appetite changes, withdrawing from other people, or needing lots of extra company, and can be overwhelming.

KEY CRYSTALS
—

Amethyst—Wear an amethyst crystal as its energy can help support you as you deal with the physical, emotional, and mental pain associated with grief.

Rose quartz—The gentle energies of rose quartz can soothe, calm, and reassure you as you process grief. Keep plenty of rose quartz near you for its loving vibrations and let it help release negativity and replace it with love.

Apache tear—The vibration of apache tear crystals is gentle and soft and helps ground and protect as you grieve. Hold it to help provide strength and healing.

OTHER GRID AND LAYOUT CRYSTALS

- Lithium quartz (to help lift depression)
- Amazonite (to aid communication and expression)
- Emerald (for strength dealing with grief)
- Rainbow aura quartz (for releasing buried hurt and grief)
- Lapis lazuli (for the pain of grief)
- Mookaite (for the emotional pain of loss)
- Rose quartz (for inner healing)
- Dioptase (for sorrow)

ADDITIONAL THERAPIES
—

Talking therapies such as counseling can be beneficial to help you work through your grief. Also look out for grief support groups, where you can learn from and support others in a similar situation. Art therapy, music therapy, journaling, singing, or gardening may all be beneficial.

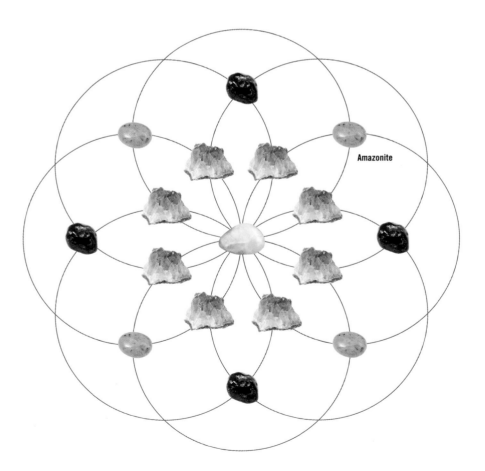

Amazonite

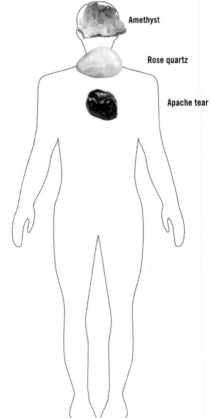

Amethyst

Rose quartz

Apache tear

SHOCK

Shock is a physical and emotional response that occurs after experiencing a traumatic event or hearing sad news about someone or something you care for. It's a normal response to something unexpected or sudden and can cause a range of physical and emotional symptoms. Shock may make you feel numb, anxious, sad, sick, nauseous, upset, panicky, or jittery, and you may not be able to think straight. The effects will ease gradually but may take some time as you take in what's happened. Practice self-care and be gentle on yourself.

KEY CRYSTALS
—

Rhodonite—Keep rhodonite in your first-aid box of crystals to reach for in times of crisis and shock. Place on the heart chakra, or make an elixir, to help calm and soothe emotional wounds.

Rose quartz—The energies of rose quartz are calming and reassuring, and it can help with inner healing, making it an ideal crystal to hold to help you deal with shock.

Obsidian—Place on the root chakra to help ground and stabilize you, mentally and physically, after experiencing shock.

OTHER GRID AND LAYOUT CRYSTALS
—

• Amethyst (for physical, mental, and emotional calming)
• Apache tear (for strength and healing)
• Dioptase (for emotional healing)
• Moonstone (to calm emotions)
• Tangerine quartz (for shock and trauma)

ADDITIONAL THERAPIES
—

Take deep breaths and try to stay calm. There are flower remedies available that are made to deal with shock—just put a few drops under your tongue. Support from friends or family is beneficial. Gardening, walking, and being outside in the fresh air and amongst nature may be helpful and give you time to process the aftereffects of shock.

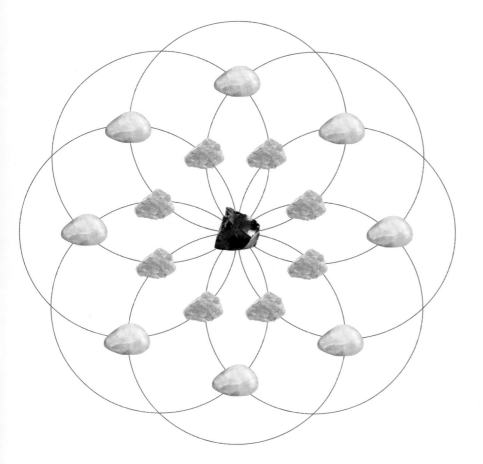

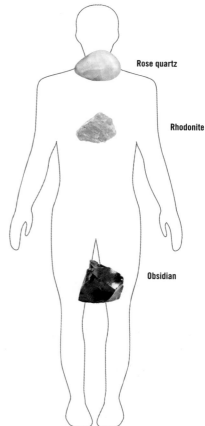

Rose quartz

Rhodonite

Obsidian

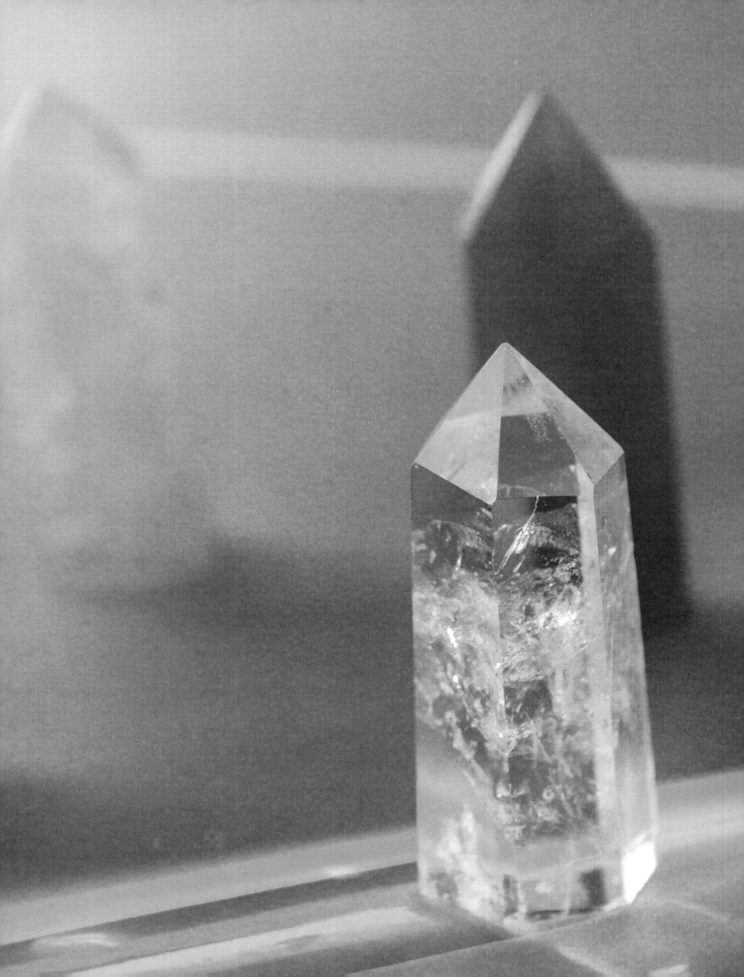

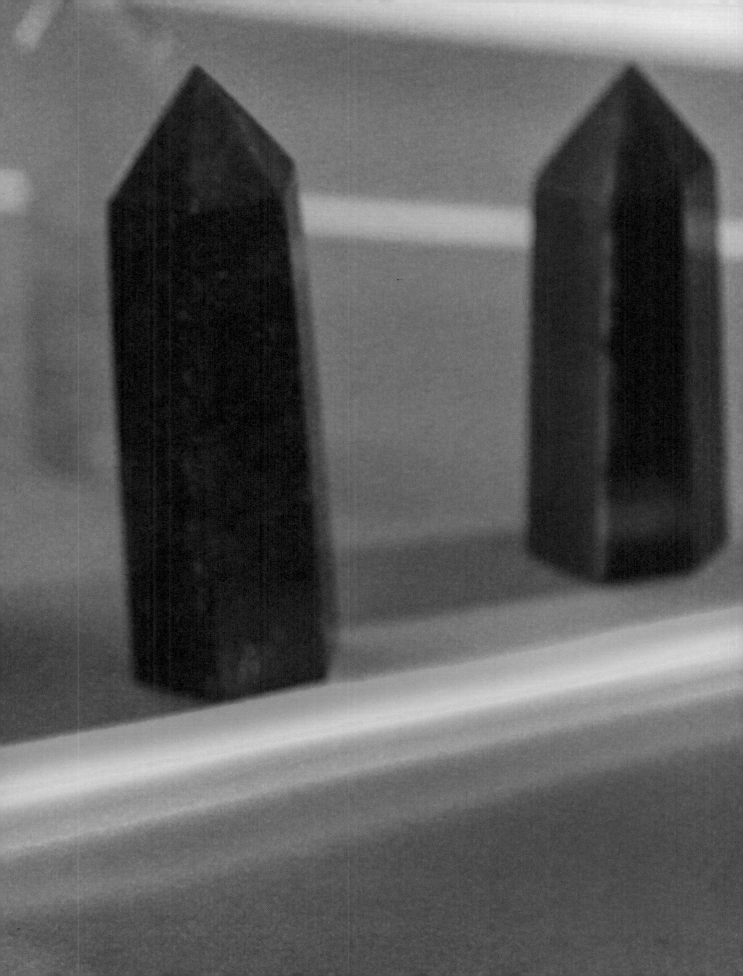

SELF-ACCEPTANCE

Self-acceptance means accepting yourself fully for who you are. It's about accepting the good and the bad and acknowledging that you're not perfect, and neither is life, but you are still a good person despite your past mistakes. Learn to be kind and compassionate to yourself, and you may find that you also manage to let go of worries, stress, and anxiety, too.

KEY CRYSTALS
—

Morganite—Place morganite on your heart chakra to boost self-love and self-acceptance. The energies of morganite are kind, comforting, and loving and can help you learn to clear negativity and view yourself in a good light.

Agate—The energy of agate promotes the importance of being your true self, so hold agate when you're working on boosting self-acceptance. It will gently nurture and support you and help keep you balanced.

OTHER GRID AND LAYOUT CRYSTALS
—

- Manganocalcite (for improved self-worth and self-acceptance)
- Chrysoprase (for acceptance of yourself and others)
- Rhyolite (to help release negative thoughts about yourself)
- Sodalite (to encourage rational thoughts)

ADDITIONAL THERAPIES
—

Meditation and mindfulness exercises may help you focus on the here and now, and aid acceptance of yourself. Try journaling your thoughts and feelings and focus on noting down positive things that you like about yourself and your achievements. Counseling may help if self-acceptance is very hard to grasp.

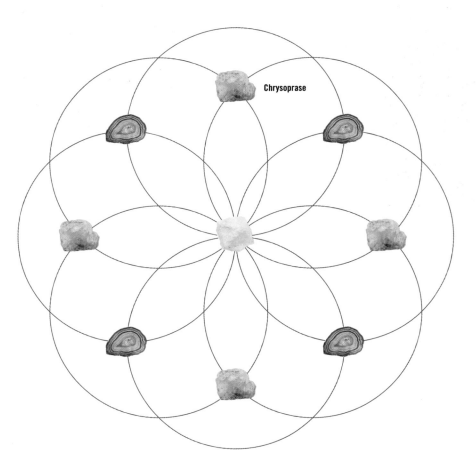

Chrysoprase

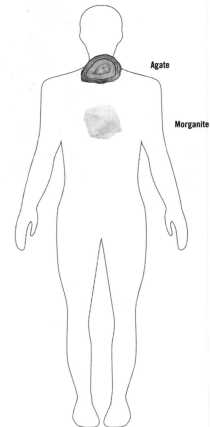

Agate

Morganite

GROUNDING

When you're grounded, you feel stable, calm, and at ease in the present moment. You're not fazed by what's going on around you, however stressful or chaotic it can be, and you feel positive and able to cope with whatever happens. When life is busy, it's easy to become distracted and dislodged from a secure, grounded feeling. It's also common for your grounded state to be knocked off-balance by healing and spiritual work, or as a result of being around lots of negative energies. Regrounding will help you get back in control and feel better.

KEY CRYSTALS
—

Hematite—Place on the root chakra to ground and stabilize you. The energies of hematite will help restore harmony to your body, mind, and spirit.

Obsidian—Place on the root chakra to help stabilize the chakras and enable you to become physically, emotionally, and mentally grounded.

Smoky quartz—Hold smoky quartz or use on the root chakra to bring back harmony and promote positivity.

OTHER GRID AND LAYOUT CRYSTALS
—

• Bloodstone (for impatience and irritability)
• Black tourmaline (for protection)
• Magnetite (for fear or anger)
• Black spinel (for stamina)
• Emerald (for strength)

ADDITIONAL THERAPIES
—

If you feel you need to be more grounded, try meditation or visualization techniques. Sit on a chair with your feet flat on the floor and imagine that you're a tree, with roots coming out from your feet that are securing you to the earth.

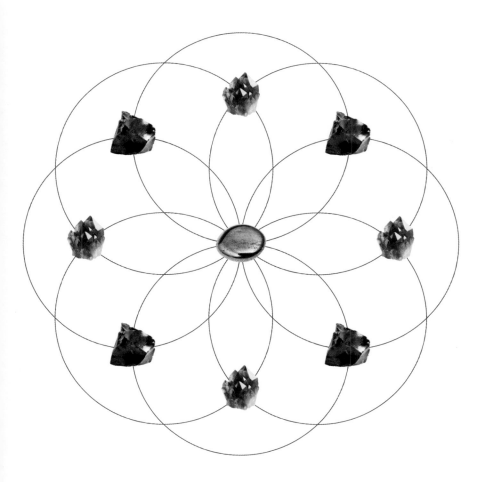

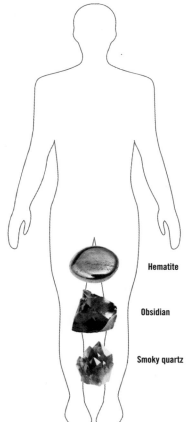

Hematite

Obsidian

Smoky quartz

SELF-CONFIDENCE

Self-confidence is the attitude you have about yourself, your skills, and your abilities. It's being positive about yourself, knowing your strengths and weaknesses, and accepting yourself for who you are. Sadly, self-confidence doesn't come naturally to everyone and events in life can batter it and make you doubt yourself. Low self-confidence can be caused by being in a critical environment, being too harsh in your judgement of yourself, having unrealistic expectations, and being afraid of failure.

KEY CRYSTALS
—

Chrysoberyl—The energies of chrysoberyl have a strong air of confidence that you can soak up. Place on the crown chakra to boost feelings of self-confidence and see the good in yourself.

Hematite—Place hematite on the root chakra. As well as grounding you, it can help boost self-confidence by bringing your thoughts down to earth and focusing on the reality.

OTHER GRID AND LAYOUT CRYSTALS
—

• Carnelian (to ground and anchor you in reality)
• Citrine (to cleanse, re-energize, and fill you with positivity)
• Garnet (for confidence and energy)
• Red tiger's eye (for motivation)
• Manganocalcite (for positivity, self-esteem, and self-confidence)

ADDITIONAL THERAPIES
—

If you're hampered by low self-confidence, individual or group-based talking therapies could help you to reevaluate your thinking. You may also find it beneficial to use journaling techniques to note down your positive qualities and what makes you feel good about yourself.

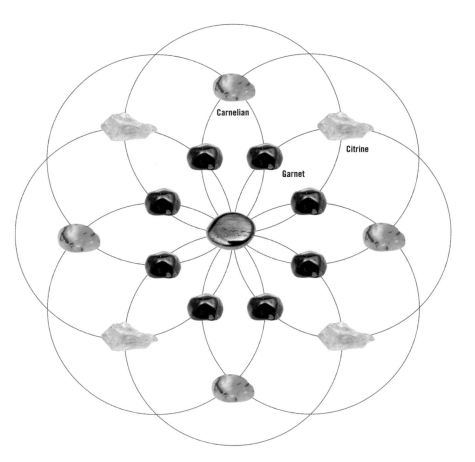

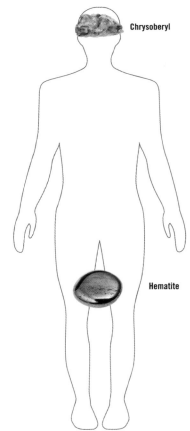

COURAGE

If you have courage, you have the inner strength and ability to do things that scare or frighten you. Courage can take many forms, and what seems courageous to one person may seem perfectly normal and not an issue to someone else. It doesn't matter what other people think, though, being courageous is all about your ability to be brave and tackle the situations, events, or people that you find scary or intimidating. It's about rising above the fear and being willing to face it head on.

KEY CRYSTALS
—

Agate—The calming energies of agate will help keep you balanced and boost the courage you need in any given situation. Keep agate in your pocket.

Aquamarine—The energies of aquamarine are inherently calming and stress-free and are ideal to hold or surround yourself with when you need a boost of courage. Aquamarine could help calm your mind of unwanted thoughts, give support, and encourage you to face your fears.

OTHER GRID AND LAYOUT CRYSTALS

- Carnelian (for vitality and strength)
- Beryl (to calm the mind, reduce stress, and promote courage)
- Bloodstone (to calm the mind and help you face fears)
- Citrine (to reduce self-criticism)
- Ruby (for protection)
- Topaz (for emotional support)

ADDITIONAL THERAPIES
—

Utilizing the art of positive affirmations can help to reinforce your ability to overcome negativity, unleash your inner strength, and do something that takes courage. Write yourself some positive affirmations—for example, "I am positive, strong, and courageous," or "I'm glad to have the chance to show my courage." Print them out and stick them where you'll see them daily. Keep repeating them until they become second nature.

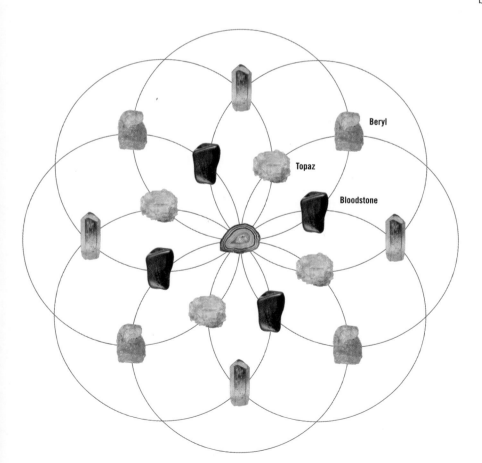

Beryl

Topaz

Bloodstone

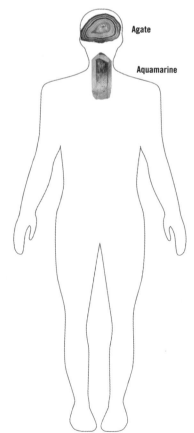

Agate

Aquamarine

MENTAL CLARITY

If you have mental clarity, you're blessed with a clear and focused state of mind that isn't clouded by worries, indecision, brain fog, or endless "what if?" questions. If you don't have mental clarity, you're likely to be your own worst inner critic, letting yourself get distracted from goals or intentions and talking yourself out of doing things. Mental clarity helps gives you focus and direction—it's easier to get things done and prioritize tasks, and it can help you push through worries and doubts. Mental clarity can also help you feel happy, at ease, and content with your life and the hand it has dealt you.

KEY CRYSTALS
—

Amazonite—The energies of amazonite are soothing and comforting and ideal for washing away negative thoughts, doubts, and worries. Place on the heart or throat chakra to help clear unwanted thoughts from your head and provide a more balanced outlook.

Ametrine—Wear ametrine as a pendant on a necklace. The energies of ametrine promote clarity of mind, aid concentration and clear thought, and help you persevere with plans.

OTHER GRID AND LAYOUT CRYSTALS
—

- Apatite (for motivation)
- Blue fluorite (for clear, orderly thoughts)
- Apophyllite (to release mental blockages)
- Charoite (for decision-making)
- Clear topaz (for problem-solving)
- Turquoise (to purify, balance, and align)
- Atacamite (for clarity of thought)

ADDITIONAL THERAPIES
—

Aromatherapy essential oils, such as rosemary, peppermint, and lemon, can aid clarity, so add them to an aromatherapy oil burner to help clear your mind. Acupuncture may be useful for clearing the meridians and letting energy flow freely around your body.

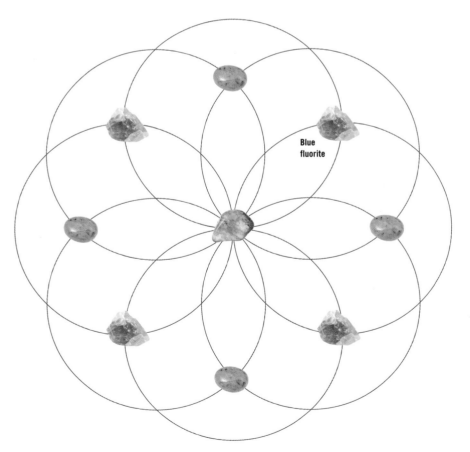

Blue fluorite

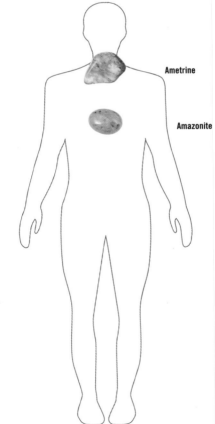

Ametrine

Amazonite

UNCONDITIONAL LOVE

Unconditional love is the ability to love someone or something else freely and without accepting anything else in return. You only see the good in them and totally accept someone for who they are, whatever their earthly flaws. It's affection without any limitations, and you feel strongly that you only want the best for them and for them to be happy—even if that means without you being in their lives. Unconditional love is often described as the love a mom has for her newborn baby. Studies have shown that unconditional love can have a positive effect on mental and emotional health.

KEY CRYSTALS
—

Rose quartz—Place rose quartz around a room or wear a rose quartz pendant near your heart chakra. The soothing, calming, and love-filled energies of rose quartz are perfect for promoting unconditional love. It will help purify and open the heart and teach you to be more loving in all areas of your life.

Manganocalcite—Place this pink calcite crystal on your heart chakra to promote feelings of unconditional love.

Morganite—Place on the heart chakra to encourage compassion, joy, and unconditional love to flow through you with confidence.

OTHER GRID AND LAYOUT CRYSTALS

- Charoite (to release negative energy)
- Pink danburite (to link your heart and mind)
- Kunzite (for protection and expression of feelings)
- Hiddenite (to awaken and attract unconditional love)
- Magnesite (for overcoming challenges of unconditional love)
- Prehnite (for protection and divine energy)

ADDITIONAL THERAPIES
—

If you have issues stopping you embracing unconditional love, talking therapies such as counseling or psychotherapy could help you get to the root of the problem.

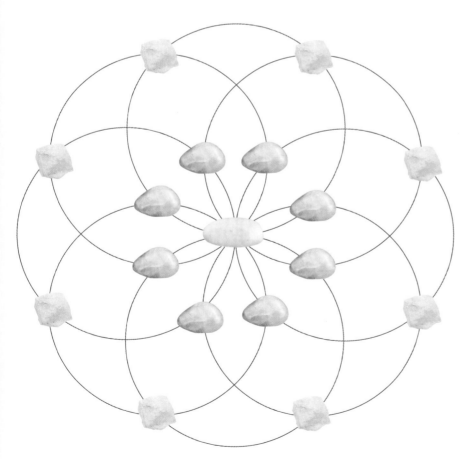

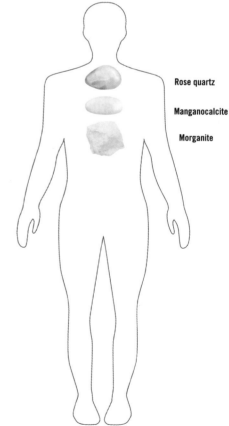

Rose quartz

Manganocalcite

Morganite

COMMUNICATION

Communication is the ability to express yourself and deliver effective messages. Communication can be verbal or nonverbal—verbal involves talking face to face to individuals or groups, whereas nonverbal refers to the communication signals you give out from your gestures, actions, what you look like, and your body language. If you're effective at communication, you're confident in what you're doing, how you're delivering the message, and being sure that your intended audience will understand what you're saying. Communication skills don't always come naturally and can be hampered by self-doubt, worry, and lack of confidence, especially when they involve speaking to groups.

KEY CRYSTALS
—

Turquoise—Place on the throat chakra to release blockages and help you to express yourself clearly.

Aquamarine—Hold or place on the throat chakra to boost courage and provide protection when speaking. Its calming energies will help reduce stress and clear your mind of unwanted negative thoughts so you can focus on delivering your message.

OTHER GRID AND LAYOUT CRYSTALS
—

• Apophyllite (to calm, relieve stress, and release negativity)
• Celestite (for inner peace and strength)
• Blue fluorite (for orderly thought and clear communication)
• Labradorite (to calm an overactive mind and dispel fears)
• Blue lace agate (to help articulation of words)

ADDITIONAL THERAPIES
—

Chakra meditations could be used to help remove blockages and negative energy from your body. Improved communication skills and confidence at speaking in front of people can be learned through therapists, either on an individual basis or in a group format.

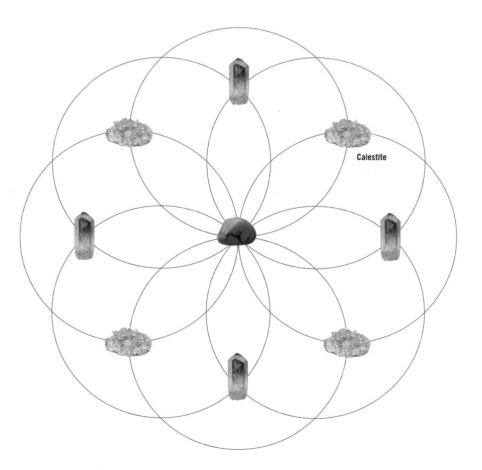

Calestite

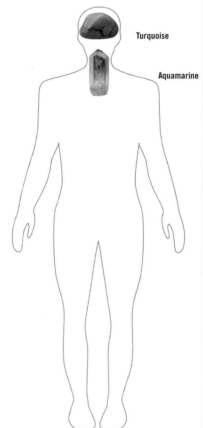

Turquoise

Aquamarine

RENEWING POSITIVITY

Positivity is the art of being optimistic and upbeat about situations, events, people, or other occurrences in life. It's not always easy being positive, and levels of positivity naturally ebb when negative circumstances occur or things don't work out as well as you'd hoped. Spending time focusing on renewing positivity is highly beneficial. Being positive can make you feel better in yourself—mentally, physically, and emotionally—and it can make you a better and happier person to be around.

KEY CRYSTALS

—

Carnelian—Place on the root chakra to release blockages, improve vitality, and remove fear and negativity from your life.

Dioptase—Place dioptase over the heart chakra, as this crystal can help promote a feeling of living positively, of banishing fear and negative emotions, and focusing on making the best of the here and now.

OTHER GRID AND LAYOUT CRYSTALS

—

• Clear quartz (to raise energy)
• Rose quartz (for reassurance)
• Topaz (for vibrance, energy, and joy)
• Emerald (for strength)
• Howlite (to still the mind)
• Pyrite (to help you overcome feelings of inertia and reinstate positivity in your life)
• Opal (to amplify positivity)

ADDITIONAL THERAPIES

—

Use positive affirmations to reinforce your positivity. Write down your affirmations and repeat them daily, until they become second nature. It's also worth keeping a journal of positive thoughts and things that have happened in your life, so that you can look back on it for inspiration if your positivity wanes.

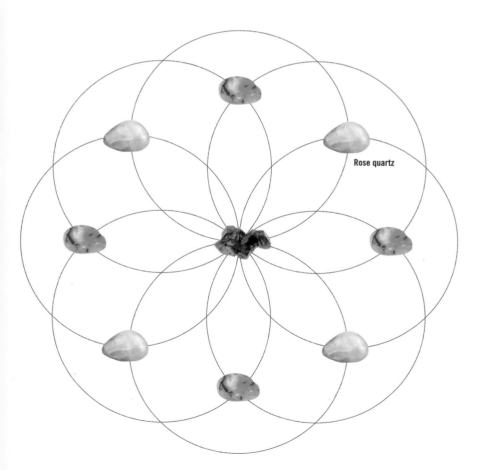

Rose quartz

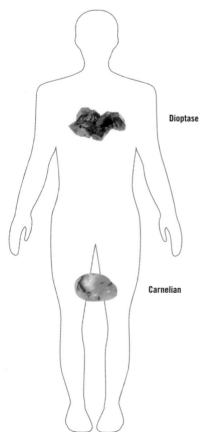

Dioptase

Carnelian

COPING WITH CHANGE

Nothing ever stays the same, however much you'd love it to. Things are constantly changing and evolving, although it may not always feel like it's for the better. Even though you may take small changes in your stride and hardly notice the effects, big changes can have more of an impact and throw you off-kilter. Initial ways of handling changes may be to pretend and deny that they're happening, but this approach doesn't do you any good mentally or emotionally in the long run. Instead, it's better for your health to try to cope with change, adapt to differences, and accept them for what they are.

KEY CRYSTALS
—

Lepidolite—Hold or wear lepidolite to help you cope with changes going on in your life. The crystal may help make transitions smoother and help your acceptance of the situation.

Danburite—Place on the heart chakra to heal and help you come to terms with changes. The energies of the crystal are calming and reassuring and can help you adapt and accept new situations.

OTHER GRID AND LAYOUT CRYSTALS
—

• Bloodstone (to ground you, dispel fear, and aid courage)
• Aquamarine (to reduce stress and quieten worries)
• Iolite (to help release negativity)
• Morganite (for compassion and joy)
• Ocean jasper (for quiet strength)
• Rhyolite (to uplift and aid cheerfulness)

ADDITIONAL THERAPIES
—

Maintaining some form of schedule is important as you're going through changes—at the very least, try to exercise regularly, eat a healthy diet, and get fresh air. Depending on the changes in question, there may be support groups available. Use journaling to make a note of all the positive aspects that could arise as the result of change and use positive affirmations to help train your mind to accept it.

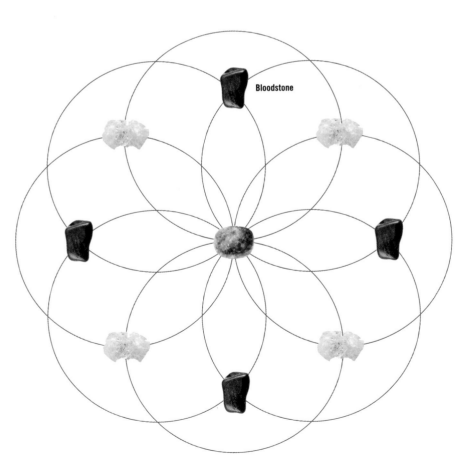

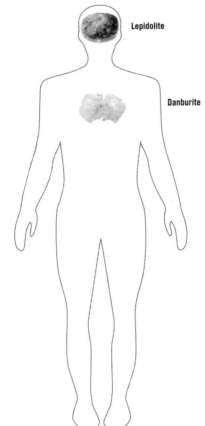

FORGIVENESS

Forgiveness is the act of being able to consciously and deliberately forgive someone or something that's happened. Holding grudges and being bitter about things that have happened won't do you any good healthwise, either physically, mentally, or emotionally. It will cause symptoms such as stress, worry, anxiety, anger, and despair—all emotions that can eat you up inside and leave you feeling worse. By practicing forgiveness, you consciously accept what's happened and move on from the situation.

KEY CRYSTALS

—

Apache tear—The vibration of apache tear crystals is gentle and soft and helps ground and protect you as you release forgiveness. Hold it to help provide strength and healing.

Rose quartz—Surround yourself with rose quartz to soothe, calm, and reassure you that love and forgiveness is a better path than anger.

OTHER GRID AND LAYOUT CRYSTALS

—

• Chrysoprase (for trust and security as you practice forgiveness)
• Manganocalcite (to help you forgive and leave things in the past)
• Rhodonite (to help balance the emotions)
• Rutilated quartz (for releasing negative energy)
• Selenite (for deep peace)
• Rainbow aura quartz (to help you forgive and release buried hurt)

ADDITIONAL THERAPIES

—

Counseling and psychotherapy could be useful to help you work through difficult issues in your past, bring emotions to the surface, and help you learn to forgive. Therapies such as acupuncture or reflexology may help to release blockages in meridians, which may in turn aid your healing process. If you find it difficult to express emotions, try journaling, creating artwork, or music therapy to express yourself in other ways.

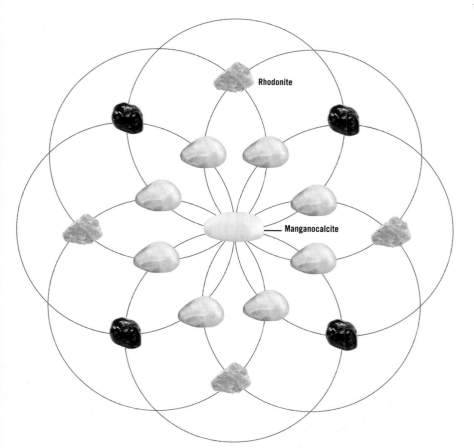

Rhodonite

Manganocalcite

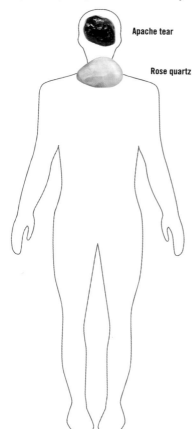

Apache tear

Rose quartz

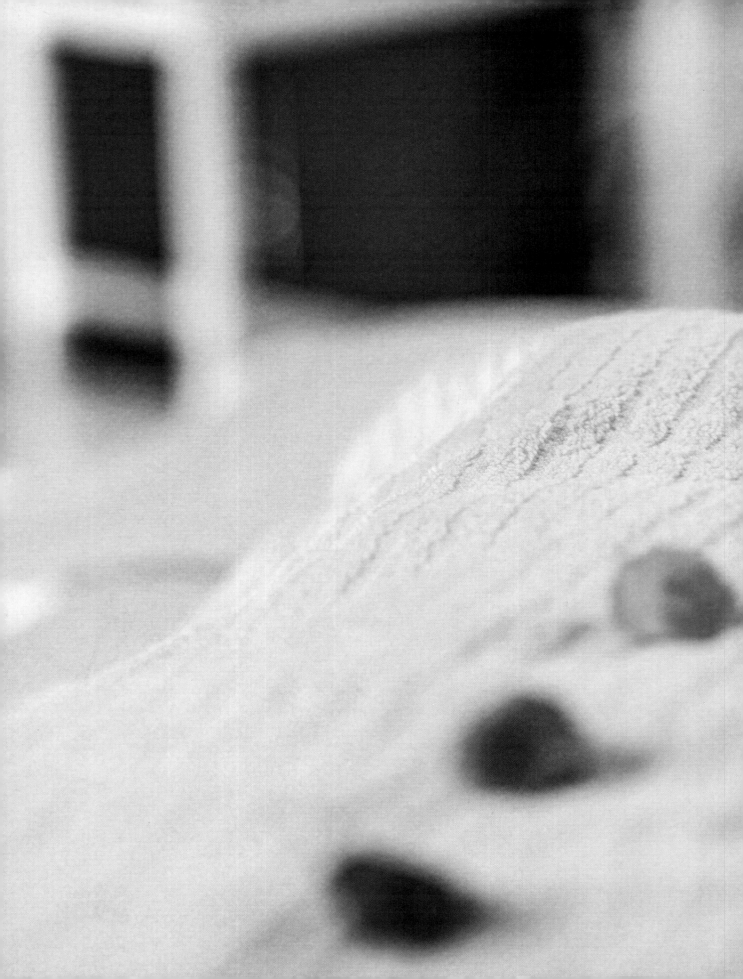

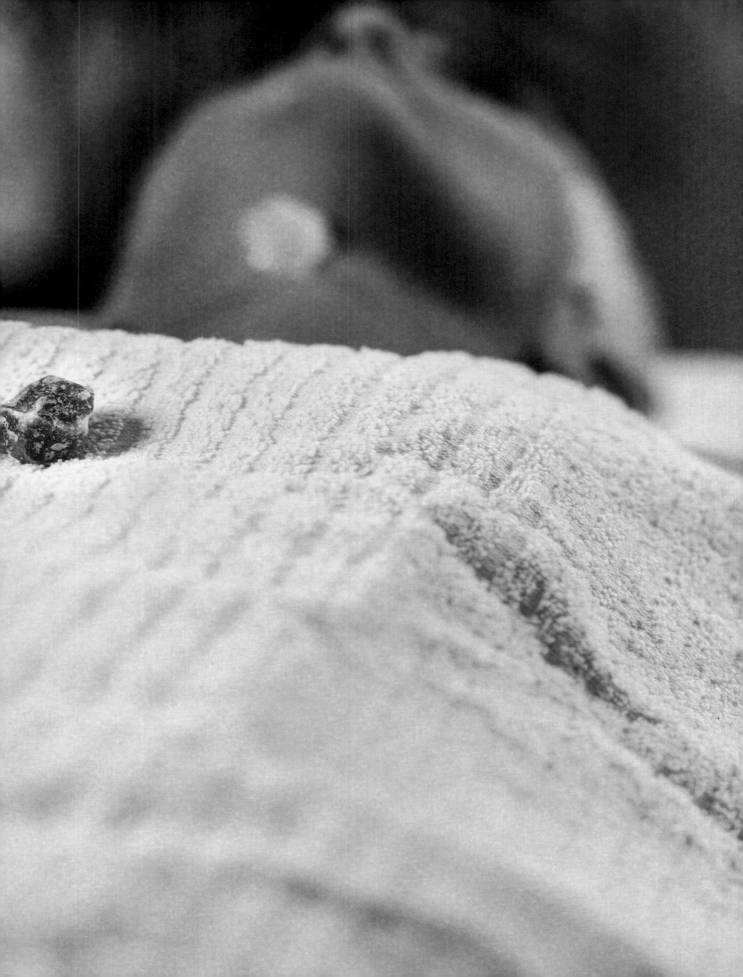

ALIGNMENT

If your aura is out of alignment, you might not feel your usual self. You may feel sluggish, fatigued, and under the weather and be more affected by negative energies and views. Your aura is strongly connected to your chakras and if one is out of alignment, the chances are the other system is, too. Realignment is a bit like giving your aura a health checkup—it will help sort out the problems and little niggles and get things working more efficiently again.

KEY CRYSTALS
—

Kyanite—If your aura needs aligning, use a kyanite crystal wand to first re-activate all your chakras. Working from the base chakra upward, rotate your kyanite crystal in a clockwise direction over each chakra. When all your chakras are fully reactivated, run the kyanite over your aura, using a smoothing motion, to realign all the layers.

Jasper—Use jasper to help realign all your chakras. Place on each chakra, one at a time, or use multiple jasper crystals, one on each of the chakras in one go.

OTHER GRID AND LAYOUT CRYSTALS
—

• Amazonite (to help block geopathic stress and electromagnetic pollution, which may pull the aura out of alignment)
• Labradorite (to help realign the etheric and physical bodies)
• Magnetite (to help alignment)
• Black tourmaline (to ground you)
• Aqua aura quartz (to realign your physical, mental, emotional, and spiritual bodies)

ADDITIONAL THERAPIES
—

A chakra meditation can be useful, where you focus on cleansing and detoxifying each chakra in turn. You could also try an aura creative visualization, where you imagine smoothing down all the layers of your aura so they realign perfectly and gradually see the colors come back to life.

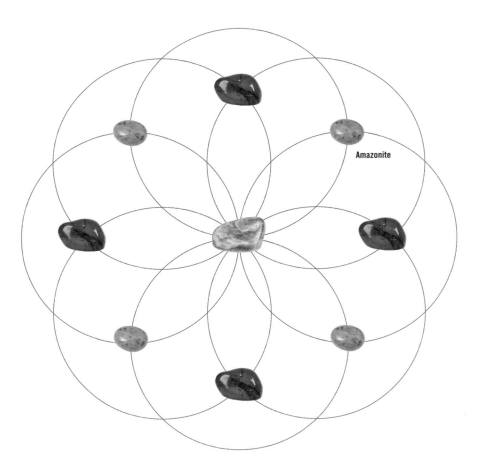

Amazonite

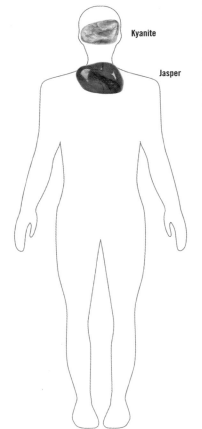

Kyanite

Jasper

CLEANSING

Your aura is sensitive and can easily pick up negative energies from other people—their emotions and experiences. Just as you need to cleanse and refresh your crystals after using them, so too does your aura need cleansing now and again. Cleansing will keep it in tip-top condition and help you feel better. When your aura is uncleansed, the colors can darken, the shine will fade, and you can feel dull and lacking in vitality. You may also feel unexpected emotions, such as frustration, doubt, stress, or anxiety.

KEY CRYSTALS
—

Ametrine—Use the harmonizing power of ametrine to cleanse your aura. It will help release negativity, clear blockages, and boost clarity. Place it on the solar plexus for the best results.

Charoite—Place on the crown chakra to cleanse your aura of negative emotions, particularly if you're feeling frustrated or stressed.

Aqua aura quartz—Hold in your hand and visualize the energies of aqua aura quartz cleaning, clearing, and cleansing your aura. When your aura is fully cleansed with aqua aura quartz, you'll be free of negativity and more strongly spiritually aligned.

OTHER GRID AND LAYOUT CRYSTALS
—

• Chevron amethyst (to cleanse and clear the aura or debris)
• Apophyllite (to calm and reduce stress)
• Green fluorite (to cleanse and neutralize the aura)
• Andradite garnet (to cleanse, clear, and expand the aura)
• Rutilated quartz (to cleanse and energize the aura)
• Brown spinel (for aura cleansing)
• Topaz (to help your aura become clear, vibrant, and filled with positive energy)

ADDITIONAL THERAPIES
—

Meditation and creative visualization techniques are ideal to use alongside crystals as you work on cleansing your aura. What you have on the inside affects the outside, too, so drink plenty of water to hydrate and cleanse your body, eat a nutritious diet, and develop healthy lifestyle habits to help keep your aura in good condition.

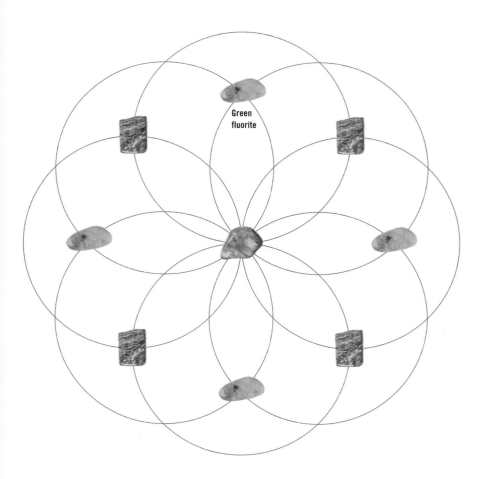

Green fluorite

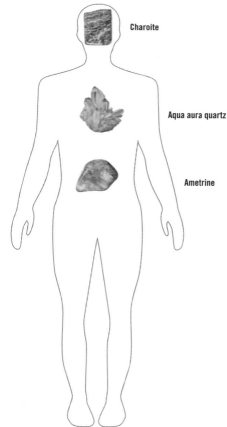

Charoite

Aqua aura quartz

Ametrine

STRENGTHENING

Sometimes your aura could do with an extra boost of strength. This is similar to how there are times when physically, mentally, or emotionally you need extra support. It may be that you're going through difficult times, facing extra stresses and pressures, or dealing with a lot of negativity in your life. When your aura is restrengthened, it will give you an extra layer of auric protection and have a positive impact on your ability to cope with stress and negativity. Think of it like an extra-strong layer of armor protecting you from harm.

KEY CRYSTALS
—

Mahogany obsidian—Place on the sacral and solar plexus chakras to help stabilize and strengthen your aura.

Pyrolusite—Hold or surround yourself with pyrolusite if someone is trying to mentally or emotionally manipulate you. It will help strengthen your aura and give you the energy to defend yourself against unwanted manipulation.

OTHER GRID AND LAYOUT CRYSTALS
—

• Lithium quartz (to heal and deflect negativity)
• Danburite (to strengthen the link to higher realms)
• Herkimer diamond (to detoxify)
• Iolite (to reenergize the aura)
• Selenite (for protection, peace, and calm)
• Apophyllite (to calm and reduce stress)

ADDITIONAL THERAPIES
—

Use creative visualization techniques to improve your overall positivity and boost the strength of your aura. Acupuncture may help clear blocked meridians in your body, boosting your auric strength.

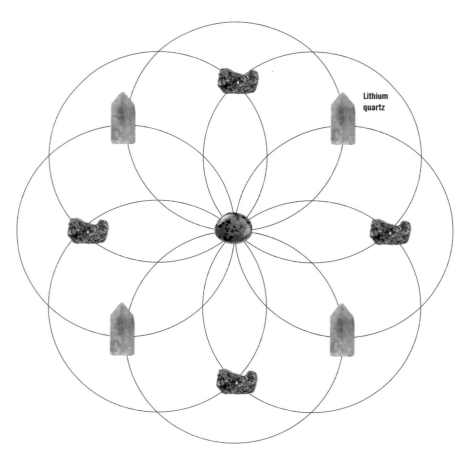

Lithium quartz

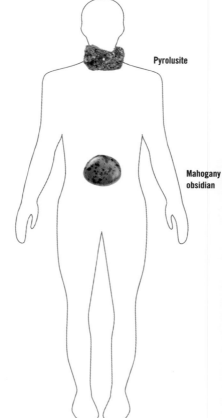

Pyrolusite

Mahogany obsidian

LEAKAGE

Aura leakage is where your energy leaks out of your auric field and it's caused by absorbing too much negative energy. For example, your aura becomes clogged up and congested by excessive stress, emotional pain, and discomfort, toxic environments, poor diet, lack of exercise, and bad lifestyle choices. It can also be caused if you're very highly sensitive and are affected too much by other people's words, actions, feelings, and thoughts. A leaky aura can become toxic and make you feel very out of sorts, mentally, physically, and emotionally.

KEY CRYSTALS
—

Kunzite—Use kunzite to help draw out toxins in your aura, make it whole again, and reinstate a feeling of love and clarity.

Black tourmaline—Keep black tourmaline near you in a room, or in your pockets, to help you remain grounded and protect your aura from leakage. It will help deflect negative energies and keep your aura whole.

Black tourmaline with mica—A crystal with the addition of mica will enable negative energies from psychic attack attempts to be bounced back to the sender.

OTHER GRID AND LAYOUT CRYSTALS
—

• Lithium quartz (to heal and deflect negativity)
• Herkimer diamond (to detoxify your aura of negative energies)
• Iolite (to reenergize your aura)
• Selenite (to promote protection, peace, and calm)
• Black tourmaline (for grounding)
• Rutilated quartz (to cleanse and energize the aura)

ADDITIONAL THERAPIES
—

Use intuitive methods to visualize the areas of your aura where energy is leaking from and fix the holes. Imagine smoothing and filling the holes, so energy can no longer escape. Focus on adopting a healthy lifestyle, including healthy eating and exercise habits.

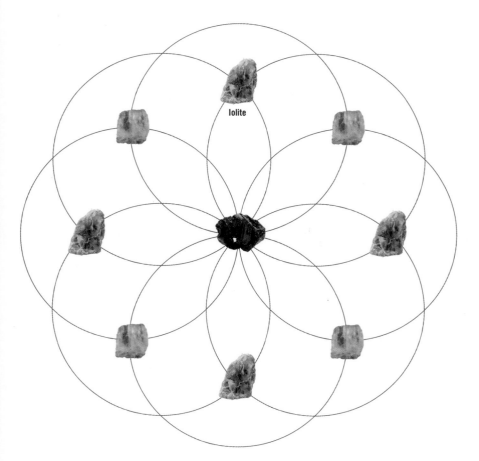

Iolite

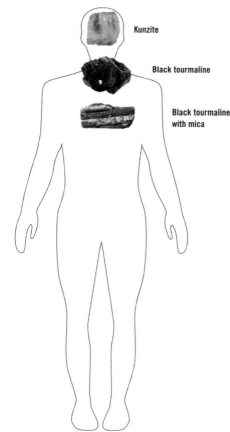

Kunzite

Black tourmaline

Black tourmaline with mica

CREATIVITY

Creativity is the art of coming up with new, original, and imaginative ideas and notions and turning them into reality. If you have a creative mind, you're likely to think in different ways from someone who doesn't—there are no limitations on your imagination and you can go above and beyond to develop new ideas and concepts. Being creative is all about trying new things, breaking free of traditional ways or means of doing things, and seeing things in a different light. While some people are naturally gifted at enhancing creativity, it's a skill that can be fine-tuned and developed.

KEY CRYSTALS
—

Cerussite—Surround yourself with cerussite, as this crystal can help balance the left and right sides of your brain and encourage creativity.

Lapis lazuli—This is a stone of self-expression, so it is perfect to help enhance creativity. Wear lapis lazuli, particularly around the area of your throat chakra, and let its energies help you express yourself in a creative manner.

Tiger's eye—If your creative spark is feeling blocked, use tiger's eye to release it. Place on the third eye chakra or hold it in your hand and let the energies of tiger's eye release blockages and let creativity flow.

OTHER GRID AND LAYOUT CRYSTALS

- Aventurine (to enhance creativity)
- Ametrine (to connect the physical with the higher consciousness and trigger creative ideas)
- Stilbite (to boost powers of creativity)
- Alexandrite (to promote creativity)
- Bloodstone (to boost creative intuition)
- Chalcedony (to bring the mind, body, and spirit into harmony)
- Chrysocolla (for inspiration)
- Herkimer diamond (to energize and enliven)

ADDITIONAL THERAPIES
—

Being outside in nature can help spark creativity—walk by the ocean, in fields, a park, or in a forest and absorb the sounds and sights of the natural world. Scents can also inspire, so try burning aromatherapy essential oils and seeing what effects different scents have on your ideas.

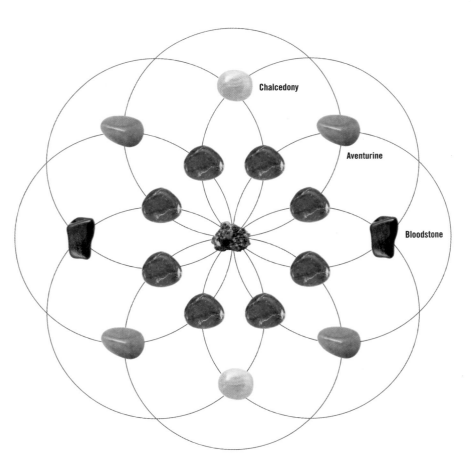

Chalcedony

Aventurine

Bloodstone

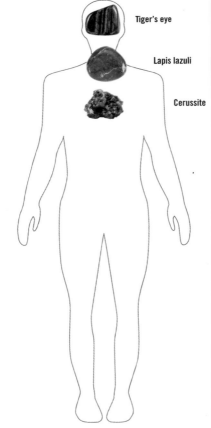

Tiger's eye

Lapis lazuli

Cerussite

INTUITION

Intuition is the ability to instinctively know and understand something without consciously knowing why. It's that gut feeling you have about something when you just "know." Intuition bridges the gap between your conscious and subconscious mind and it can take you by surprise when it suddenly pops its head up like an inner voice calling to you. It's easy to ignore the feeling if you don't logically understand why you think that, but learning to listen to your intuition could help with better decision-making and help you avoid toxic people or negative situations.

KEY CRYSTALS
—

Magnetite—Hold magnetite to strengthen positive energies, help you become more balanced, and learn to trust your intuition. Placed on the root chakra it can help to ground you for spiritual work.

Pietersite—Place on the third eye chakra to enhance your spiritual abilities and open up the ability to be more intuitive.

Amethyst—Place amethyst under your pillow at night and it could promote the ability to have more intuitive dreams.

OTHER GRID AND LAYOUT CRYSTALS
—

• Apophyllite (to help stimulate intuition)
• Danburite (for enhancing intuition)
• Fluorite (to heighten intuitive abilities)
• Iolite (to aid intuitive insight)
• Lapis lazuli (to help open the third eye)
• Moonstone (to close the gap between the conscious and unconscious mind)
• Selenite (to increase vibrations and create a better state to open intuition)
• Sodalite (to help link logic and intuition)
• Stilbite (for creative intuition and protection)

ADDITIONAL THERAPIES
—

Practicing regular meditation and learning to still your mind so you can hear the small voice within is a great way of learning to listen to and trust your intuition. Walking in nature and letting your mind be calm and quiet can also trigger moments of clarity. Use journaling to write down intuitive thoughts and trust your own abilities.

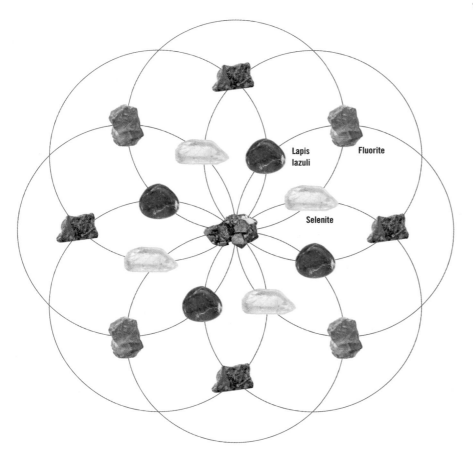

Lapis lazuli

Fluorite

Selenite

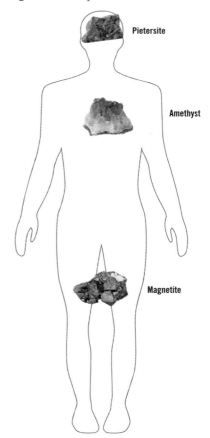

Pietersite

Amethyst

Magnetite

MEDITATION

Meditation is the art of stilling your mind, becoming calm and relaxed, and increasing your awareness. Traditional meditation techniques focus not on controlling your mind, but on giving yourself time and space to connect with it. When you master the art of meditation you can learn, grow, and harness its inner innate power. It takes time, perseverance, and concentration to learn to not let your mind wander from focusing on something as simple as your breathing, but it can be highly beneficial to your mental, emotional, physical, and spiritual health to do so.

KEY CRYSTALS
—

Aquamarine—Hold aquamarine while you meditate, as it can have a very calming effect on your mind and help you clear unwanted thoughts.

Azurite—Surround yourself with azurite, as this crystal could support you as you enter a meditative state.

Amethyst—Place on your third eye chakra for spiritual wisdom and insight as you meditate.

Magnesite—Place on the third eye chakra for increased peace and wisdom.

OTHER GRID AND LAYOUT CRYSTALS
—

• Apophyllite (links the body with the mind)
• Chrysocolla (to aid meditation)
• Kunzite (good to use if you find it hard to meditate)
• Kyanite (to encourage high vibrational energies)
• Boji stone (high vibrational energy, but grounding, too)
• Clear quartz (for clarity of mind)
• Yellow calcite (for deep relaxation and spiritual connections)
• Lavender smithsonite (to help reach higher states of consciousness)

ADDITIONAL THERAPIES
—

If you find it hard to clear your mind of all thoughts when attempting to meditate, practice with mindfulness instead. This enables you to focus on specific things and is a good way of building up to full-blown meditation. Try walking meditations outside in nature. Relaxing music can help calm your mind, as can aromatherapy essential oils such as lavender or bergamot.

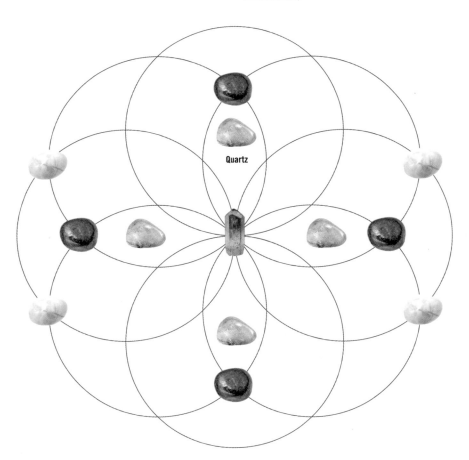

Quartz

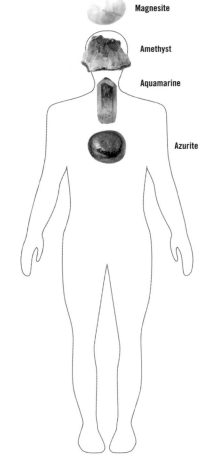

Magnesite

Amethyst

Aquamarine

Azurite

COMMUNION WITH SPIRITS

Communicating with spirits, otherwise known as mediumship, psychic work, or clairvoyancy, involves opening yourself up to the higher spiritual realms and reaching out to communicate with spirits. It can take various forms and different tools may be used to enhance communication, such as crystal balls, Ouija boards, or divination cards. Communion with spirits isn't something to be taken lightly—you need to ensure you are fully aware of what you're doing and have effectively grounded yourself, as some of the energies you encounter may be overwhelming. Not all spirits are good entities.

KEY CRYSTALS
—

Aquamarine—Hold aquamarine to promote a desire to open up your clairvoyant abilities.

Magnesite—Place on the third eye chakra to help get you into a deeply relaxed state for communicating with spirits.

Fluorite—For spiritual protection while connecting with spirits, hold fluorite. It will heighten spiritual connections whilst offering an essential layer of protection.

OTHER GRID AND LAYOUT CRYSTALS
—

• Amethyst (to enhance psychic skills)
• Cherry opal (to enhance spiritual connections)
• Dumortierite (to aid in the development of psychic work)
• Angelite (for channeling spirits)
• Kyanite (to aid psychic abilities)
• Herkimer diamond (for spiritual grounding)
• Moonstone (to enhance psychic skills)
• Hematite (to ground and protect)
• Labradorite (to raise consciousness, strengthen faith, and aid clairvoyance)
• Blue jade (for peace and reflection as you commune with spirits)

ADDITIONAL THERAPIES
—

Practicing relaxation and meditation can help you relax the body and open the mind, and learning to trust your intuition can be useful, too. Chakra and aura-cleansing techniques can be beneficial before and after communing with spirits.

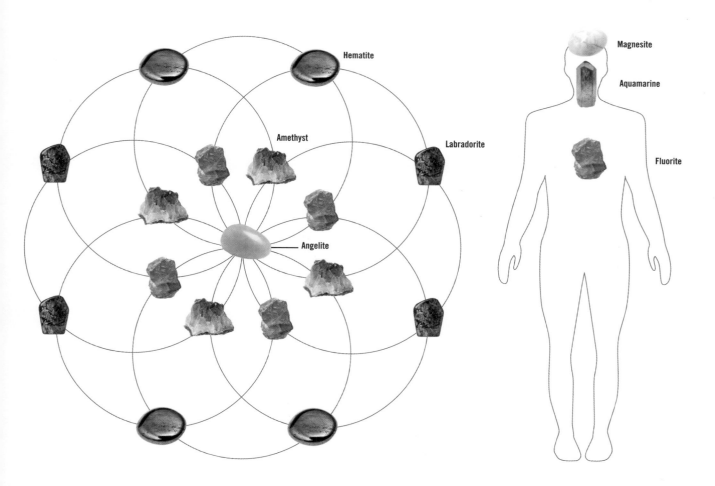

Hematite

Amethyst

Labradorite

Angelite

Magnesite

Aquamarine

Fluorite

POLLUTION

Exposure to pollution can have an effect on your health—physically, mentally, and emotionally. It can dull your aura, clog your chakras, and generally affect the normal functioning of your body, mind, and spirit. There are different types of pollution, including air, water, and noise pollution, as well as more subtle energy pollution. If you're exposed to high levels of pollution, the effects can come on quickly over days, whereas the effects of low levels will gradually build up over time.

KEY CRYSTALS
—

Aquamarine—Make a crystal gem elixir using the indirect method and spray it around your aura to ward off pollution and negative energies.

Turquoise—Wear as jewelry or place around you to help purify the energy surrounding you and ward off the effects of pollution. Turquoise is useful for helping to remove electromagnetic smog and to protect you from environmental pollutants.

OTHER GRID AND LAYOUT CRYSTALS

- Amethyst (to protect)
- Bloodstone (to cleanse and ground)
- Blue lace agate (to calm, heal, and surround you with peace)
- Opal (to dispel pollution)
- Beryl (for filtering out pollution)
- Amazonite (for electromagnetic pollution)
- Malachite, polished (to dispel pollution)

ADDITIONAL THERAPIES
—

Holistic therapies such as acupuncture can help keep your meridians open and flowing, so pollution doesn't impact you too much. If air quality is an issue at home, try an air purifier to help purify the air you're breathing in.

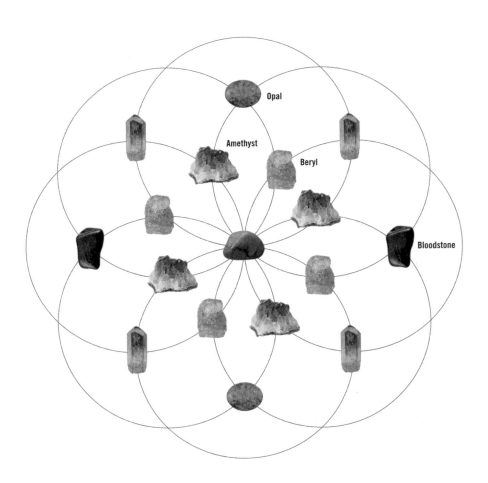

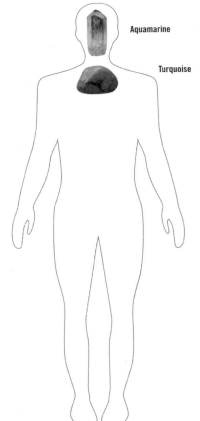

Aquamarine

Turquoise

RADIATION

Radiation is energy that is emitted in the form of electromagnetic waves or rays containing particles. There are some naturally occurring minerals in the ground, soil, and water, plus radon, a naturally occurring gas that contains elements of radioactivity and gives off small amounts of radiation. When you're at high altitudes, such as on a mountain, you can be exposed to high levels of cosmic rays. Human technology, such as x-ray machines, radiotherapy treatments, and the generation of nuclear power, all give off radiation, too. Exposure to too much radiation can cause symptoms such as fatigue, muscle and joint pain, insomnia, and concentration and memory issues.

KEY CRYSTALS
—

Amazonite—Wear as jewelry to protect yourself from the effects of radiation. The crystal may also help to filter away unwanted elements.

Black tourmaline—Place on the root chakra to protect the aura and the body from the unwanted effects of radiation. It will help ground you and dispel negativity.

Herkimer diamond—Position between yourself and the source of radiation to protect from radioactivity.

OTHER GRID AND LAYOUT CRYSTALS
—

• Sodalite (to clear the mind, body, and spirit)
• Smoky quartz (to neutralize the effects of radiation)
• Malachite, polished (to soak up radiation)
• Fluorite (to clean and stabilize the body, mind, and spirit)
• Hematite (to protect against electromagnetic fields)

ADDITIONAL THERAPIES
—

Natural remedies such as spirulina and chlorella may be beneficial to counteract the effects of radiation exposure (the Russians are said to have used them after the Chernobyl nuclear power disaster).

Taking probiotics may help by restoring the right levels of healthy bacteria into your body, and acupuncture could help restore balance. Bathing in magnesium salts may help cleanse your body and adding buckwheat to your diet may offer some benefits.

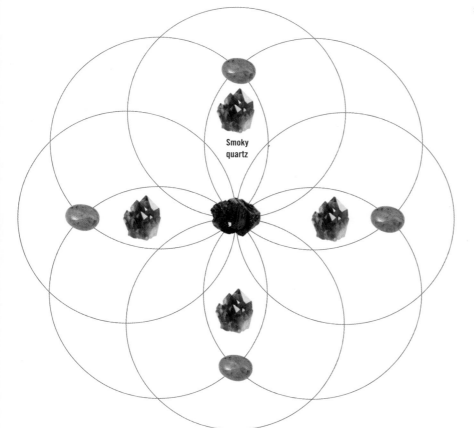

Smoky quartz

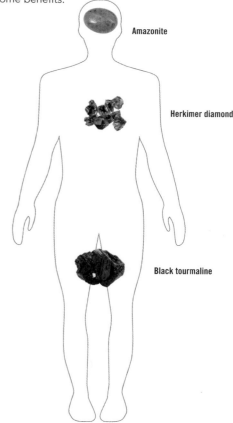

Amazonite

Herkimer diamond

Black tourmaline

OTHERS' OPINIONS

There may be times when other people have strong opinions and are intent on directing them toward you, whether you want to hear them or not. It can be hard to deal with constant verbal dialogue, especially when others' opinions are not in harmony with yours. It can be emotionally and mentally draining, leaving you feeling fatigued, stressed, and perhaps even in doubt of your own true feelings and views.

KEY CRYSTALS

—

Opal—Wear opal if you're on the receiving end of unwanted opinions from other people. Opal can act like a shield, bouncing back the unwanted views and sending them back to their source.

Black tourmaline—Shield yourself mentally, physically, and emotionally from the unwanted opinions of others with black tourmaline. This protective crystal will help ground and strengthen you.

OTHER GRID AND LAYOUT CRYSTALS

- Amber (to clear away negativity)
- Blue calcite (to ease stress and anxiety)
- Ruby (to harness your own power and help you stand by your beliefs)
- Amethyst (to emotionally protect yourself)
- Amazonite (to dispel negative views)
- Chrysocolla (to help you stay true to your views and opinions)

ADDITIONAL THERAPIES

—

Use creative visualization techniques to imagine a strong shield surrounding you and the other person, or people, and your body covered in pure white, impenetrable light. If the opinions being directed your way are very toxic, perhaps even add in a fierce jaguar patrolling your shield to ward off unwanted views. Before being in contact with people with strong views, meditating, grounding, and centering yourself can be beneficial.

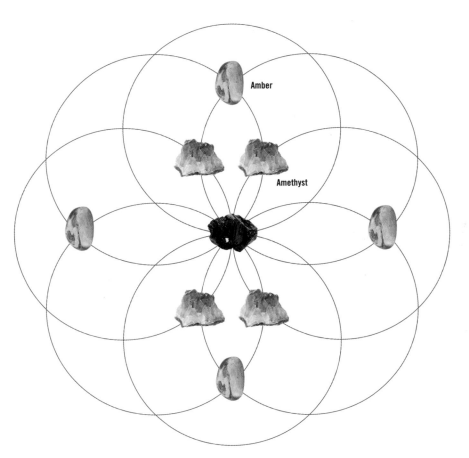

Amber

Amethyst

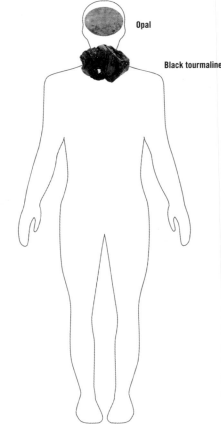

Opal

Black tourmaline

PSYCHIC ATTACK

A psychic attack is a mental assault made by someone using negative power, and these can be consciously or unconsciously made. For example, someone harboring strong feelings of negativity and anger toward you and releasing the feelings unconsciously can have an impact on you. Negative energies are draining. If you're under psychic attack, you're likely to feel fatigued, experience insomnia, have a heaviness over you, feel like you can't function as normal, believe that things keep going wrong, or suffer one infection after another. Psychic attacks can sometimes create a form of psychic cord linking the attacker to you—and unless you're able to cut that cord or deflect the negative energy without it harming you, the effects will continue.

KEY CRYSTALS
—

Amethyst—Wear as jewelry or surround yourself with amethyst, as it can help dispel attempts at psychic attacks. The crystal is powerful and protective, transforming negativity into positivity.

Black tourmaline—Place black tourmaline around your body to ground and protect you from psychic attack.

Black tourmaline with mica—A crystal with the addition of mica will enable negative energies from psychic attack attempts to be bounced back to the sender.

OTHER GRID AND LAYOUT CRYSTALS
—

• Black obsidian (to repel negative forces)
• Green chlorite (to help fight off a psychic attack)
• Labradorite (for a barrier against negativity)
• Apache tear (to absorb negativity and protect from psychic attacks)
• Black kyanite (to cut psychic cords)
• Jet (to protect from dark forces)
• Smoky quartz (to ground you)

ADDITIONAL THERAPIES
—

Do things that make you feel good and fill you with joy, gratitude, faith, hope, and happiness. Cleanse your environment with sage. Use meditations and visualizations to surround yourself with a pure white light that protects you at all times. Use chakra and aura healing methods to clear blockages and strengthen your personal energy systems.

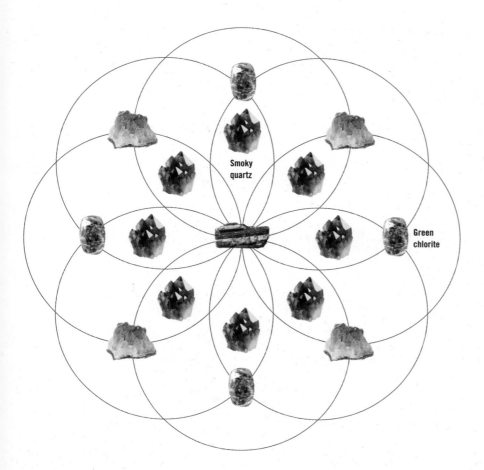

Smoky quartz

Green chlorite

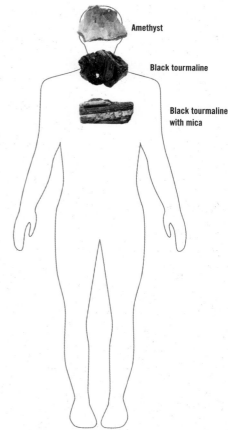

Amethyst

Black tourmaline

Black tourmaline with mica

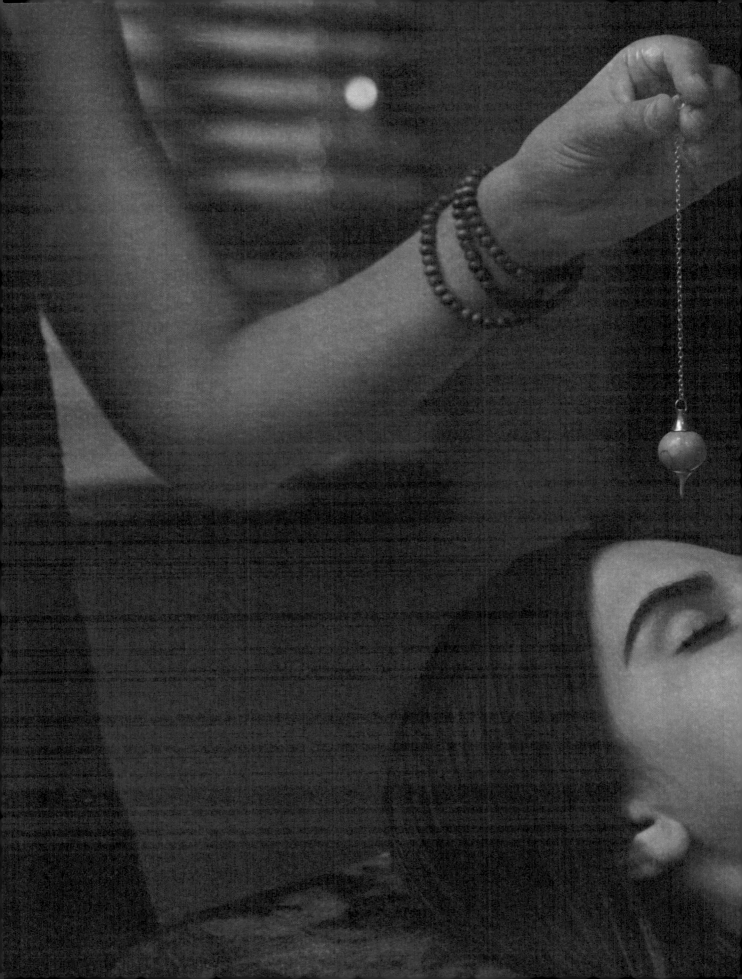

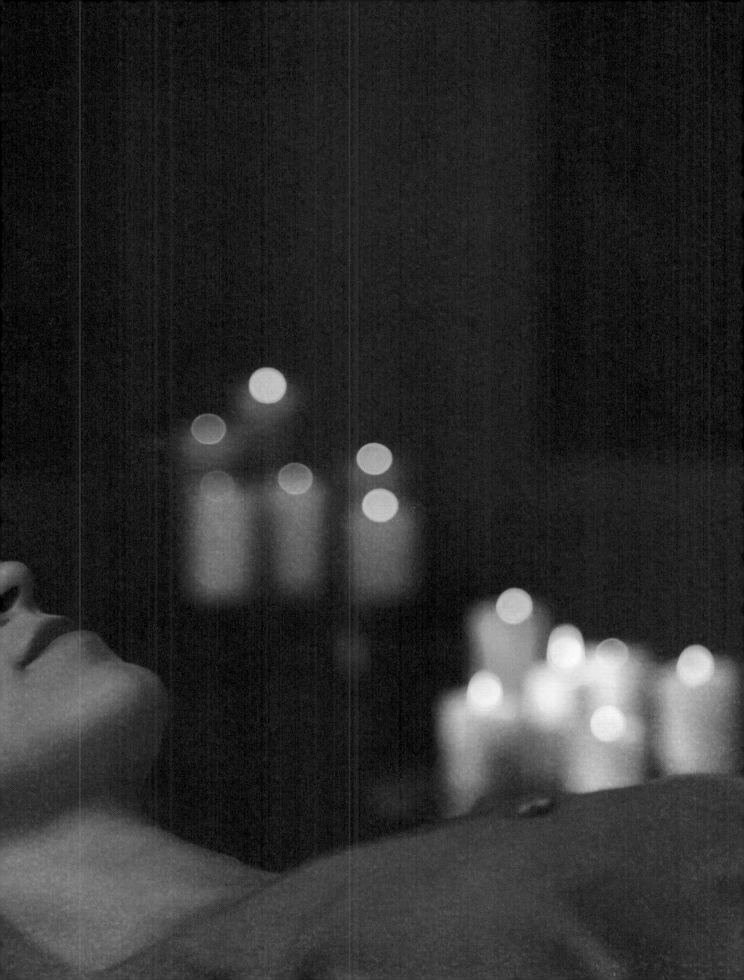

REFERENCE

PART FOUR

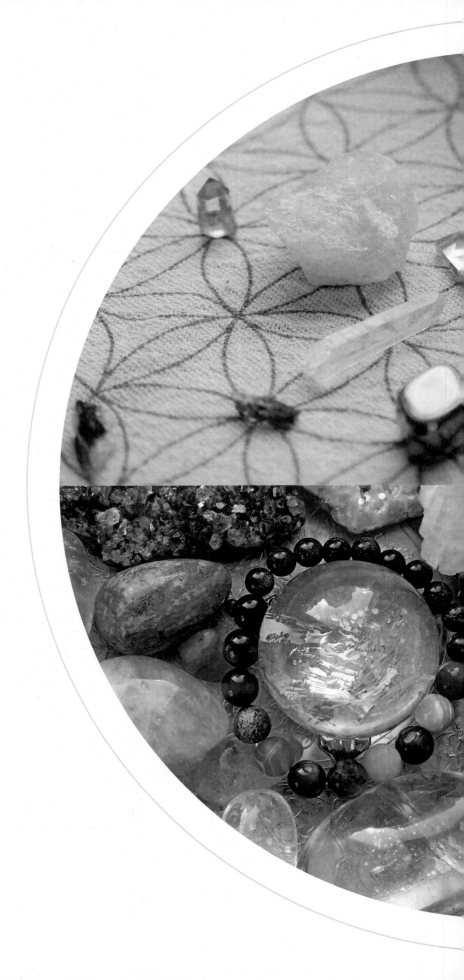

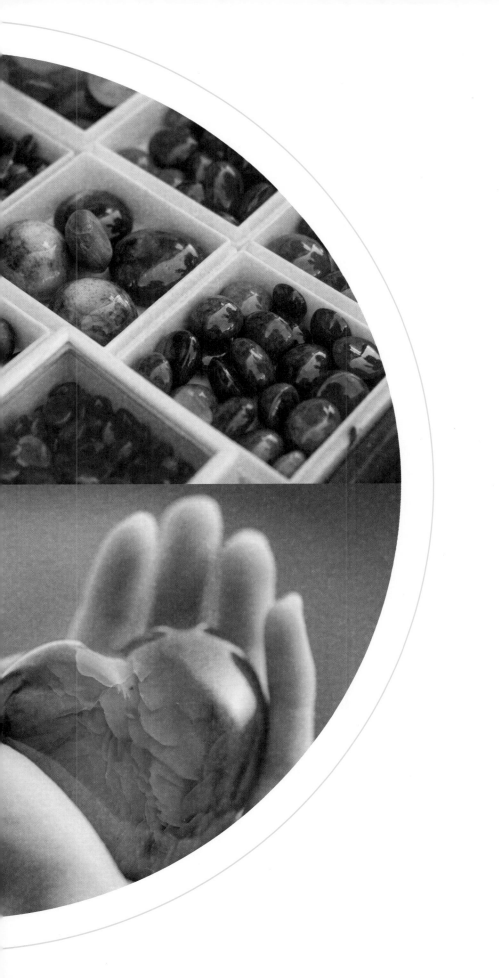

CRYSTAL GRID TEMPLATES

Crystal grids can be created from a range of different symbols and can be as basic or complicated as you wish. You can use simple geometric shapes or special symbols that you know and love as the basis for laying out crystal grids.

To get you started and help inspire you, here are some crystal grid templates that you could use. As you practice with creating grids, your crystals can be placed directly onto the grids on these pages, or you could copy or trace them out onto another sheet of paper so you can lay them flat and keep them in place more efficiently.

If you're feeling creative, you can also use these layout ideas as the basis to inspire your own grid designs. Extra circles or geometric shapes can easily be added to create new patterns, or you could draw your own from scratch. Be guided by your intuition and see what works and feels right for you!

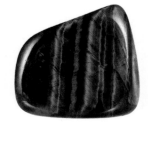

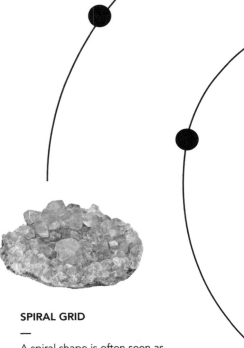

SPIRAL GRID

—

A spiral shape is often seen as representing creativity, but it can be much more.

Spiritually, a spiral can be a symbol of a connection with the divine and the path you travel to reach it. It also has connections with nature—shells are typically this shape. However you view a spiral shape, space your crystals out along the lines and curves to create your spiral grid layout.

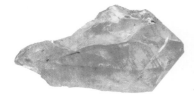

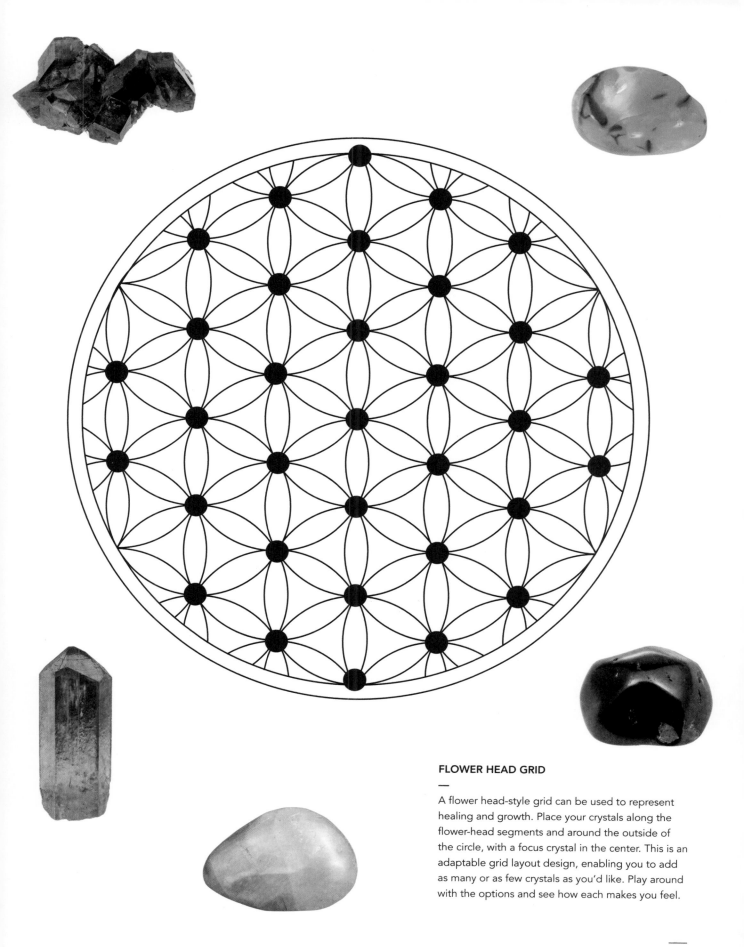

FLOWER HEAD GRID

—

A flower head-style grid can be used to represent healing and growth. Place your crystals along the flower-head segments and around the outside of the circle, with a focus crystal in the center. This is an adaptable grid layout design, enabling you to add as many or as few crystals as you'd like. Play around with the options and see how each makes you feel.

STAR OF DAVID GRID

—

The Star of David, sometimes known as the Hexagram of Solomon, is an ancient Jewish symbol formed from two triangles linked together. It makes a strong geometric statement, often representing stability and togetherness.

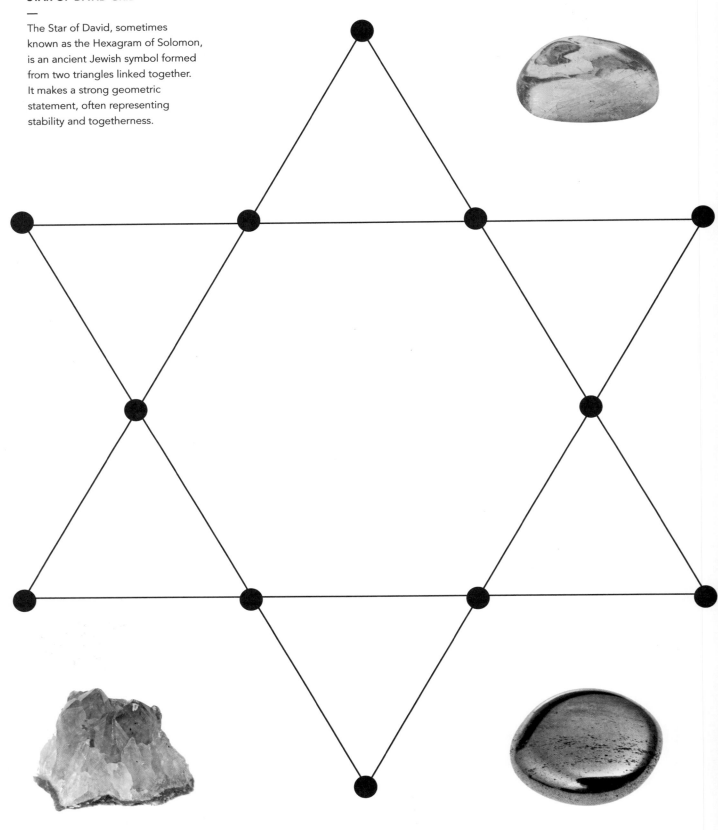

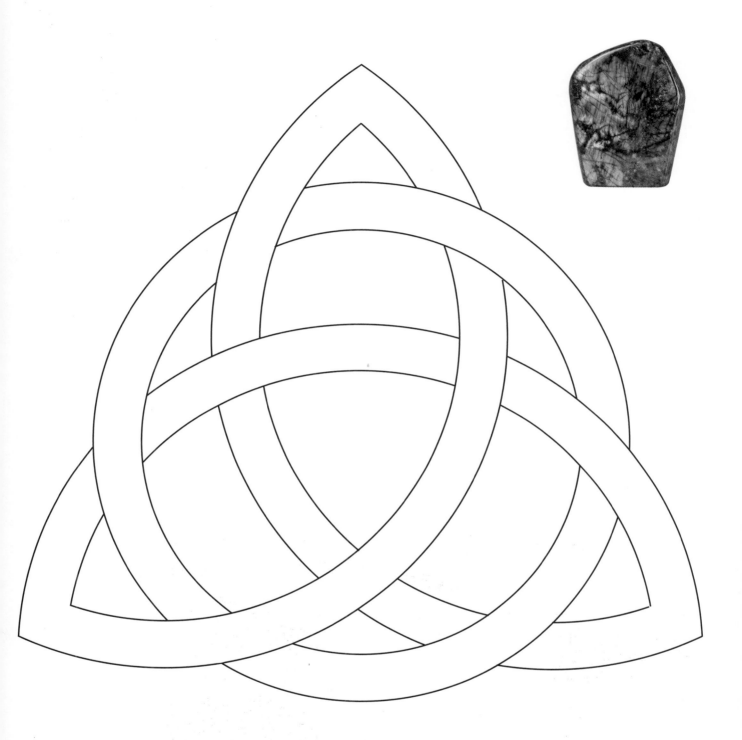

THE TRIQUETRA GRID
—

The triquetra symbol, also known as the Trinity Knot, is one of the most well-known Celtic symbols. It represents the power and unity of three—be it three elements (air, water, and earth), the three cycles of life (life, death, and rebirth), elements of time (past, present, and future), or representing a family (mother, father, and child). If you feel drawn to this ancient Celtic symbol, it could be an ideal choice to use as a grid layout.

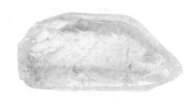

HOLISTIC HEALTH ORGANIZATIONS

United States and Canada

Academic Consortium for Integrative
Medicine & Health
www.imconsortium.org

American Holistic Health Association
www.ahha.org

American Holistic Nurses Association
www.ahna.org

American Society of Alternative Therapists
www.asat.org

The Canadian College of Holistic Health
www.cchh.org

Foundation for Alternative and Integrative
Medicine
www.faim.org

Natural Health Practitioners of Canada
www.nhpcanada.org

National Association of Holistic Health
Practitioners
www.nahhp.com

National Center for Complementary and Integrative Health
www.nccih.nih.gov

Natural Medicines–Therapeutic Research Center
www.naturalmedicines.therapeuticresearch.com

United Kingdom

Affiliation of Crystal Healing Organisations
www.crystal-healing.org

British Complementary Medicine Association
www.bcma.co.uk

Complementary Therapists Association
www.ctha.com

Federation of Holistic Therapists
www.fht.org.uk

The Complementary Medical Association
www.the-cma.org.uk

The General Regulatory Council
for Complementary Therapies
www.grcct.org

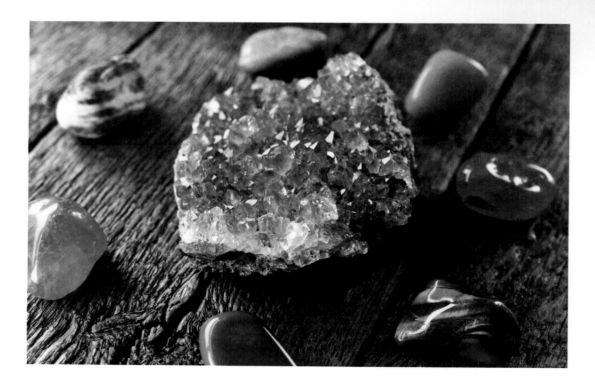

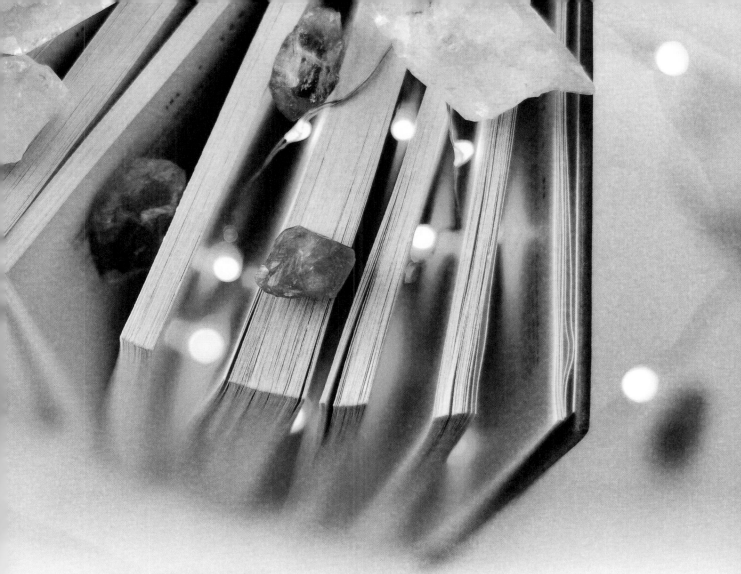

FURTHER READING

Chakra Healing, Margarita Alcantara
(Althea Press, 2017)

Crystals for Beginners, Karen Frazier
(Althea Press, 2017)

Crystal Prescriptions, Judy Hall
(John Hunt Publishing, 2006)

Energy Medicine, Donna Eden
(Piatkus Books, 2008)

Intuitive Studies, Gordon Smith
(Hay House, 2012)

Meditation with Intention, Anusha Wijeyakumar
(Llewellyn Publications, 2021)

Mindfulness, Mark Williams and Danny Penman
(Piatkus Books, 2011)

My Pocket Tai Chi
(Adams Media, 2018)

The Book of Crystal Grids, Philip Permutt
(CICO Books, 2017)

*The Crystal Bible / The Crystal Bible 2
/ The Crystal Bible 3*, Judy Hall
(Godsfield Press, 2009, 2009, 2012)

The Crystal Code, Tamara Driessen
(Ballantyne Books, 2018)

The Crystal Healer, Philip Permutt
(CICO Books, 2016)

The Life-Changing Power of Intuition, Emma Lucy Knowles
(Pop Press, 2021)

The Little Book of Chakras, Patricia Mercier
(Gaia, 2017)

Unblocked, Margaret Lynch Raniere and David Raniere
(Hay House, 2021)

You Are a Rainbow: Essential Auras, Emma Lucy Knowles
(Pop Press, 2020)

GLOSSARY

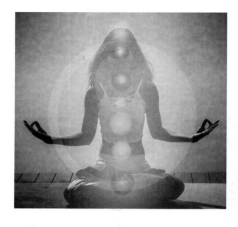

Aura
The aura is an invisible energy field that surrounds all living things, including animals and human beings. Some people are able to see auras, and their colors can be used to interpret health and vitality.

Biofeedback
The method by which a person can learn to control their bodily functions by monitoring their brain waves, muscles, blood pressure, breathing, and more.

Chakra
A chakra is an invisible spiritual energy center that's located within your body. The word chakra comes from ancient Sanskrit, where it translates to mean "wheel" or "disk," and chakras can be thought of as like a spinning wheel of energy.

Double terminated crystal
A double terminated crystal is one that has points at either end. It can be a useful addition to your crystal collection, as energy can be both directed into the body and drawn away from it at the same time.

Electromagnetic field
An electromagnetic field is an invisible field of radiation produced by electric or magnetic devices. For example, devices such as cell phones, radar systems, electric trams, power lines, microwave ovens, pylons, and x-ray machines.

Etheric body
The etheric body is another name for the aura that surrounds the human body.

Geopathic stress
Geopathic stress is the idea that the earth gives off energy vibrations and it can be disturbed by things going on underground, such as pipes, geological faults, underground water, and power lines. It's thought that the energy disturbances can have a negative impact on human health and well-being, as well as potentially affect buildings.

Gridding
Gridding is the art of laying out crystals in a pattern or grid to create a more focused and potentially more powerful healing technique.

Grounding
Grounding is a technique where you consciously connect yourself to the earth. It helps give a firm foundation for crystal work, meditation, or other holistic therapies.

Kundalini
Kundalini is an inner energy or ultimate life force. The idea of kundalini comes from many esoteric traditions and belief systems, including Hinduism and Buddhism, where it's regarded as being like a "coiled snake."

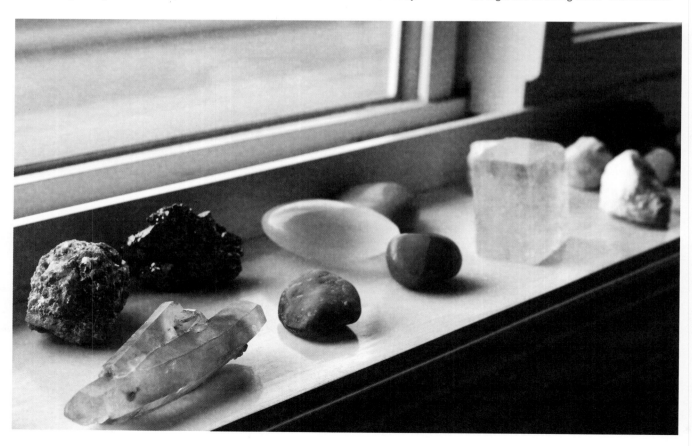

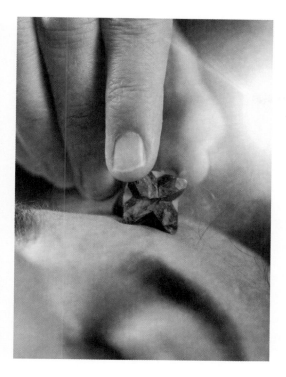

Planetary grid

The planetary grid is the idea that a grid of geometric patterns exist that map the Earth. At points where certain grids intersect and form into a matrix, there may be strong energy centers. Often these energy centers are located at sacred sites such as Stonehenge, in England, or Machu Picchu, in Peru.

Psychic attack

A psychic attack is a form of mental assault made by someone using negative power. A psychic attack can be made consciously or unconsciously, and the negative energies emitted can have a detrimental effect on physical, mental, emotional, and spiritual health.

Kundalini is believed to start at the base of the spine, but when it's awakened, it can rise up through the body and the chakras to the top of the head.

Meridian

A meridian is a term that originates from traditional Chinese medicine and refers to an energy channel in the body. The meridians are used within therapies such as acupuncture and acupressure, where needles or gentle pressure are used to unblock meridians and get energy flowing freely again.

Merkaba

A merkaba is a symbolic geometric star shape made up of two intersecting tetrahedrons. Merkaba comes from the Hebrew word for chariot and means "light spirit body."

Occlusion

An occlusion is a mineral deposit found within a crystal. It can be seen as looking like spots or cloudy patches.

Qi

Qi—pronounced "chee"—is a vital form of life energy. The idea of qi originates from traditional Chinese medicine, where it's believed that blockages or deficiencies in qi relate to physical, mental, and emotional health issues.

Subtle energy field

A subtle energy field is the term used to describe an invisible layer of energy that surrounds all living things.

Tumbled crystals

Tumbled crystals are small crystals that have been polished in a special tumbling machine so that their surfaces become smooth and glossy.

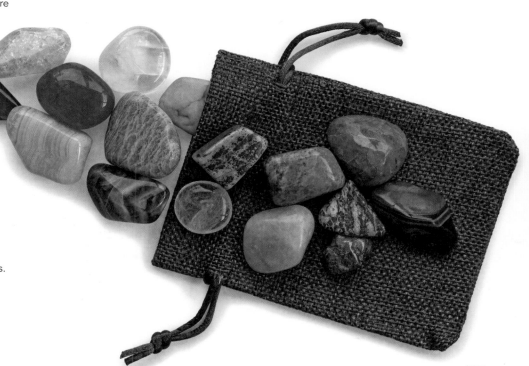

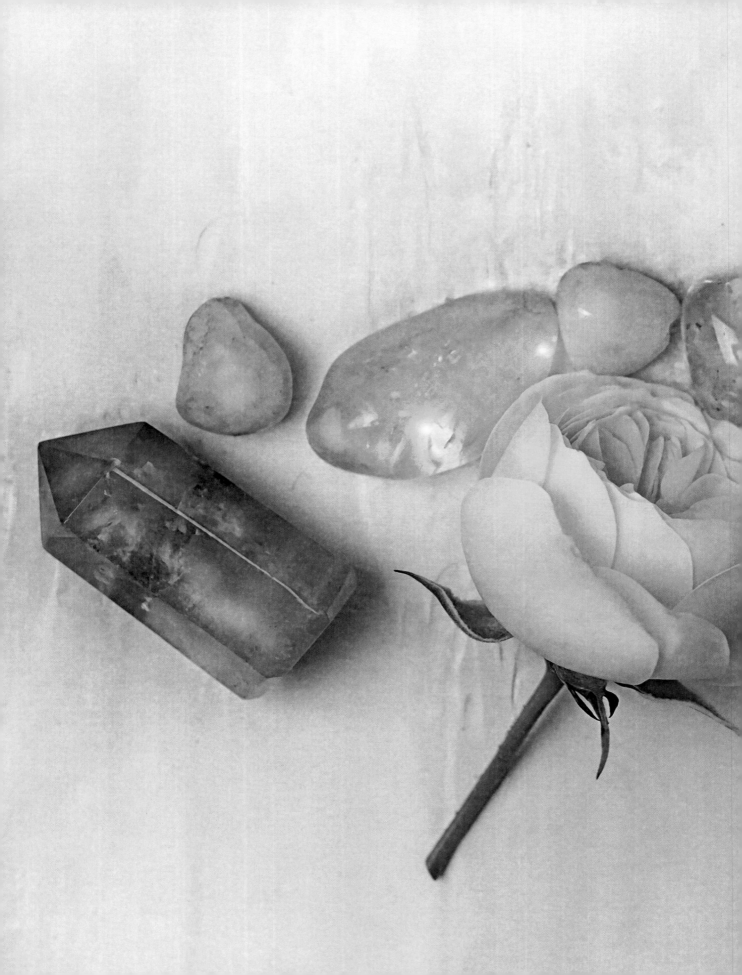

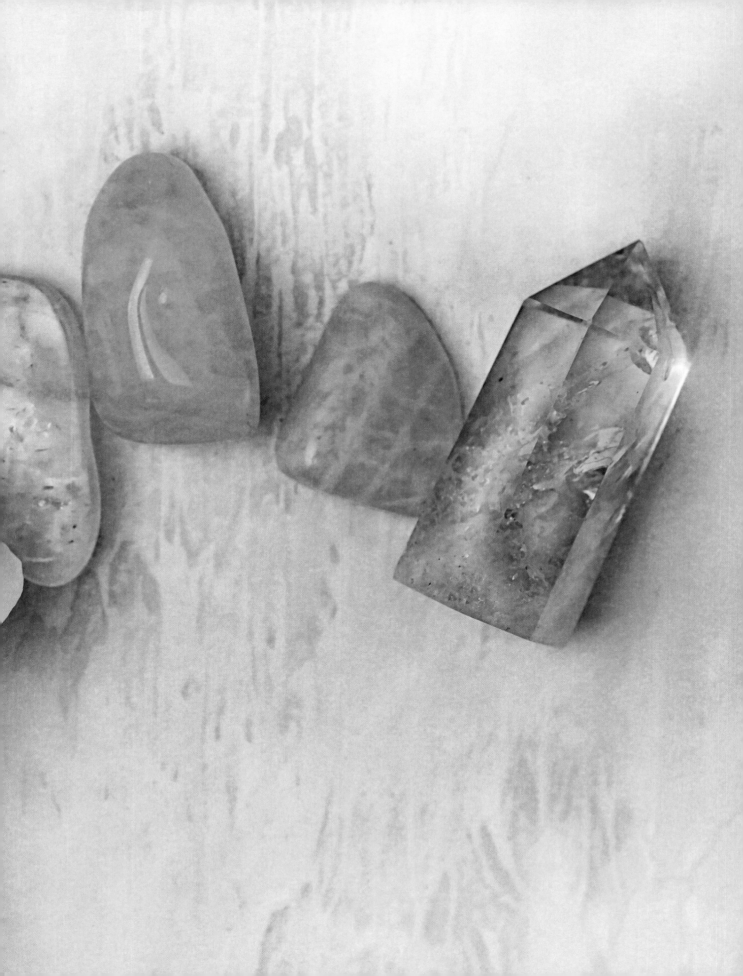

INDEX

Page references in **bold** indicate main entry.
Page references in *italics* indicate images.

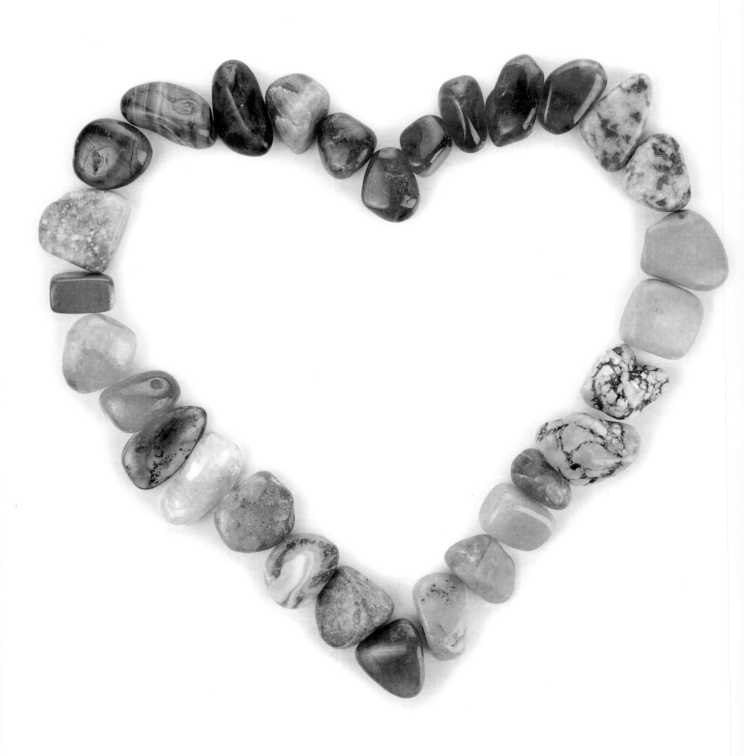